60 HIKES WITHIN 60 MILES

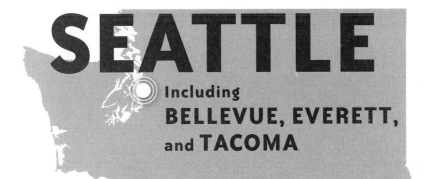

SEATTLE

Including
BELLEVUE, EVERETT,
and **TACOMA**

THIRD EDITION

Andrew Weber and
Bryce Stevens

MENASHA RIDGE PRESS
Birmingham, Alabama

60 Hikes Within 60 Miles: Seattle

Library of Congress Cataloging-in-Publication Data

Names: Weber, Andrew, 1971- author. | Stevens, Bryce, 1969-
Title: 60 hikes within 60 miles, Seattle : including Bellevue, Everett, and
    Tacoma / Andrew Weber and Bryce Stevens.
Other titles: Sixty hikes within sixty miles, Seattle
Description: Third edition. | Birmingham, AL : Menasha Ridge Press, 2016.
Identifiers: LCCN 2016018983 | ISBN 9781634040181 (paperback)
Subjects: LCSH: Hiking—Washington (State) —Seattle Region—Guidebooks. |
    Seattle Region (Wash.) —Guidebooks. | BISAC: TRAVEL / United States / West
    / Pacific (AK, CA, HI, NV, OR, WA). | SPORTS & RECREATION / Hiking. |
    HEALTH & FITNESS / Healthy Living.
Classification: LCC GV199.42.W22 W47 2016 | DDC 796.5109797/72—dc23
LC record available at https://lccn.loc.gov/2016018983
ISBN: 978-1-63404-018-1; eISBN: 978-1-63404-019-8

Cover design by Scott McGrew
Text design by Annie Long
Cover photo © Andrew Weber
Front cover: View from Mailbox Peak
Back cover (left to right): Billy Frank Jr. Nisqually National Wildlife Refuge; Barclay Lake, Stone Lake, and Eagle Lake; Bare Mountain; and Greider Lakes
All back cover and interior photos, unless otherwise noted, by Andrew Weber and Bryce Stevens
Maps by Andrew Weber, Bryce Stevens, and Scott McGrew

MENASHA RIDGE PRESS
An imprint of AdventureKEEN
2204 1st Ave. S., Suite 102
Birmingham, AL 35233
800-443-7227, fax 205-326-1012

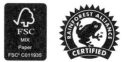

Visit menasharidge.com for a complete listing of our books and for ordering information. Contact us at our website, at facebook.com/menasharidge, or at twitter.com/menasharidge with questions or comments. To find out more about who we are and what we're doing, visit our blog, blog.menasharidge.com.

DISCLAIMER

This book is meant only as a guide to select trails in the Seattle area and does not guarantee hiker safety in any way—you hike at your own risk. Neither Menasha Ridge Press nor Andrew Weber or Bryce Stevens is liable for property loss or damage, personal injury, or death that result in any way from accessing or hiking the trails described in the following pages. Please be aware that hikers have been injured in the Seattle area. Be especially cautious when walking on or near boulders, steep inclines, and drop-offs, and do not attempt to explore terrain that may be beyond your abilities. To help ensure an uneventful hike, please read carefully the introduction to this book, and perhaps get further safety information and guidance from other sources. Familiarize yourself thoroughly with the areas you intend to visit before venturing out. Ask questions, and prepare for the unforeseen. Familiarize yourself with current weather reports, maps of the area you intend to visit, and any relevant park regulations.

Overview

Other cities in the 60 Hikes Within 60 Miles series:

Albuquerque

Atlanta

Baltimore

Boston

Chicago

Cincinnati

Cleveland

Dallas and Fort Worth

Denver and Boulder

Harrisburg

Houston

Los Angeles

Madison

Minneapolis and St. Paul

Nashville

New York

Philadelphia

Phoenix

Pittsburgh

Richmond

Sacramento

Salt Lake

San Antonio and Austin

San Diego

San Francisco

St. Louis

Washington, D.C.

Table of Contents

Acknowledgments

THIS BOOK WOULD NOT BE POSSIBLE without the tireless efforts of countless volunteers, employees, and representatives from a host of organizations, including The Mountaineers, Washington State Trails Association, Washington Department of Natural Resources, U.S. Forest Service, National Park Service, and various county and city departments of parks and recreation, who make the Seattle-area trail system one of the finest in the world. Nor would it be possible without the museum staff and the amateur and professional historians and archivists who allowed me to share and learn from their passions in order to bring the rich history of the Pacific Northwest to life. Their contributions to this book were immeasurable, even though they are almost certainly unaware of what they've done. Special thanks also go to Harlee Case and Larry and Nonnie Crook for providing me the time and space I needed to work.

Finally, I would like to express my boundless gratitude to my friends and family and especially my wonderful wife, Heather, and two sons, Bennett and Russell, who provided unlimited patience, tolerance, and support while this project was underway. And I would like to thank the entire staff at Menasha Ridge Press, who presented Bryce and me with this unique opportunity and guided the work to completion. Without their leadership, this book would never have made it out of the wilderness.

—Andrew Weber

I WOULD LIKE TO THANK EVERYONE who has joined me on excursions in the past, making these outdoor adventures fun and memorable. These good friends and family members have explored Washington with me on foot, mountain bikes, sea kayaks, snowshoes, skis, snowboards, motorcycles, parachutes, and even bungee cords. Thanks to these people, I have the knowledge base required to assemble a variety of hikes in the parks and mountains around the wonderful city of Seattle.

Finally, my greatest thanks go to those who wanted to hike with me while researching this book but stayed at home most of the time—my patient wife, Julie, and my adventurous sons, Kyle and Andrew.

—Bryce Stevens

Foreword

WELCOME TO MENASHA RIDGE PRESS'S 60 Hikes Within 60 Miles, a series designed to provide hikers with the information they need to find and hike the very best trails surrounding metropolitan areas.

Our strategy was simple: First, find a hiker who knows the area and loves to hike. Second, ask that person to spend a year researching the most popular and very best trails around. And third, have that person describe each trail in terms of difficulty, scenery, condition, elevation change, and all other categories of information that are important to hikers. "Pretend you've just completed a hike and met up with other hikers at the trailhead," we told each author. "Imagine their questions; be clear in your answers."

Authors Andrew Weber and Bryce Stevens have selected 60 of the best hikes in and around the Seattle metropolitan area. From the driftwood-strewn shores of Puget Sound to the snowy heights of the Cascade Mountains, Weber and Stevens provide hikers (and walkers) with a great variety of hikes—and all within roughly 60 miles of Seattle.

You'll get more out of this book if you take a moment to read the Introduction, which explains how to read the trail listings. The "Topo Maps" section on page 4 will help you understand how useful topos are on a hike and will also tell you where to get them. And though this is a where-to, not a how-to, guide, readers who have not hiked extensively will find the "Introduction" of particular value.

As much for the opportunity to free the spirit as to free the body, let these hikes elevate you above the urban hurry.

All the best,
The Editors at Menasha Ridge Press

Preface

SEATTLE IS CONNECTED TO THE OUTDOORS like few other places in the world. On a clear day, either or both the Cascade and Olympic Mountains can be seen from just about any high point in the city. Advertising for the Space Needle, arguably Seattle's most prominent man-made attraction, emphasizes its view of distant Mount Baker rather than of the downtown area nearby. Whenever the seemingly endless gray days of winter lead to speculation on the suitability of Seattle as a place to live, it can take only a glimpse of Mount Rainier to remind people why they choose to make their homes here. "The mountain is out," locals say, when Rainier emerges from the clouds to make such an appearance, as if greeting an old friend who has been away.

Not surprisingly for a place so in love with the natural environment, reams of paper and gallons of ink have been consumed in an effort to catalog Washington's trails. This could well lead someone to ask whether anyone really needs another Washington hiking guidebook. Aren't there enough already?

Many celebrated trails in Washington are nowhere near Seattle at all, far outside any reasonable range for a day trip from the city. What has been lacking—and is now available here—is a true Seattle hiking guidebook.

From easy walks in local city parks to demanding hikes and scrambles in the mountains, there is something here for everyone. Within this book's modest 60-mile radius, beaches, tide pools, old-growth forests, high peaks, swimming holes, alpine meadows, lakes, glaciers, and more invite exploration. Many of the things to be found on the featured trails are obvious: forests, rivers, and mountains. But there are more-subtle treasures, too, in historical and cultural gems. Walk a few steps down a path traveled by the pioneers and feel a link with history unavailable in any museum. Or take a cursory glance at many Washington maps for an introduction to the Chinook language, which predates the settlers by centuries and provides names for countless geographic features. Even veteran hikers are sure to make some new discoveries and find something in this book they didn't already know about. Or maybe you need a good reason to revisit some old favorites and see how familiar places have changed over time.

The most important message this book can send is that wilderness is not only found way out there; it's also right here, for those who know where to look. Islands in Puget Sound, the lowlands of South King County, and the Kitsap Peninsula—all worthy of visits in their own right and good places to escape the crowds—are just a few of the quietly overlooked hiking destinations highlighted within these pages.

There is also no reason summer needs to be viewed as the one-and-only hiking season. Plenty of trails are open year-round and offer special seasonal attractions. Who can forget a waterfall at its maximum flow when it crests after a week of winter rain? Or an ancient forest at its most evocative when thick fog lends an otherworldly atmosphere to the giant trees? This guidebook shows the way.

ABOUT THE HIKES

If Seattle stood at the center of a plain, a 60-mile circle could be drawn to encompass all the hikes in this book. The resulting overview map might resemble a pepperoni pizza, with the featured trails distributed evenly around the city. However, the Seattle region has a rugged and interesting topography, bounded by Puget Sound to the west and the Cascade Mountains to the east, preventing any such easy apportionment of the 60 Hikes Within 60 Miles promised by the title.

Accordingly, although the hikes described are generally scattered over a wide area, there are a few places where they are concentrated, as dictated by the necessities of the landscape. It is also an unfortunate geographic reality that the peaks of the Olympics, despite beckoning Seattle from only 40 miles away, are nonetheless too remote for inclusion. Although it is blessed with some magnificent trails, the Olympic Peninsula requires several hours to reach by road, ferry, or both, and therefore had to be left out.

Of the featured 60 hikes, approximately one-third are located in urban or suburban areas, another third are in rural areas, and the remaining third are in the wilderness. About 40 can be hiked year-round, including many in the mountains.

If you hiked one trail from this book each week without fail, regardless of weather or other commitments, it would take you more than a year to complete them all. And that doesn't even take into consideration the destinations that frequently include multiple hiking options. In the era of ever-escalating gas prices, this book provides great opportunities for outdoor recreation within about an hour's drive.

Thankfully, the same terrain that restricts where trails can be found also makes hiking here unique and rewarding. If the waters of Puget Sound largely limit the number of hikes to the west of the city, the ones that are available are nonetheless exceptional. The remaining hikes in this book—the vast majority—run in a broad arc on the eastern side of the urban area, stretching from Mount Rainier in the south to the Boulder River Wilderness in the north.

Seattle Parks

The hikes in this group definitively prove that it is not necessary to venture far from home to find a good trail. You can't help but be amazed at the natural attractions to be discovered here, practically in your own backyard. Many parks preserve pieces of the landscape like it used to be, before urban development began. Some, such as Schmitz Preserve Park and Seward Park, still harbor stands of old-growth forest. Carkeek Park and Discovery Park both offer great beach access.

Bellevue and the Eastside

Despite the rapid growth of Bellevue and the suburban area, many great natural pockets remain on the Eastside, from Saint Edward State Park and O. O. Denny Park on the shores of Lake Washington to the panoramic heights of the Issaquah Alps. Mercer Slough Nature Park and Redmond Watershed Preserve both feature interesting wetlands and the wildlife that goes with it, while the many trails on Cougar, Squak, and Tiger Mountains provide the closest hikes to Seattle with a "big-mountain" feel. The interesting industrial history of the region can also be found, awaiting discovery along Coal Creek.

I-90 and the Snoqualmie Pass Area

Snoqualmie Pass is the first area most people think of for hiking near Seattle. That's no surprise, given that the trail up Mount Si is a virtual rite of passage for anyone who's ever laced up a pair of hiking boots in the Puget Sound region. The I-90 corridor serves as a grand gateway to the Cascade Mountains, where towering peaks such as Granite, Defiance, Mailbox, and Teneriffe challenge all comers and provide commensurate rewards in the form of great views from their summits for hikers tough enough to reach them. If that's not enough, many of the waterfalls that inspired the name *Cascades* are in abundance along the trails around Snoqualmie Pass, and they are the main attractions at places such as Twin Falls and Franklin Falls.

Kitsap Peninsula and the Islands

Most hikers who look out over Puget Sound are inevitably drawn to the Olympic Mountains, distracted from the treasures at their feet by the prominent peaks on the horizon. Whidbey Island's untamed shoreline offers up two wild beaches, at Useless Bay and Ebey's Landing, the latter also providing great views over the Strait of Juan de Fuca from its stunning high-bluff trail. A similar taste of the island life is also available just to the west of Seattle on Bainbridge and Vashon, each with a unique hiking experience only a short ferry ride away. On the Kitsap Peninsula, the horseshoe-shaped Hood Canal reaches its end at the ecologically rich Theler Wetlands. Kitsap is also home to Green Mountain, an exceptional high point on the generally low-lying terrain between the Olympic Peninsula and the mainland. The peak provides a great view over much of the sound from an unusual perspective that few people see. And unique Blake Island Marine State Park presents a special challenge and reward for those intrepid enough to journey across the water.

North of Seattle

For residents of the cities north of Seattle, Stevens Pass is a local version of Snoqualmie Pass, complete with easy access along US 2. Both passes have their own distinct flavor and attractions, though. Unlike Snoqualmie, where hikers can ascend the significant mountains with relative ease, few trails reach the top of the sharp and forbidding peaks around Stevens, whose summits are best left to serious climbers. Hikers should be content to view jagged Baring Mountain and Mount Index from the Heybrook Ridge Lookout or the shores of Lake Serene, one of the finest swimming holes in the Cascades. The region's rich pioneer history also awaits exploration along trails that feel like tours through a living museum, particularly as you experience the remnants of a once-mighty railroad on the fascinating Iron Goat Trail.

The town of Granite Falls serves as entry portal to the rugged mountains of northern Snohomish County. With no suitable crossing to the east, the only road that manages significant penetration into the area is forced to bend back on itself, creating the Mountain Loop Highway. Yet the mountains here are accessible on foot, allowing hikers to reach great locations that cars cannot. Magnificent groves of old-growth forest populate the areas near Heather Lake; Boulder River Trail runs deep into the wilderness of the same name. The hike up Mount Pilchuck is a true Puget Sound classic, culminating in a spectacular view of the entire region from the summit lookout.

South of Seattle

Lacking any easily recognizable landmarks, the region encompassed by southern King County, Pierce County, and the lower end of Puget Sound is often overlooked by hikers. Yet this "forgotten frontier" does offer some worthy trails and an eclectic mix of outdoor attractions. Point Defiance features interesting history alongside great views of the South Sound, not to mention some old-growth trees, also the main attraction at Federation Forest State Park. Bird-watchers will love the Billy Frank Jr. Nisqually National Wildlife Refuge. And the Mud Mountain Dam and Recreation Area provides an interesting look at the White River (and man's attempts to control it), while Pinnacle Peak stands like a lone sentinel above the surrounding flatlands, a geologic oddity demanding further investigation.

Words cannot do justice to the natural wonders that pervade the area around Washington's most famous landmark, Mount Rainier. Ancient forests, thundering waterfalls, and giant glaciers are just a few of the spectacular features to be found throughout the 236,000 acres that make up Mount Rainier National Park. Head to the aptly named Spray Falls to see one of the most beautiful waterfalls in the state, and continue up to the high alpine meadows at Spray Park for an unforgettable wildflower display. Just to the north, the view from the top of Tolmie Peak makes the mountain and its massive ice floes seem close enough to touch.

Get Out and Explore on Your Own

Tell someone you are writing a guidebook—a hiking guidebook of all things—and you are sure to be flooded with advice, questions, and ideas. Everyone has something to say, and Seattle residents invariably show their passion for the outdoors in the strength of their opinions. You must include this hike, someone's favorite; you cannot include that other one, the secret hike no one knows about. You have to write in this particular style, or use a photo from this vantage point, or include these features on the map.

Beneath all of the advice lies a not-too-well-hidden subtext: Who are you to write a guidebook for me? And indeed, the question is a good one. Every individual has a unique experience on the trails, the product of countless factors such as physical fitness, personal preference, and even one's mood on a given day. Nobody owns the trails, and we are all free to enjoy them in our own way—and this is the reason most of us go hiking in the first place. No guidebook could hope to capture all of the ways people experience the outdoors, and none should even try.

I was reminded of this on a hike one cloudy Mother's Day, when I stumbled across a half dozen moms with several bottles of champagne and a basket of strawberries escaping six husbands and who knows how many kids at a secluded viewpoint in the Issaquah Alps. A guidebook might have led them to the spot, but it certainly didn't tell them this was the thing to do when they got there.

Let these audacious women be your inspiration, and use this book as a sampler for your own adventures; it is nothing more than a brief introduction to hiking in the Pacific Northwest. No one could ever hope to produce an exhaustive accounting of the vast outdoor resources to be found in this remarkable corner of the planet—or tell you how they should be enjoyed, which is the best reason to go exploring on your own. Make the most of this unique, wonderful region. There is no place like it anywhere else in the world.

60 Hikes by Category

Hike Categories

- ✓ Mileage
- ✓ Difficulty
- ✓ Running
- ✓ Kid-Friendly
- ✓ Dogs*
- ✓ Solitude

REGION Hike Number/Hike Name	page	Mileage	Difficulty	Running	Kid-Friendly	Dogs*	Solitude
SEATTLE PARKS							
1 Camp Long	16	1.1	E		✓	✓	
2 Carkeek Park and Beach	21	3.5	E–M		✓	✓‡	
3 Discovery Park and Beach	26	3.0	E–M	✓	✓	✓‡	
4 Schmitz Preserve Park	31	1.0	E		✓	✓	
5 Seward Park	35	4.6	E	✓	✓	✓‡	
6 Washington Park Arboretum and Foster Island	39	3.5	E		✓	✓‡	
7 Woodland Park and Green Lake Park	44	1.3	E	✓	✓	✓	
BELLEVUE AND THE EASTSIDE							
8 Coal Creek Natural Area	52	6.0	E–M	✓	✓	✓	
9 Cougar Mountain: Wilderness Peak Loop	57	3.5	M	✓	✓	✓	
10 Evans Creek Preserve	61	3.0	E–M	✓	✓	✓	
11 Mercer Slough Nature Park	65	2.1	E		✓	✓	
12 O. O. Denny Park	70	1.0	E		✓	✓	✓
13 Redmond Watershed Preserve	74	4.6	E–M	✓	✓		
14 Saint Edward State Park	78	2.5	M	✓	✓	✓	
15 Squak Mountain State Park: Double Peak Loop	82	6.7	M			✓	
16 Tiger Mountain: Chirico Trail	87	4.0	M		✓	✓	
17 Tiger Mountain: Poo Poo Point Trail	91	7.0	D	✓		✓	
18 Tiger Mountain: West Tiger Three Loop	96	5.1	M–D	✓		✓	
19 Tolt River–John MacDonald Park	101	2.0–2.3	E–M		✓	✓	

REGION Hike Number/Hike Name	page	Mileage	Difficulty	Running	Kid-Friendly	Dogs*	Solitude
I-90 AND THE SNOQUALMIE PASS AREA							
20 Annette Lake and Asahel Curtis Nature Trail	108	0.75–6.0	E–D	✓	✓	off-leash	
21 Bare Mountain	112	7.0	D			✓	✓
22 Dirty Harry's Peak and Balcony Trail	117	7.5	D			✓	✓
23 Franklin Falls and Old Snoqualmie Pass Wagon Road	122	2.0	E		✓	✓	
24 Granite Mountain Lookout Tower	126	8.0	D			✓	
25 Ira Spring Trail to Mason Lake, Mount Defiance, and Bandera Mountain	130	6.5–10.0	M–D	✓		✓	
26 Little Si	135	4.0	M			✓	
27 Mailbox Peak	139	10.0	D			✓	
28 McClellan Butte	144	9.0	D	✓		✓	
29 Middle Fork Snoqualmie River Trail	149	6.0–10.0	M	✓		off-leash	
30 Mount Si	154	8.0	D	✓		✓	
31 Mount Teneriffe and Teneriffe Falls	159	5.6–8.0	M–D			✓	
32 Rattlesnake Ledge and Rattlesnake Mountain	164	4.0–8.8	M–D			✓	
33 Twin Falls Natural Area and Olallie State Park	169	2.5	M	✓	✓	✓	
KITSAP PENINSULA AND THE ISLANDS							
34 Bainbridge Island: Gazzam Lake Nature Preserve	176	2.0–5.0	E–M	✓	✓	✓	
35 Blake Island Marine State Park	181	3.0	E		✓	✓	✓
36 Ebey's Landing State Park and National Historical Reserve	186	3.5	M		✓	✓	
37 Green Mountain State Forest	191	4.0–7.7	M–D	✓		✓	
38 Hood Canal and Theler Wetlands	196	2.8	E		✓		
39 Useless Bay Park and Double Bluff Beach	201	4.0	E		✓	off-leash†	✓
40 Vashon Island: Point Robinson and Maury Island Marine Park	205	1.5–3.0	E–M		✓	off-leash	✓

*Dogs allowed on leash unless otherwise noted.

† Dogs allowed off-leash after the first 500 feet (they must be leashed up to that point).

‡ Dogs allowed on leash in most areas but not allowed in others.

REGION Hike Number/Hike Name	page	Mileage	Difficulty	Running	Kid-Friendly	Dogs*	Solitude
NORTH OF SEATTLE							
41 Barclay Lake, Stone Lake, and Eagle Lake	212	4.5–7.5	E–D	✓	✓	✓	✓
42 Boulder River Trail	217	2.0–8.4	E–M	✓	✓	✓	✓
43 Greider Lakes	221	8.6	D			✓	✓
44 Heather Lake	226	5.25	M	✓	✓	✓	
45 Heybrook Ridge and Lookout Tower	230	2.8	M		✓	✓	
46 Iron Goat Trail	234	6.0	M	✓	✓	✓	
47 Lake Serene and Bridal Veil Falls	240	3.4–7.4	D			✓	
48 Lime Kiln Trail	245	4.8–6.4	E–M	✓	✓	✓	✓
49 Meadowdale Beach County Park	250	2.5	E–M		✓	✓	
50 Mount Pilchuck State Park	254	5.0	M	✓		✓	
51 Spencer Island Natural Wildlife Reserve	258	4.0	E		✓		
52 Wallace Falls State Park	263	4.0–5.4	M–D	✓	✓	✓	
SOUTH OF SEATTLE							
53 Billy Frank Jr. Nisqually National Wildlife Refuge	270	4.7	E–M		✓		
54 Federation Forest State Park	275	4.0	E		✓	✓	
55 Flaming Geyser State Park	280	0.4–1.7	E–M		✓	✓	
56 Mount Rainier National Park: Mowich Lake, Eunice Lake, and Tolmie Peak Lookout	285	6.0	M	✓			
57 Mount Rainier National Park: Spray Falls and Spray Park	290	4.5–7.0	M–D	✓	✓		
58 Mud Mountain Dam and White River Trail	295	6.5	M	✓	✓	off-leash	✓
59 Pinnacle Peak County Park: Cal Magnusson Trail	300	2.0	M		✓	✓	
60 Point Defiance Park	304	4.3	E	✓	✓	✓	

*Dogs allowed on leash unless otherwise noted.

† Dogs allowed off-leash after the first 500 feet (they must be leashed up to that point).

‡ Dogs allowed on leash in most areas but not allowed in others.

More Hike Categories

✓ Busy	✓ Waterfalls	✓ Rivers/Streams
✓ Urban	✓ Lake	✓ Scenic

REGION Hike Number/Hike Name	page	Busy	Urban	Waterfalls	Lake	Rivers/Streams	Scenic
SEATTLE PARKS							
1 Camp Long	16	✓	✓				
2 Carkeek Park and Beach	21	✓	✓				✓
3 Discovery Park and Beach	26	✓	✓				✓
4 Schmitz Preserve Park	31		✓				
5 Seward Park	35	✓	✓		✓		✓
6 Washington Park Arboretum and Foster Island	39	✓	✓		✓		
7 Woodland Park and Green Lake Park	44	✓	✓		✓		
BELLEVUE AND THE EASTSIDE							
8 Coal Creek Natural Area	52	✓	✓	✓			
9 Cougar Mountain: Wilderness Peak Loop	57	✓				✓	
10 Evans Creek Preserve	61	✓					
11 Mercer Slough Nature Park	65	✓	✓			✓	✓
12 O. O. Denny Park	70		✓				
13 Redmond Watershed Preserve	74	✓	✓				
14 Saint Edward State Park	78	✓	✓		✓		
15 Squak Mountain State Park: Double Peak Loop	82						
16 Tiger Mountain: Chirico Trail	87	✓					
17 Tiger Mountain: Poo Poo Point Trail	91						
18 Tiger Mountain: West Tiger Three Loop	96	✓			✓		
19 Tolt River–John MacDonald Park	101					✓	
I-90 AND THE SNOQUALMIE PASS AREA							
20 Annette Lake and Asahel Curtis Nature Trail	108	✓			✓		
21 Bare Mountain	112			✓			✓
22 Dirty Harry's Peak and Balcony Trail	117						✓

REGION Hike Number/Hike Name	page	Busy	Urban	Waterfalls	Lake	Rivers/Streams	Scenic
I-90 AND THE SNOQUALMIE PASS AREA (*continued*)							
23 Franklin Falls and Old Snoqualmie Pass Wagon Road	122	✓		✓		✓	✓
24 Granite Mountain Lookout Tower	126	✓					✓
25 Ira Spring Trail to Mason Lake, Mount Defiance, and Bandera Mountain	130	✓		✓	✓		✓
26 Little Si	135	✓					✓
27 Mailbox Peak	139	✓					✓
28 McClellan Butte	144						✓
29 Middle Fork Snoqualmie River Trail	149					✓	
30 Mount Si	154	✓					✓
31 Mount Teneriffe and Teneriffe Falls	159			✓			✓
32 Rattlesnake Ledge and Rattlesnake Mountain	164	✓			✓		
33 Twin Falls Natural Area and Olallie State Park	169	✓		✓		✓	
KITSAP PENINSULA AND THE ISLANDS							
34 Bainbridge Island: Gazzam Lake Nature Preserve	176				✓		
35 Blake Island Marine State Park	181						✓
36 Ebey's Landing State Park and National Historical Reserve	186						✓
37 Green Mountain State Forest	191						
38 Hood Canal and Theler Wetlands	196	✓					✓
39 Useless Bay Park and Double Bluff Beach	201						✓
40 Vashon Island: Point Robinson and Maury Island Marine Park	205						✓
NORTH OF SEATTLE							
41 Barclay Lake, Stone Lake, and Eagle Lake	212	✓			✓		✓
42 Boulder River Trail	217			✓		✓	✓
43 Greider Lakes	221				✓		
44 Heather Lake	226	✓			✓		✓
45 Heybrook Ridge and Lookout Tower	230						✓

REGION Hike Number/Hike Name	page	Busy	Urban	Waterfalls	Lake	Rivers/Streams	Scenic
46 Iron Goat Trail	234						✓
47 Lake Serene and Bridal Veil Falls	240	✓		✓	✓		✓
48 Lime Kiln Trail	245					✓	
49 Meadowdale Beach County Park	250	✓	✓			✓	
50 Mount Pilchuck State Park	254	✓					✓
51 Spencer Island Natural Wildlife Reserve	258		✓			✓	✓
52 Wallace Falls State Park	263	✓		✓		✓	
SOUTH OF SEATTLE							
53 Billy Frank Jr. Nisqually National Wildlife Refuge	270	✓				✓	✓
54 Federation Forest State Park	275					✓	
55 Flaming Geyser State Park	280					✓	
56 Mount Rainier National Park: Mowich Lake, Eunice Lake, and Tolmie Peak Lookout	285	✓			✓		✓
57 Mount Rainier National Park: Spray Falls and Spray Park	290	✓		✓			✓
58 Mud Mountain Dam and White River Trail	295					✓	
59 Pinnacle Peak County Park: Cal Magnusson Trail	300	✓					
60 Point Defiance Park	304	✓	✓				✓

More Hike Categories

✓ Historical Sites	✓ Wildflowers	✓ Viewpoints
✓ Bird-Watching	✓ Old-Growth Forest	✓ Year-Round

REGION Hike Number/Hike Name	page	Historical Sites	Bird-Watching	Wildflowers	Old-Growth Forest	Viewpoints	Year-Round
SEATTLE PARKS							
1 Camp Long	16	✓					✓
2 Carkeek Park and Beach	21					✓	✓
3 Discovery Park and Beach	26	✓				✓	✓
4 Schmitz Preserve Park	31				✓		✓
5 Seward Park	35				✓	✓	✓
6 Washington Park Arboretum and Foster Island	39		✓				✓
7 Woodland Park and Green Lake Park	44		✓				✓
BELLEVUE AND THE EASTSIDE							
8 Coal Creek Natural Area	52	✓					✓
9 Cougar Mountain: Wilderness Peak Loop	57						✓
10 Evans Creek Preserve	61						✓
11 Mercer Slough Nature Park	65	✓	✓				✓
12 O. O. Denny Park	70				✓		✓
13 Redmond Watershed Preserve	74						✓
14 Saint Edward State Park	78						✓
15 Squak Mountain State Park: Double Peak Loop	82	✓				✓	✓
16 Tiger Mountain: Chirico Trail	87					✓	✓
17 Tiger Mountain: Poo Poo Point Trail	91					✓	✓
18 Tiger Mountain: West Tiger Three Loop	96					✓	✓
19 Tolt River–John MacDonald Park	101					✓	✓
I-90 AND THE SNOQUALMIE PASS AREA							
20 Annette Lake and Asahel Curtis Nature Trail	108				✓		
21 Bare Mountain	112				✓	✓	
22 Dirty Harry's Peak and Balcony Trail	117	✓				✓	

REGION Hike Number/Hike Name	page	Historical Sites	Bird-Watching	Wildflowers	Old-Growth Forest	Viewpoints	Year-Round
I-90 AND THE SNOQUALMIE PASS AREA (*continued*)							
23 Franklin Falls and Old Snoqualmie Pass Wagon Road	122	✓				✓	
24 Granite Mountain Lookout Tower	126			✓		✓	
25 Ira Spring Trail to Mason Lake, Mount Defiance, and Bandera Mountain	130			✓		✓	
26 Little Si	135					✓	✓
27 Mailbox Peak	139			✓		✓	
28 McClellan Butte	144				✓	✓	
29 Middle Fork Snoqualmie River Trail	149						✓
30 Mount Si	154					✓	
31 Mount Teneriffe and Teneriffe Falls	159					✓	
32 Rattlesnake Ledge and Rattlesnake Mountain	164					✓	✓
33 Twin Falls Natural Area and Olallie State Park	169						✓
KITSAP PENINSULA AND THE ISLANDS							
34 Bainbridge Island: Gazzam Lake Nature Preserve	176		✓				✓
35 Blake Island Marine State Park	181	✓					✓
36 Ebey's Landing State Park and National Historical Reserve	186	✓	✓	✓		✓	✓
37 Green Mountain State Forest	191			✓		✓	✓
38 Hood Canal and Theler Wetlands	196		✓				✓
39 Useless Bay Park and Double Bluff Beach	201						✓
40 Vashon Island: Point Robinson and Maury Island Marine Park	205	✓	✓				✓
NORTH OF SEATTLE							
41 Barclay Lake, Stone Lake, and Eagle Lake	212	✓		✓			
42 Boulder River Trail	217				✓		✓
43 Greider Lakes	221				✓		
44 Heather Lake	226				✓		

REGION Hike Number/Hike Name	page	Historical Sites	Bird-Watching	Wildflowers	Old-Growth Forest	Viewpoints	Year-Round
NORTH OF SEATTLE (*continued*)							
45 Heybrook Ridge and Lookout Tower	230					✓	
46 Iron Goat Trail	234	✓		✓		✓	
47 Lake Serene and Bridal Veil Falls	240	✓			✓		
48 Lime Kiln Trail	245	✓					✓
49 Meadowdale Beach County Park	250						✓
50 Mount Pilchuck State Park	254	✓				✓	
51 Spencer Island Natural Wildlife Reserve	258	✓	✓				✓
52 Wallace Falls State Park	263				✓	✓	✓
SOUTH OF SEATTLE							
53 Billy Frank Jr. Nisqually National Wildlife Refuge	270	✓	✓			✓	✓
54 Federation Forest State Park	275				✓		
55 Flaming Geyser State Park	280	✓					✓
56 Mount Rainier National Park: Mowich Lake, Eunice Lake, and Tolmie Peak Lookout	285			✓		✓	
57 Mount Rainier National Park: Spray Falls and Spray Park	290			✓		✓	
58 Mud Mountain Dam and White River Trail	295			✓		✓	✓
59 Pinnacle Peak County Park: Cal Magnusson Trail	300						✓
60 Point Defiance Park	304	✓			✓	✓	✓

Introduction

WELCOME TO *60 Hikes Within 60 Miles: Seattle.* If you're new to hiking or even if you're a seasoned trekker, take a few minutes to read the following introduction. We'll explain how this book is organized and how to get the best use of it.

How to Use This Guidebook

THE OVERVIEW MAP, MAP KEY, AND MAP LEGEND

Use the overview map on the inside front cover to assess the general location of each hike's primary trailhead. Each hike's number appears on the overview map, on the map key facing the overview map, and in the table of contents. As you flip through the book, a hike's full profile is easy to locate by watching for the hike number at the top of each page. The book is organized by region, as indicated in the table of contents. A map legend that details the symbols found on trail maps appears on the inside back cover.

REGIONAL MAPS

The book is divided into regions, and prefacing each regional section is an overview map of that region. The regional map provides more detail than the overview map does, bringing you closer to the hike.

HIKE PROFILES

Each hike contains seven or eight key items: a brief description of the trail, a key at-a-glance box, GPS coordinates, directions to the trail, a trail map, an elevation profile (if the change in elevation is 100 feet or more), and a trail description. Many also include a note on nearby activities. Combined, the maps and information provide a clear method to assess each trail from the comfort of your favorite reading chair.

IN BRIEF

Think of this section as a taste of the trail, a snapshot focused on the historical landmarks, beautiful vistas, and other sights you may encounter on the hike.

Key At-a-Glance Information

The information in the key at-a-glance boxes gives you a quick idea of the statistics and specifics of each hike.

DISTANCE & CONFIGURATION The length of the trail from start to finish (total distance traveled) and a description of what the trail might look like from overhead. Trails can be loops, out-and-backs (trails on which one enters and leaves along the same path), figure eights, or a combination of shapes. There may be options to shorten or extend the hikes, but the mileage corresponds to the described hike. Consult the hike description to help you decide how to customize the hike for your ability or time constraints.

DIFFICULTY　　The degree of effort an average hiker should expect on a given hike. For simplicity, the trails are rated as easy, moderate, or difficult.

SCENERY　　A short summary of the attractions offered by the hike and what to expect in terms of plant life, wildlife, natural wonders, and historical features.

EXPOSURE　　A quick check of how much sun you can expect on your shoulders during the hike.

TRAFFIC　　Indicates how busy the trail might be on an average day. Trail traffic, of course, varies from day to day and season to season. Weekend days typically see the most visitors. Other trail users that you may encounter on the trail are also noted here.

TRAIL SURFACE　　Indicates whether the trail surface is paved, rocky, gravel, dirt, boardwalk, or a mixture of elements.

HIKING TIME　　The length of time it takes to hike the trail. A slow but steady hiker will average 2–3 miles an hour, depending on the terrain.

ACCESS　　A notation of any fees or permits that may be needed to access the trail or park at the trailhead. Trails administered by the U.S. Forest Service require a Northwest Forest Pass (NW Forest Pass) for parking; a day pass is $5, and the annual pass is $30. Some sites allow you to self-issue a day pass at the trailhead, but if you plan to hike frequently each year, it is certainly worth buying the annual pass. Both passes can be purchased from national forest offices, outdoor retailers, and other local vendors; they are also available online at discovernw.org. The pass is good for national forest sites in both Washington and Oregon, covering most of the Cascade Range.

Parking at trails administered by the State of Washington through several agencies, including Washington State Parks and the Department of Natural Resources (DNR), requires a Washington State Discover Pass. A day pass is $10 and an annual pass is $30. Like the NW Forest Pass, some locations allow you to self-issue a day pass at the trailhead, but if you plan to hike frequently, the annual pass is a better option. Passes are available at state park offices and regional headquarters, outdoor retailers, other local vendors, and online at discoverpass.wa.gov.

Mount Rainier National Park requires an entrance fee of $25, which covers everybody in one vehicle for seven days. An annual pass to the park costs $50. Both options are available at the park entrance stations during normal park business hours. More information on hours and fees for the park is available online at nps.gov/mora.

City and county parks typically do not require any permits or parking fees, though this is always subject to change.

WHEELCHAIR TRAVERSABLE   Notes whether the trail is wheelchair compatible.

MAPS   Here you'll find a list of maps that show the topography of the trail, including Green Trails Maps and United States Geological Survey (USGS) topo maps. Green Trails Maps, with their signature green trails overlaid onto easy-to-read topographic backgrounds, are a local favorite for hiking in the Washington Cascades. The maps are usually scaled at 1:69,500, making them less detailed than typical USGS maps, but they do show a large area, which can still be helpful in the backcountry and along the trails. They are also good for identifying nearby peaks and other prominent geographic landmarks. Some of the most recently published Green Trails Maps cover the Issaquah Alps and North Bend area peaks, including Cougar and Squak Mountains, Tiger Mountain, Rattlesnake Mountain, and Mount Si Natural Resources Conservation Area (map numbers 203S, 204S, 205S, and 206S, respectively). These maps are especially useful because the scale is 1:24,000 and because they are more current than the USGS maps.

The USGS names listed in this section are for the applicable USGS 7.5-minute quadrangle maps (1:24,000 scale). Many of these maps are out of date, so roads or trails may not be shown in the current location, if they are shown at all. However, the topographic detail of the 7.5-minute series is nonetheless extremely valuable for backcountry navigation. See the section on topo maps (page 4) for more information on reading them.

FACILITIES   What to expect in terms of restrooms and water at the trailhead or nearby.

DOGS   Status of whether or not dogs are allowed on the trail and, if so, whether a leash is required.

CONTACT   Phone numbers and websites, where applicable, for up-to-date information on trail conditions.

LOCATION   The city in which the trail is located.

COMMENTS   Provides you with those extra details that don't fit into any of the above categories.

DESCRIPTIONS

The trail description is the heart of each hike. Here, the authors provide a summary of the trail's essence and highlight any special traits the hike has to offer. The route is clearly outlined, including landmarks, side trips, and possible alternate routes along the way. Ultimately, the hike description will help you choose which hikes are best for you.

NEARBY ACTIVITIES

Look here for information on nearby activities or points of interest. This includes nearby parks, museums, restaurants, or even a brewpub where you can get a well-deserved beer after a long hike. Note that not every hike has a listing.

TRAIL MAPS

A detailed map of each hike's route appears with its profile. On each of these maps, symbols indicate the trailhead, the complete route, significant features, facilities, and topographic landmarks such as creeks, overlooks, and peaks.

ELEVATION PROFILES

For trails with significant changes in elevation, the hike description will contain a detailed elevation profile that corresponds directly to the trail map. This graphical element provides a quick look at the trail from the side, enabling you to visualize how the trail rises and falls. On the diagram's vertical axis, or height scale, the number of feet indicated between each tick mark lets you visualize the climb. To avoid making flat hikes look steep and steep hikes appear flat, varying height scales provide an accurate image of each hike's climbing challenge. Elevation profiles for loop hikes show total distance; those for out-and-back hikes show only one-way distance.

GPS INFORMATION

In addition to highly specific trail outlines, this book also includes the latitude (north) and longitude (west) coordinates for each trailhead. The latitude–longitude grid system is likely quite familiar to you, but here's a refresher, pertinent to visualizing the coordinates.

Imaginary lines of latitude—called parallels and approximately 69 miles apart from each other—run horizontally around the globe. Each parallel is indicated by degrees from the equator (established to be 0°): up to 90°N at the North Pole and down to 90°S at the South Pole.

Imaginary lines of longitude—called meridians—run perpendicular to lines of latitude and are likewise indicated by degrees. Starting from 0° at the Prime Meridian in Greenwich, England, they continue to the east and west until they meet 180° later at the International Date Line in the Pacific Ocean. At the equator, longitude lines also are approximately 69 miles apart, but that distance narrows as the meridians converge toward the North and South Poles.

In this book, latitude and longitude are expressed in degree–decimal minute format, using the NAD83 datum. For example, the coordinates for Hike 1, Camp Long (page 16), are as follows:

N47° 33.329' W122° 22.509'

For more on GPS technology, visit usgs.gov.

TOPO MAPS

The maps in this book have been produced with great care. When used with the route directions in each profile, the maps are sufficient to direct you to the trail and guide you on it. However, you will find superior detail and valuable information in the USGS 7.5-minute series topographic maps.

Topo maps are available online in many locations. At mytopo.com, for example, you can view and print topos of the entire Unites States free of charge. Online services, such as trails.com, charge annual fees for additional features such as shaded relief, which makes the topography stand out more. If you expect to print out many topo maps each year, it might be worth paying for shaded-relief topo maps. The downside to USGS topos is that many of them are outdated, having been created 20–30 years ago. But they still provide excellent topographic detail. Of course, Google Earth (earth.google.com) does away with topo maps and their inaccuracies—replacing them with satellite imagery and its inaccuracies. Regardless, what one lacks, the other augments. Google Earth is an excellent tool whether you have difficulty with topos or not.

If you're new to hiking, you might be wondering, "What's a topographic map?" In short, a topo indicates not only linear distance but elevation as well, using contour lines. Contour lines spread across the map like dozens of intricate spiderwebs. Each line represents a particular elevation; at the base of each topo, a contour's interval designation is given. If the contour interval is 20 feet, then the distance between each contour line is 20 feet. Follow five contour lines up on the same map, and the elevation has increased by 100 feet.

Let's assume that the 7.5-minute series topo reads "Contour Interval 40 feet," that the short trail we'll be hiking is 2 inches in length on the map, and that it crosses five contour lines from beginning to end. What do we know? Well, because the linear scale of this series is 2,000 feet to the inch (roughly 2.75 inches representing 1 mile), we know that our trail is approximately 0.8 mile long (2 inches are 4,000 feet). But we also know that we'll be climbing or descending 200 vertical feet (five contour lines are 40 feet each) over that distance. And the elevation designations written on occasional contour lines will tell us if we're heading up or down.

In addition to the places listed in Appendixes A and B, you'll find topos at major universities and some public libraries, where you might try photocopying what you need. But if you want your own and can't find them locally, visit nationalmap.gov or store.usgs.gov.

Allocating Time

On flat or slightly undulating terrain, the authors averaged 3 miles per hour when hiking. That speed drops in direct proportion to the steepness of a path, and it does not reflect the many pauses and forays off-trail in pursuit of yet another viewpoint, wildflower, or photograph. Give yourself plenty of time. Few people enjoy rushing through a hike, and fewer take pleasure in bumping into trees after dark. Remember, too, that your pace naturally slackens over the back half of a long trek.

Weather

As you can see from the table on the next page, which lists average daily temperatures by month for the Seattle–Tacoma area, the average highs never reach 80°F, and the average lows are well above the freezing point. However, this does not mean that it can't get very

SEATTLE-TACOMA AVERAGE DAILY TEMPERATURES BY MONTH 30-YEAR AVERAGE					
	JAN	**FEB**	**MAR**	**APR**	**MAY**	**JUN**
HIGH	46° F	50° F	53° F	58° F	64° F	70° F
LOW	36° F	37° F	39° F	42° F	47° F	52° F
	JUL	**AUG**	**SEP**	**OCT**	**NOV**	**DEC**
HIGH	75° F	76° F	70° F	60° F	51° F	46° F
LOW	55° F	56° F	52° F	46° F	40° F	36° F

hot on some summer days or uncomfortably cold on some winter days, especially at higher elevations. What it does mean is that most of the year you can hike without dealing with extreme temperatures—though you might get wet.

For better or worse, Seattle is nearly synonymous with rain. Yet that perception is surely due to the high number of overcast and drizzly days each year, rather than the actual measured rainfall of about 39 inches. On average, Seattle gets less rain than Miami, Atlanta, Houston, Boston, New York, Philadelphia, Indianapolis, and Washington, D.C. However, Seattle beats all those cities when totaling the number of annual rainy days (around 160). You are most likely to get wet in Seattle October–March. December is the wettest month, with about 6 inches of accumulated precipitation each year, on average; and July is the driest, with less than 1 inch.

Summer days in the Puget Sound region can be hot on occasion, but typically the air doesn't feel as humid as it does in many other parts of the United States. This is a particular benefit to hiking around Seattle, because heat plus humidity can spell danger when one is exercising outdoors. Use common sense when hiking on hot days, and rest in the shade if necessary. Stay hydrated by drinking water throughout the hike, and you will minimize any chance of heat-related illness.

In the winter months, the Cascade Range is typically buried under a blanket of snow. This includes the higher-elevation hikes along I-90, US 2, and Mountain Loop Highway, as well as those in Mount Rainier National Park. The foothills, including the Issaquah Alps, do get snow in the winter, but it rarely lingers for more than a week or two. That is why this book contains 40 hikes that are considered accessible year-round, even though some of the trails may be snow-covered part of the year. Usually these trails are still hikable in snowy conditions, which may, in fact, be the best time of the year to explore them. If you want to find solitude and experience a different outdoor setting, then venture a couple miles from any trailhead when there is snow on the ground. Just keep in mind that trails may be muddy and slippery under these conditions. Dress warmly and be prepared with the 10 essentials. (See "The 10 Essentials" section on page 8.)

Seattle's spring and fall are mild and pleasant. When it's not raining, these are great days to be outside. Spring blooms and fall leaves make the scenery spectacular, and the trails of the Cascades are usually clear of snow by late June, so nearly every trail in this book should be hikable by then, except in the most extreme years. Think that never happens? The winter of 2007–08 saw record snows across much of the region, rendering many popular trails unusable until July or even August. The winter of 2014–15 was just the opposite, with record low snowfall, making some seasonal trails available year-round.

Water

"How much is enough? One bottle? Two? Three? But think of all that extra weight!" Well, one simple physiological fact should convince you to err on the side of excess when it comes to deciding how much water to pack: A hiker working hard in 90ºF heat needs approximately 10 quarts of fluid every day—that's 2.5 gallons (12 large water bottles or 16 small ones). In other words, pack along one or two bottles even for short hikes.

Serious backpackers hit the trail prepared to purify water found along the route. This method, while less dangerous than drinking it untreated, comes with risks. Purifiers with ceramic filters are the safest but are also the most expensive. Many hikers pack along the slightly distasteful tetraglycine hydroperiodide (also known as iodine tablets, sold under the names Potable Aqua, Coughlan's, and others).

Probably the most common waterborne bug that hikers face is *Giardia,* which may not affect you until one to four weeks after ingestion. It will have you passing noxious rotten-egg-smelling gas, vomiting, shivering with chills, and living in the bathroom. But there are other parasites to worry about that are harder to kill than *Giardia,* including *E. coli* and *Cryptosporidium.*

For most people, the pleasures of hiking make carrying water a relatively minor price to pay to remain healthy. If you're tempted to drink "found" water, do so only if you understand the risks involved. Better yet, hydrate prior to your hike, carry (and drink) 6 ounces of water for every mile you plan to hike, and hydrate again after you're finished.

Clothing

There is a wide variety of clothing from which to choose. Basically, use common sense and be prepared for anything. If all you have are cotton clothes when a sudden rainstorm comes along, you'll be miserable, especially in cooler weather. It's a good idea to carry along a light wool sweater or some type of synthetic apparel (polypropylene, Capilene, Thermax, and so on) as well as a hat.

Be aware of the weather forecast and its tendency to be wrong. Always carry raingear. Thunderstorms can come on suddenly in the summer. With appropriate raingear, a normally crowded trail can be a wonderful place of solitude. Do, however, remain aware of the dangers of lightning strikes.

Footwear is another concern. Though tennis shoes may be appropriate for paved areas, some trails are rocky and rough; tennis shoes may not offer enough support. Waterproofed or not, boots should be your footwear of choice. Sport sandals are more popular than ever, but these leave much of your foot exposed, leaving you vulnerable to hazardous plants and thorns or the occasional piece of glass.

The 10 Essentials

One of the first rules of hiking is to be prepared for anything. The simplest way to be prepared is to carry the "10 Essentials." In addition to carrying the items listed below, you need to know how to use them, especially navigation items. Always consider worst-case scenarios such as getting lost, hiking back in the dark, breaking gear (for example, finding a broken hip strap on your pack or a water filter plugged), twisting an ankle or sustaining some other serious injury, and encountering thunderstorms or inclement conditions. The items listed below don't cost a lot of money, don't take up much room in a pack, and don't weigh much, but they might just save your life.

➢ Water: durable bottles and water treatment, such as iodine or a filter

➢ Map: preferably a topo map and a trail map with a route description

➢ Compass: a high-quality compass

➢ First aid kit: a good-quality kit including first aid instructions (see details below)

➢ Knife: a multitool device with pliers is best

➢ Light: flashlight or headlamp with extra bulbs and batteries

➢ Fire: windproof matches or lighter and fire starter

➢ Extra food: You should always have food in your pack when you've finished hiking.

➢ Extra clothes: rain protection, warm layers, gloves, warm hat

➢ Sun protection: sunglasses, lip balm, sunblock, sun hat

First Aid Kit

A typical first aid kit may contain more items than you might think necessary. These are just the basics. Prepackaged kits in waterproof bags are available (Atwater Carey and Adventure Medical Kits make a variety of kits). Even though there are quite a few items listed here, they pack down into a small space:

Ace bandages or Spenco joint wraps

Acetaminophen and/or ibuprofen

Antacid (for stomach upset)

Antibiotic ointment (Neosporin or the generic equivalent)

Band-Aids

Benadryl or the generic equivalent, diphenhydramine (an antihistamine, in case of allergic reactions)

Butterfly-closure bandages

Emergency mylar space blanket (for shock victims and emergency shelter)

Epinephrine in a prefilled syringe (for those known to have severe allergic reactions to such things as bee stings)

First aid manual

Gauze (one roll and a half dozen 4-by-4-inch compress pads)

Hydrogen peroxide or iodine swabs

Insect repellent

Moistened towelettes and antiseptic wipes

Moleskin/Spenco Second Skin

Needle or safety pin

Triangle bandage (has many first aid uses, such as to make a sling or tourniquet)

Tweezers

Whistle (more effective in signaling rescuers than your voice is)

Pack the items in a waterproof bag such as a zip-top bag.

Animal and Plant Hazards

BLACK BEARS

It's unlikely that you will meet a bear on any of these trails; there are still very few in Washington, and in most cases, the bear will detect you first and leave. Should you encounter a bear, here is some advice, based on suggestions from the National Park Service:

➢ Stay calm.

➢ Move away, talking loudly to let the bear discover your presence.

➢ Back away while facing the bear.

➢ Avoid eye contact.

➢ Give the bear plenty of room to escape; bears will rarely attack unless they are threatened or provoked.

➢ Don't run or make sudden movements; running will provoke the bear, and you cannot outrun a bear.

➢ Do not attempt to climb trees to escape bears, especially black bears. The bear will pull you down by the foot.

➢ Fight back if you are attacked. Black bears have been driven away when people have fought back with rocks, sticks, binoculars, and even their bare hands.

MOSQUITOES

Though it's not a common occurrence, individuals can become infected with the West Nile virus by being bitten by an infected mosquito. Culex mosquitoes, the primary variety that can transmit West Nile virus to humans, thrive in urban rather than in natural areas.

They lay their eggs in stagnant water and can breed in standing water that remains for more than five days. Most people infected with West Nile virus have no symptoms of illness, but some may become ill, usually 3–15 days after being bitten.

Due to its cooler summers and lower humidity, the Seattle area doesn't have a lot of mosquitoes. However, if you plan on hiking near an area with stagnant water, you may want to wear protective clothing, such as long sleeves, long pants, and socks. Loose-fitting, light-colored clothing is best. Spray clothing with insect repellent. Remember to follow the instructions on the repellent and to take extra care with children.

POISON IVY, POISON OAK, AND POISON SUMAC

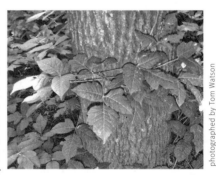

Recognizing poison ivy, oak, and sumac and avoiding contact with them is the most effective way to prevent the painful, itchy rashes associated with these plants. Poison ivy ranges from a thick, tree-hugging vine to a shaded ground cover, 3 leaflets to a leaf; poison oak occurs as either a vine or shrub, with 3 leaflets as well; and poison sumac flourishes in swampland, each leaf containing 7–13 leaflets. Urushiol, the oil in the sap of these plants, is responsible for the rash.

Poison ivy

Usually within 12–14 hours of exposure (but sometimes much later), raised lines and/or blisters will appear, accompanied by a terrible itch. Refrain from scratching because

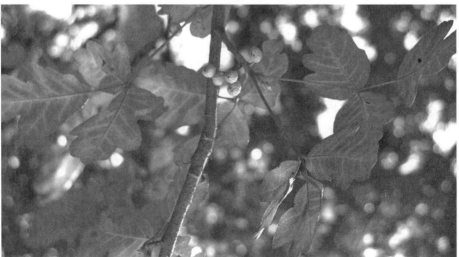

Poison oak

bacteria under fingernails can cause infection, and you will spread the rash to other parts of your body. Wash and dry the rash thoroughly, applying a calamine lotion or other product to help dry the rash. If itching or blistering is severe, seek medical attention. Remember that oil-contaminated garments, pets, or hiking equipment can easily cause an irritating rash on you or someone else, so wash not only any exposed parts of your body but also clothes, gear, and pets.

SNAKES

The most common snakes you'll encounter in and west of the Cascades are nonpoisonous garter snakes. The only venomous snake in Washington is the western rattlesnake, but sightings of these pit vipers are generally infrequent, occurring most often in dry, rocky, or exposed zones during the warmest months of the year. The standard advice for hiking in rattlesnake territory is as follows:

> ➢ Don't put your hands or feet where you can't see them—say, at the top of a rock outcrop, or in tall grass or a log pile.
> ➢ Be extra cautious in hot weather, when snakes are more active.
> ➢ Scan the trail continuously as you hike.
> ➢ Keep kids from running ahead on the trail. Bites to children are more severe than those to adults.

Should you encounter a rattlesnake, its body language will reveal its mood. A coiled rattler is primed for a strike, while a relaxed rattler is more sanguine. If the snake is within striking distance, stand motionless and wait for it to calm down and move on. Taking small, slow steps backward is another smart strategy. If you're out of immediate range, you can either skirt the snake or wait for it to move. Some people believe tapping the ground with a stick—from a safe distance, rather than in the snake's face—will encourage the snake to move on.

STINGING NETTLES

Stinging nettles are common in disturbed areas, moist woodlands, and partially shaded trails. The toothed leaves are oval, ribbed, and covered with hairs. When you brush past stinging nettles, sharp, tiny spines covering the leaves and stems penetrate your skin and release histamine and formic acid. The result is an itchy rash relieved only with hydrocortisone creams and cool compresses.

TICKS

Ticks like to hang out in the brush that grows along trails. Ticks, which are arachnids and not insects, need a host on which to feast in order to reproduce. The ticks that light onto you while hiking will be very small, sometimes so tiny that you won't be able to spot them. The two primary varieties, deer ticks and dog ticks, both need a few hours of actual attachment before they can transmit any disease they may harbor. Ticks may settle in shoes, socks, or hats, and they may take several hours to actually latch on. The best strategy is to visually check every half hour or so while hiking, do a thorough check before you get in the car, and then, when you take a posthike shower, do an even more thorough check of your entire body. Also, throw clothes into the dryer for 10 minutes when you get home, and be sure to check your pet for any hitchhikers. Ticks that haven't attached are easily removed but not easily killed. If you pick off a tick in the woods, just toss it aside. If you find one on your body at home, dispatch it and then send it down the toilet. For ticks that have embedded, removal with tweezers is best.

The blacklegged deer tick is the culprit behind Lyme disease. Experts advocate abundant repellent containing permethrin on footwear and pant legs because the nymphal stage blacklegged tick often lurks in dead leaves, and ticks rarely climb higher than 18–24 inches off the ground. They can grab on to your shoes and are quite quick to climb up. Get more information from the American Lyme Disease Foundation at aldf.com.

Hiking with Children

No one is too young for a hike in the woods or through a city park. Be mindful, though. Flat, short trails are best with an infant. Toddlers who have not quite mastered walking can still tag along, riding on an adult's back in a child carrier. Use common sense to judge a child's capacity to hike a particular trail, and always keep in mind the possibility that the child will tire quickly and need to be carried.

When packing for the hike, remember the needs of the child as well as your own. Make sure children are adequately clothed for the weather, have proper shoes, and are protected from the sun with sunscreen. Kids dehydrate quickly, so make sure you have plenty of fluid for everyone.

Hikes suitable for children (Kid-Friendly) are indicated in the table on pages xiv–xvi.

Trail Etiquette

Whether you're on a city, county, state, or national park trail, always remember that great care and resources (from both nature and from your tax dollars) have gone into creating these trails. Treat the trail, wildlife, and fellow hikers with respect.

➤ Hike on open trails only. Respect trail and road closures (ask if not sure), avoid possible trespass on private land, and obtain all permits and authorization as required. Also, leave gates as you found them or as marked.

➤ Leave only footprints. Be sensitive to the ground beneath you. This means staying on the existing trail and not blazing any new trails. Be sure to pack out what you pack in. No one likes to see the trash someone else has left behind.

➤ Never spook animals. An unannounced approach, a sudden movement, or a loud noise startles most animals. Surprised animals can be dangerous to you, to others, and to themselves. Give them plenty of space and time to adjust to your presence.

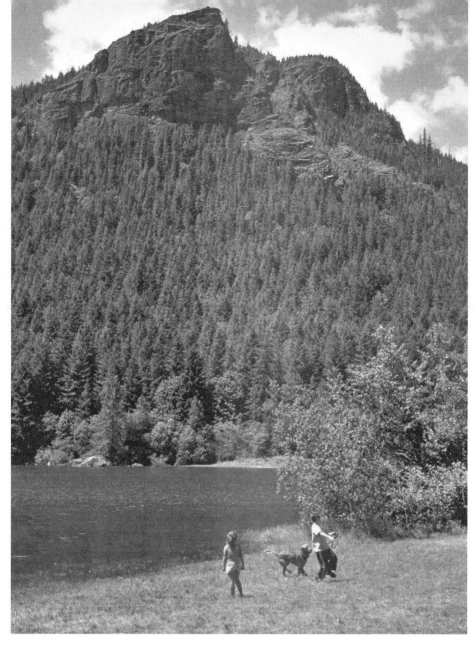

Rattlesnake Mountain from Rattlesnake Lake (see page 164)

> ➤ Plan ahead. Know your equipment, your ability, and the area in which you are hiking—and prepare accordingly. Be self-sufficient at all times; carry necessary supplies for changes in weather or other conditions (see "The 10 Essentials" on page 8). A well-executed trip is a satisfaction to you and to others.

> ➤ Be courteous to other hikers, bikers, or equestrians you encounter on the trails.

SEATTLE PARKS

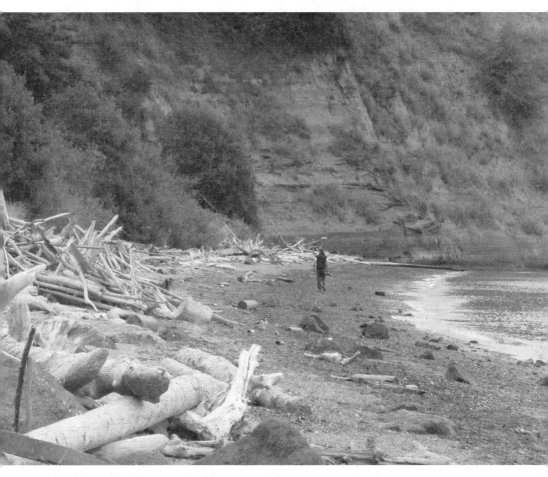

South Beach at Discovery Park (see page 26)

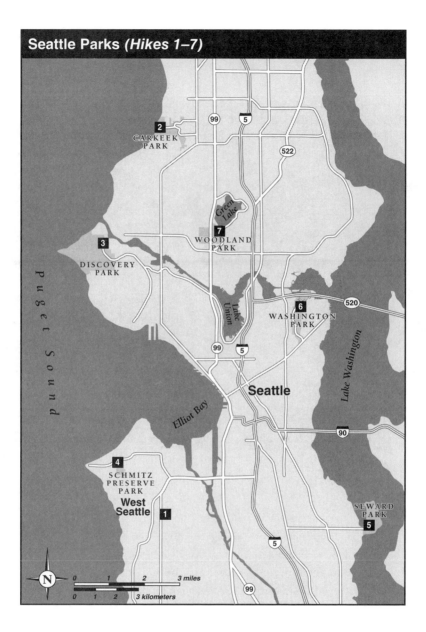

Seattle Parks *(Hikes 1–7)*

CARKEEK
PARK

Green
Lake

WOODLAND
PARK

DISCOVERY
PARK

Lake
Union

WASHINGTON
PARK

Lake Washington

Puget Sound

Seattle

Elliot Bay

SCHMITZ
PRESERVE
PARK

West
Seattle

SEWARD
PARK

N

0   1   2   3 miles

0   1   2   3 kilometers

1 Camp Long

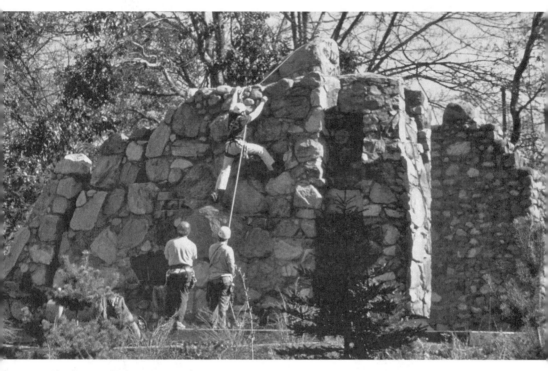

Climbers on Schurman Rock

In Brief

Originally established as an outdoor training ground for the Boy Scouts, Camp Long has grown into one of West Seattle's premier parks. Ever since the scouting facilities were opened to the general public in 1984, everyone has been welcome to hike the trails, camp in the shelters, and even climb on famous Schurman Rock, where many serious Cascade mountaineers first tested and developed their skills.

Description

At just less than 70 acres, Camp Long is far from a significant park if measured by size alone. Yet, as the old saying goes, good things come in small packages. For density of attractions, few parks can match this often-overlooked West Seattle reserve.

All outings at Camp Long should start at the visitor center. Built by the Works Progress Administration (WPA) during the Great Depression, the structure was modeled

16

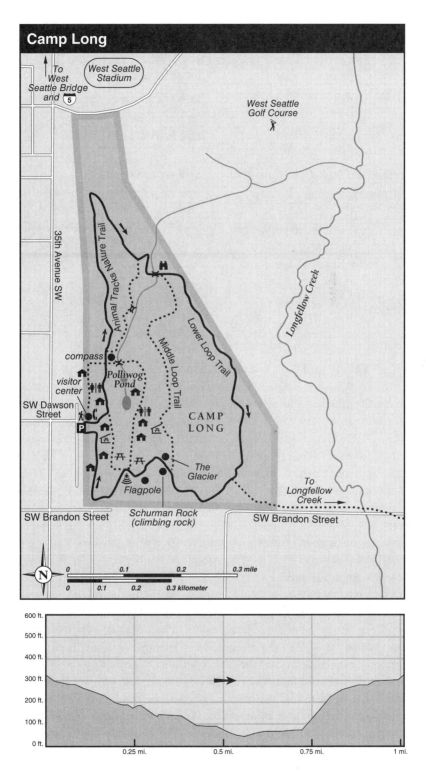

Camp Long

DISTANCE & CONFIGURATION: 1.1-mile loop with many side-trip options	**FACILITIES:** Toilets and water at visitor center
DIFFICULTY: Easy	**DOGS:** Allowed on-leash
SCENERY: Picturesque pond, stream, and fields; seasonal views of Seattle	**CONTACT:** 206-684-7434; seattle.gov /parks/environment/camplong.htm
EXPOSURE: Mostly shaded	**LOCATION:** 5200 35th Ave. SW, Seattle, WA 98126
TRAFFIC: Moderate	
TRAIL SURFACE: Dirt, gravel, paved	**COMMENTS:** Historical Boy Scout camp with old lodge and cabins for rent, climbing rock, and glacier-roping practice course. To rent one of the cabins or shelters, the Environmental Learning Center, or the fire circle, contact the Camp Long office; information on open hours, equipment rentals, and climbing classes on Schurman Rock is also available.
HIKING TIME: 1–2 hours	
ACCESS: Hikable year-round, Tuesday– Sunday, 10 a.m.–6 p.m.; no fee for parking or trail access	
WHEELCHAIR TRAVERSABLE: Yes, on Rolling Hills Trail and the service road	
MAP(S): USGS *Seattle South*	

after Oregon's Multnomah Falls Lodge, which was completed more than a decade earlier in 1925; the heavy stones used in construction at Camp Long had once paved Seattle's E. Madison Street, which was being resurfaced at the time.

Growing right next to the lodge door is an interpretive garden of native plants, modeling a forest-edge plant community typical of the area. Ecologists call this type of environment an ecotone, the meeting of two different landscapes to create a particularly high diversity of species. (The same phenomenon occurs in oceans, where unusual densities of marine life congregate where warm and cold currents mix.) Many of the plants visible in Camp Long's ecotone can also be seen in the interior of the park.

Inside the visitor center, you'll find information on the history and natural environment of the park in a series of helpful displays. The facility also features a great hall (to the left of the entrance) that is often used for educational gatherings and also hosts the occasional wedding or other ceremony.

An easily completed loop around the perimeter of Camp Long on a series of named trails provides the best hiking option. To get started, circle around the back of the visitor center and pass by several of the camping cabins. Much like the lodge itself, these buildings were built by the WPA, using reclaimed materials from around the city as part of an environmental recycling ethic that the camp continues to promote today.

Head down a gentle slope toward Polliwog Pond, then turn left along the service road next to the water to find the beginning of Animal Tracks Nature Trail, in front of the number-seven cabin (also known as St. Helens). Here you should look for a giant stone compass sunk into the ground, another WPA project built to help young Boy Scouts develop wilderness-navigation skills.

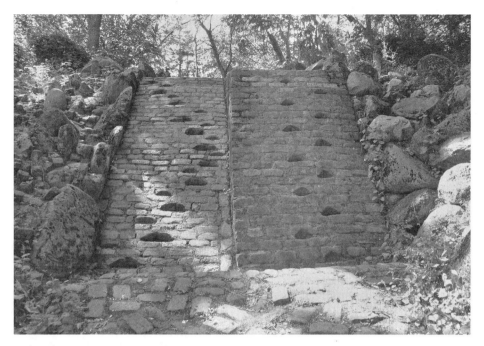

The Glacier

Animal Tracks Nature Trail, which follows a ridge to the northern end of the park, offers seasonal views of downtown Seattle, the docks at Harbor Island, and the Space Needle through gaps in the trees in winter. (The forest is a mix of red alder, big-leaf maple, and various other species, including western red cedar, although there is no old growth; the understory is characterized by sword ferns, ivy, Oregon grape, and blackberry bushes.) The trail bends sharply around to the right at its northern point and heads downhill. Stay to the left at a junction with Middle Loop Trail (the general rule for hiking the perimeter in the clockwise) and cross a tributary of Longfellow Creek, the outflow from the wetlands next to the pond you saw at the outset.

At a second junction, stay left again to join Lower Loop Trail, which runs along the eastern edge of the park closest to the West Seattle Golf Course. Red foxes, frequently spotted on the nearby golf course grounds, can sometimes be observed here as well.

Shortly before Lower Loop Trail ends, a narrow, unmarked trail heads into the trees to the left. This junction connects Camp Long to Longfellow Creek Trail, a 4-mile-long urban creek corridor through West Seattle; it provides an option for anyone wishing to add to their total hiking distance, although the route frequently travels along roads and sidewalks.

Past the junction, the trail climbs a short hill to reach the bottom of The Glacier, a manufactured-rock surface where climbers are likely to be practicing their rope and ice-travel techniques. The Glacier is an add-on to Schurman Rock, just up the stone steps to the left, which tends to be the focus of more-advanced climbing and belaying activity.

Schurman Rock is named for Camp Long cofounder and scout leader Clark Schurman, who envisioned creating a climbing surface that emulated many types of rocks and challenges typical of the Olympic and Cascade ranges, and for whom Camp Schurman on Mount Rainier's Emmons Glacier is also named. Completed in 1939, Schurman was the first artificial climbing rock in North America and has served as the staging ground for many great young climbers who later moved on to bigger things. The rock got a major face-lift in 2003, thanks to a consortium of public and private outdoor groups, so it will continue to help train climbers long into the future. In fact, some of them may be practicing on the day of your hike, making the picnic tables and grassy area next to the rock a great place to relax and watch them at work. When you are ready to wrap up your hike, cross the lawn to reach the service road through the trees, and follow it back to the parking lot.

GPS TRAILHEAD COORDINATES
N47° 33.329' W122° 22.509'

From I-5 just south of downtown Seattle, take Exit 163A for West Seattle Bridge–Columbian Way. Stay to the west on the off-ramp and continue onto the West Seattle Bridge, which becomes Fauntleroy Way SW when it ascends to West Seattle. In 2.6 miles, at the first traffic light, turn left onto 35th Avenue SW and drive 0.7 mile up the hill to SW Dawson Street. At this intersection, turn left into Camp Long and continue through the gate to the parking lot on the right.

2 Carkeek Park and Beach

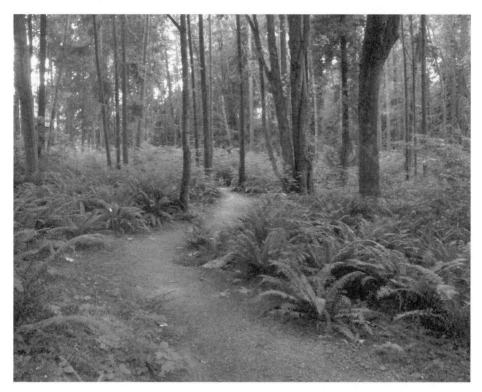

South Ridge Trail

In Brief

Occupying a stretch of Puget Sound shoreline in northwestern Seattle, Carkeek Park presents a mix of well-developed fields and play areas, an extensive network of trails, and a wide expanse of rocky beach to explore. High bluffs above the water allow all comers to enjoy views usually reserved for the residents of the upscale Blue Ridge neighborhood where the park is nestled.

Description

Carkeek is no secret to many Seattle residents. On any weekend in good weather, expect to compete for space on the playing fields and in the parking lot. People come here for good reason: The park has a variety of attractions, and despite the crowds, plenty of peace and solitude can be found on the trails by anyone willing to put forth a little effort.

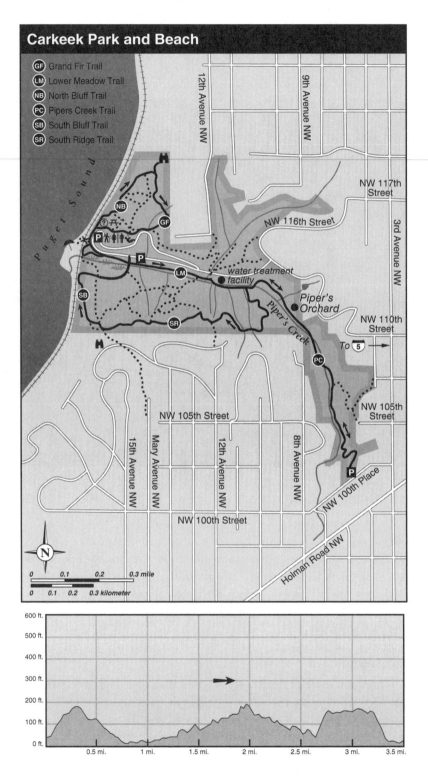

Carkeek Park and Beach

GF Grand Fir Trail
LM Lower Meadow Trail
NB North Bluff Trail
PC Pipers Creek Trail
SB South Bluff Trail
SR South Ridge Trail

DISTANCE & CONFIGURATION: 3.5-mile figure eight around the perimeter (many more trails in the park interior)	6 a.m.–10 p.m.; no fee for parking or trail access
DIFFICULTY: Easy–moderate	**WHEELCHAIR TRAVERSABLE:** Yes, on Salmon to Sound Trail, Pipers Creek Trail (from the Lower Meadow to Piper's Orchard), and Wetland Trail
SCENERY: Wildlife (salmon in Pipers Creek when spawning), woodlands, beach, and sea life	
EXPOSURE: Wooded park with many shady areas	**MAP(S):** On information board near bridge over the railroad tracks; USGS *Seattle North*
TRAFFIC: Busy often, but South Ridge trails see little traffic	**FACILITIES:** Toilets and water near the northern park play area
TRAIL SURFACE: Mixture of gravel, dirt, boardwalk, and pavement	**DOGS:** Allowed on-leash on trails but not allowed on beach
HIKING TIME: 1–2 hours, or longer with side trips	**CONTACT:** 206-684-0877; seattle.gov /parks/environment/carkeek.htm
ACCESS: Hikable year-round, daily,	**LOCATION:** 950 NW Carkeek Park Road, Seattle, WA 98177

From the entrance, the road winds through woods and fields to the upper parking lot next to the playground. If this lot is full, various other less-formal parking opportunities can be found farther along the one-way loop road. There is sure to be space somewhere.

Many visitors never venture too far beyond their cars. Adjacent to the parking lot are grass fields that host frequent volleyball, softball, and Frisbee games, and a group of public picnic areas with outdoor grills also stands nearby. A charming playground, which features a slide where kids pass through a giant salmon, will keep children occupied for hours.

Several hiking opportunities are available from the upper parking lot. Despite Carkeek's limited size, the woods north and south of the park road are interlaced with a substantial network of trails. It is possible to get disoriented with so many options, but because of the restricted space, no one will stay lost for very long. The easiest way to see the park is to explore on your own; a pamphlet with a trail map should be available at a billboard in the southwest corner of the upper parking lot, next to the beach-access bridge.

Note that Seattle Parks and Recreation is trying to decrease the number of informal trails by specifically graveling maintained trails and letting the rest return to nature, so try to stay on the official trails if you can. Bicycles are allowed only on Pipers Creek Trail. Dogs are forbidden on the beach and must be leashed at all times everywhere else.

THE BEACH

From the upper playfield, you can access Carkeek Park's beach via a footbridge that crosses some railroad tracks. Kids are sure to be delighted if a train thunders underneath, especially because the vantage offers the chance to see the speeding cars up close, and many freight trains stretch more than a mile in length.

The view west from the beach encompasses Bainbridge Island and the Kitsap Peninsula with the jagged Olympic Mountains beyond. All kinds of boats—from small daysailers to giant tankers making for the Strait of Juan de Fuca—provide perspective.

The beach sits on Puget Sound, and the water is too cold for an extended swim (though a quick dip or wade can provide relief on a hot summer day). Exploration, therefore, is the main attraction for many park users. Low tide reveals crabs, anemones, starfish, and many other small marine animals hidden in the tide pools and among the rocks. The exposed sand allows you to wander up or down the shoreline, possibly as far as Golden Gardens Park over a mile away on Shilshole Bay to the southwest.

THE NORTH BLUFF

To reach the northern side of the park, look for the North Bluff Trailhead along the fence behind the picnic tables. The gravel trail climbs quickly onto the North Bluff, where several viewpoints open above the cliff and expose the steep drop to the beach below. The trail eventually dead-ends at the North Meadow, an open grassy area on a hill with a remarkable view of the sound. Houses are visible nearby, too, as the meadow borders on private property.

Retreat a short distance and you'll find wooden stairs down to the left. Descend into darker woods, composed largely of big-leaf maples and red alders; ferns, salal, and other undergrowth cover the forest floor along the route.

Complete the obvious perimeter loop (no more than 0.7 mile) to return to the park road and your car. Various spur trails lead through the center of the loop and can be used to lengthen your hike.

PIPERS CREEK AND THE SOUTH RIDGE

The most extensive hiking opportunities at Carkeek are found on Pipers Creek Trail and the adjoining trails of the South Ridge. Pipers Creek flows through the center of the park, emptying into Puget Sound, and its namesake trail runs alongside it for about 1 mile up to an alternate park entrance.

The trail starts just below the upper parking lot; look for a footpath sign and some steps down. As with the North Bluff, there are many options here. You will know when you have reached Pipers Creek, though, and the right trail is easy to find.

A small wetland lies at the mouth of the creek. The trail surface turns to boardwalk to pass through the lowland bog, with its carpet of algae and high reeds, before returning to gravel. Chum and coho salmon run the creek to spawn in season, an amazing spectacle, given the creek's minimal flow and the heavy development nearby.

After following the edge of the grassy lower meadow for about 0.3 mile, the trail passes a small water-treatment plant, then enters a broad ravine. The second-growth forest here is similar in composition to the woods on the North Bluff, although the occasional giant stump testifies to the size of the western red cedars and western hemlocks that grew here before being cut down in the early 20th century.

Upon entering the ravine, the trail starts a gradual uphill climb. Soon some apple trees appear on the left, marking the remnants of the Piper Homestead Orchard. A. W. Piper, the land's owner, was a politician and artist who opened a bakery and candy company in 1876. He and his wife, Minna, sold produce and flowers they grew in the orchard from a wagon in Pike Place Market downtown until the property was sold and turned into a park in 1929.

The trail continues its steady ascent for another 0.5 mile until reaching the head of the ravine at the Eddie McAbee Park entrance on NW 100th Place. There is room for only a few cars here, but this side entry can be a good alternate access to the park.

Return down Pipers Creek Trail to just before the water-treatment facility and find South Ridge Trail to the left. Even on a busy summer day, you can expect to have this area of the park to yourself. This trail leads uphill to the southern edge of the ravine then winds along the top of the ridge back toward the beach. Many side paths lead off into the adjacent residential area as the trail negotiates a series of short rises. Other spurs lead back down to Pipers Creek, but it is easy to stay on the ridge.

After 0.5 mile, you will reach the South Bluff and a high overlook. There is no doubt you are at the park boundary, as you emerge from the trees and find yourself practically in someone's backyard. Find South Bluff Trail, which drops quickly through the woods along the top of the cliff. Be careful here, especially if you have children with you—the sharp drop-off to the beach and sandy tread can be hazardous. From the bottom of the South Bluff it is an easy walk back to your car.

GPS TRAILHEAD COORDINATES
N47° 42.742' W122° 22.658'

Starting on I-5 north of downtown Seattle, take Exit 173. If coming from the south, at the end of the ramp, turn left onto First Avenue NE and then turn left again at the next light onto Northgate Way, headed west. If coming from the north, head west on Northgate Way, which eventually becomes N. 105th Street and continues across WA 99. In 1.4 miles, at the next major intersection after WA 99, turn right onto Greenwood Avenue. In 0.3 mile turn left onto NW 110th Street, which soon becomes NW Carkeek Park Road. In 0.9 mile, signs guide you into the parking areas of Carkeek Park and the one-way loop road. Park in the upper lot nearest the beach or continue down to the lower parking lot.

3 Discovery Park and Beach

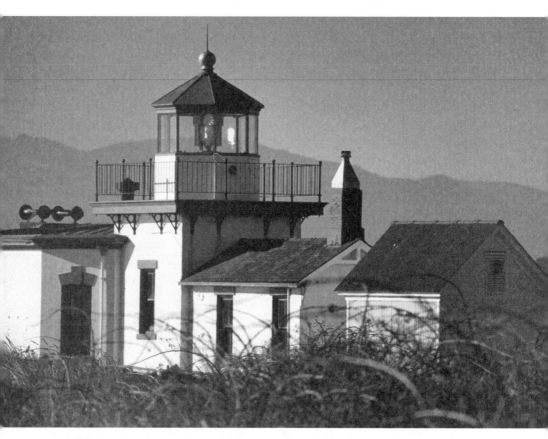

West Point Lighthouse

In Brief

Occupying a prominent point between Shilshole and Elliott Bays, this former military installation is the largest park in the city of Seattle. Blessed with 534 acres of forests, fields, bluffs, and beaches, and even a picturesque lighthouse with excellent views of northern Puget Sound, Discovery Park is a great destination for the entire family.

Description

Discovery Park has more than 10 miles of trails, including a prominently marked Loop Trail that circles most of the open fields and old military housing in the park's southern

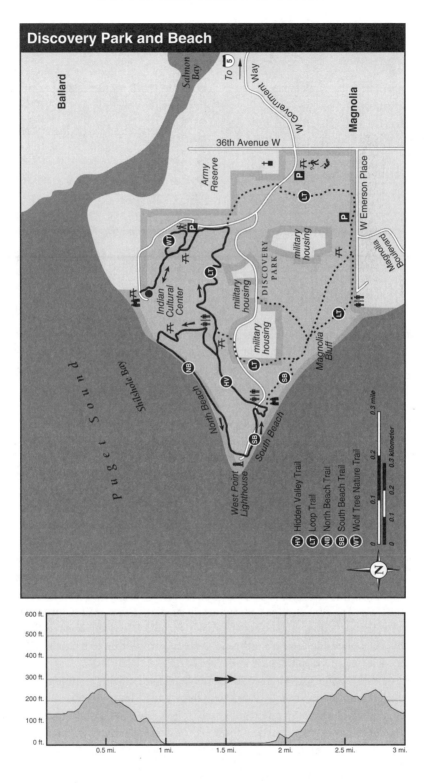

DISTANCE & CONFIGURATION: 3.0-mile loop with many options to extend the hike	**ACCESS:** Hikable year-round, daily, 4 a.m.–11:30 p.m.; no fee for parking or trail access
DIFFICULTY: Easy–moderate	**WHEELCHAIR TRAVERSABLE:** No, but the park has 5 miles of paved roads closed to vehicles.
SCENERY: Historical Fort Lawton grounds, sandy beaches, lighthouse; views of Puget Sound, Seattle, and Mount Rainier	
	MAP(S): USGS *Seattle North*
	FACILITIES: Toilets and water at trailhead
EXPOSURE: Shaded on upper trails; exposed on beach trails	**DOGS:** Allowed on-leash on trails but not allowed on beach
TRAFFIC: High	**CONTACT:** 206-386-4236; seattle.gov /parks/environment/discovery.htm
TRAIL SURFACE: Mixture of dirt, pavement, gravel, and boardwalk	
	LOCATION: 3801 Discovery Park Blvd., Seattle, WA 98199
HIKING TIME: 2–4 hours	

end. However, because this trail never reaches the beach—arguably the park's leading attraction—a better and more representative loop is described here. This hike descends through the wooded areas in the northern half of the park, travels along the beach to the lighthouse, then returns up the bluff, offering many options for further exploration along the way.

From the North Parking Lot, begin by heading west along the paved road, which is closed to vehicles. Stay on this road through the first junction at the end of the grassy picnic area, where another road branches to the left.

A second junction in the road heads up a small rise to the Daybreak Star Indian Cultural Center. Run by the United Indians of All Tribes Foundation (UIATF), this organization provides social services to American Indians. The site for the cultural center was obtained following a heated standoff between American Indian activists and the US government in spring of 1970 after the military decommissioned Fort Lawton. Bernie Whitebear, a former Green Beret and longtime advocate for American Indian causes, led a so-called invasion and occupation of the fort, arguing that the property was on historical American Indian land. The city of Seattle, however, wanted to turn Fort Lawton into a public park. After several months and significant media attention, a compromise agreement was reached, ceding 20 acres of the newly formed Discovery Park to the UIATF with a 99-year renewable lease from the city. Whitebear went on to head the UIATF for three decades, until his death in 2000 at the age of 62.

The cultural center's striking architecture blends modern and traditional American Indian design, and offers an impressive view from a high bluff out over Shilshole Bay, making it a quick and worthy side trip. Simply follow the road around to the northern side of the building—its best facade—and look for a wooden overlook platform on the far side of the lawn. From this viewpoint, the masts at Shilshole Marina resemble a forest of thin trees near the Lake Washington Ship Canal entrance; on a clear day, Mount Baker can be seen far away to the north.

After this short detour, continue back on the main road, which curves around to the left and starts heading south. About 0.25 mile past the cultural center, the official Loop Trail intersects the road. Turn right on the Loop Trail until you reach a second road, then turn right again and follow the road back to the north, to where it dead-ends. This somewhat awkward, roundabout route is the result of a landslide that washed away a better access path sometime in the past.

Go straight past the end of the road to a clearing. On the left side of the clearing is a gap in a chain-link fence with a green wooden post and a sign directing hikers to North Beach Trail. Follow this path as it descends through trees on a steep slope with some wooden stairs, bending to the right and dropping 200 feet in about 0.08 mile.

The trail turns left, above a long breakwater of heavy boulders, along the shore toward the lighthouse. Even with only moderate wind, sizable swells often crash against the rocks here, despite the short run of open water and considerable shelter provided by Bainbridge Island and the Kitsap Peninsula across Puget Sound.

After 0.5 mile, the breakwater gives way to a stretch of sandy beach below the lighthouse. The trail cuts inland, but the beach itself provides a more interesting way to get around the point, except during bad weather or at extreme high tide. Lots of shells, driftwood, and other flotsam lie on the sand, providing fun for beachcombers of all ages who search for treasures along the shore. Marine wildlife—including crabs, barnacles, starfish, and sea anemones—is frequently visible at low tide. This approach also provides excellent views of the lighthouse itself, known as the West Point Lighthouse, and its attached radar installation.

The far side of the point (where the sandy beach continues southeast for another 0.5 mile) has treasures all its own, offering interesting views of West Seattle, Mount Rainier, Puget Sound, and the Olympic Mountains. This area is known as South Beach, and it is certainly worth exploring. Be wary of the tides, though, as people have been known to get trapped here below the steep walls of Magnolia Bluff.

When you are ready to continue hiking, look for the trail heading uphill on the northern side of the lighthouse access road. The path follows the road for a few hundred yards before reaching a junction (signed for Hidden Valley Trail) across from an excellent viewpoint over South Beach from the top of the bluff.

Take Hidden Valley Trail and climb up through the woods, crossing several intersections until it ends on the park's official Loop Trail, just short of another road. Note that once you cross this road, you are back on the same short section of the Loop Trail you hiked earlier, except now you're traveling in the opposite direction.

Stay on the Loop Trail as it winds up and down through a pleasant forest for 0.5 mile and crosses two more paved roads (long closed to traffic) in one of the nicest sections of the upper park. At a third paved road, head left down the hill to return to the North Parking Lot, where you began.

To extend your hike, the best bet is to follow the official Loop Trail as far as you wish to go, potentially adding several more miles if you complete the entire circuit. Another option is to take South Beach Trail away from the beach rather than Hidden Valley Trail, as described earlier, then continue all the way around the Loop Trail counterclockwise. This will allow you to see the open southern half of the park without ever having to retrace your steps.

Nearby Activities

For more than 75 years, the Fisherman's Terminal has been the best place in Seattle to buy fresh fish straight off the boat. Nowadays, a comfortable facade and a host of eateries greet visitors to the working docks, providing multiple opportunities to sample the North Pacific catch of the day. To reach the Fisherman's Terminal, turn left from Gilman Avenue W onto W. Emerson Place and cross a bridge over the train tracks; the entrance is on the left on 19th Avenue W.

GPS TRAILHEAD COORDINATES
N47° 39.900' W122° 24.691'

From I-5 north of downtown Seattle, take Exit 169 for NE 45th Street, and drive west. Continuing west, 45th Street becomes 46th Street, then drops down into the neighborhood of Ballard and becomes Market Street. In 2.7 miles, in Ballard, go left on 15th Avenue NW and cross the Ballard Bridge. In 1.0 mile make the first right after the bridge onto W. Emerson Place, then in 0.5 mile make another right onto Gilman Avenue W. Gilman Avenue W eventually becomes W. Government Way and in 1 mile goes into the Discovery Park east entrance. Once inside the park, stay to the right and drive 0.7 mile to the North Parking Lot.

4 Schmitz Preserve Park

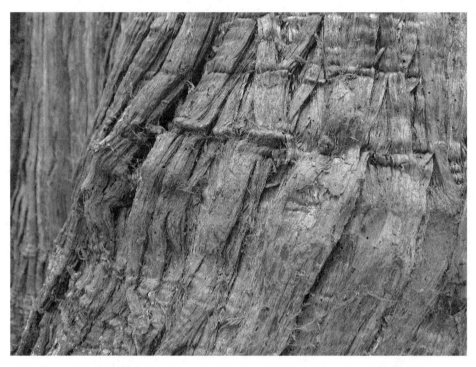

Western red cedar bark

In Brief

This unassuming little park hides a singular example of old-growth forest in the middle of the city. With a good network of trails through a quiet, secluded valley, Schmitz Preserve Park makes a great place for a quick escape to the woods, despite its limited size.

Description

A full century after it was established in 1908, Schmitz Park, originally a 30-acre parcel of land donated by Ferdinand and Emma Schmitz, remains true to its founders' intent—to be kept as an example of the local forest as it was discovered by Seattle's first settlers.

The pioneers of the Denny Party, who landed just down the hill at Alki Point in November 1851, would undoubtedly still feel at home in Schmitz, even if they would find the rest of Seattle completely unrecognizable. Ironically, the park has come to represent Seattle's past, though the name *Alki* comes from a Chinook word indicating "the future."

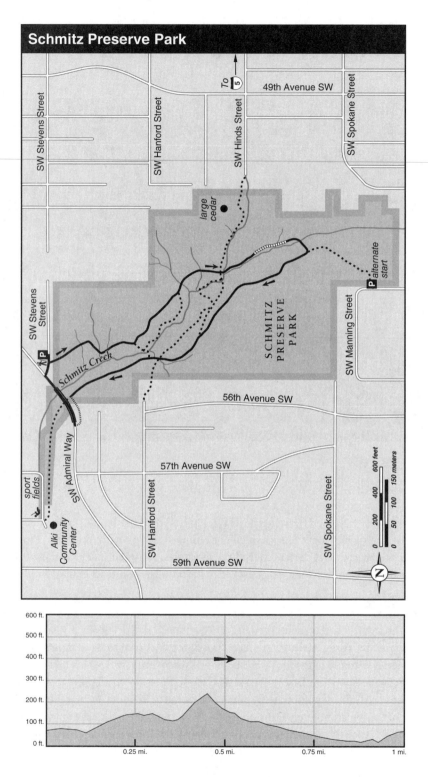

Schmitz Preserve Park

DISTANCE & CONFIGURATION: 1.0-mile loop (side-trip options)	**ACCESS:** Hikable year-round, daily, 6 a.m.–10 p.m.; no fee for parking or trail access
DIFFICULTY: Easy	
SCENERY: Old-growth forest contrasted with enormous logging stumps in an urban park; a cascading stream	**WHEELCHAIR TRAVERSABLE:** No
	MAP(S): USGS *Seattle South*
EXPOSURE: Shaded	**FACILITIES:** None
TRAFFIC: Moderate	**DOGS:** Allowed on-leash
TRAIL SURFACE: Dirt, gravel, and some boardwalk	**CONTACT:** 206-684-4075; www.seattle.gov/parks/park_detail.asp?ID=465
HIKING TIME: 1–2 hours	**LOCATION:** 5551 SW Admiral Way, Seattle, WA 98116

Now expanded to more than 50 acres, Schmitz Park continues to protect the region's natural heritage. In fact, it does such a good job that the University of Washington Forestry Department uses the park as a prime example of Pacific Northwest old-growth forest, proudly displaying it to visiting Asian forest managers. One can only hope the university's visitors will be as committed to good land stewardship as the Schmitz family was back in 1908, since the future of the global environment will undoubtedly be determined in Asia, home to more than half of the world's population and most of its fastest-growing economies. Already today, dust clouds from desertification in western China occasionally reach the US Pacific Coast, exacerbating smog and other air-pollution problems and underlining the global effects of environmental degradation.

At one time, it was possible to drive on a road to the center of the park, but that changed following a landslide in 2002. Now all cars must be parked on adjacent surface streets, although many visitors come from the surrounding communities and walk to the park from home, forgoing their cars altogether.

The trails here are unsigned but easy to follow, and there is no chance of getting lost for any length of time. A narrow loop with multiple side trails leading out to nearby streets and neighborhoods runs through the center of the park. If you mistakenly end up on one of these side trails, simply retrace your steps to rejoin the main route.

Find the trailhead above the bridge on SW Stevens Street and start hiking down the hill on the old gravel road, which soon becomes a dirt singletrack trail. Head left along Schmitz Creek to begin the clockwise loop; this small stream defines the park's central ravine and is marked by several small waterfalls along the way.

A few mammoth stumps indicate that minimal logging did occur here in the late 1800s. Nonetheless, some truly giant trees remain. A particularly impressive western red cedar, its deeply grooved bark showing the passage of time, stands on a rise on a spur trail that leaves the main trail to the left from a large intersection and eventually dead-ends at a nearby street. Watch for other ancient trees with blackened bark, revealing forest fires that swept through West Seattle in years past.

A boardwalk runs through the wetlands along the creek, winding through skunk cabbage, water parsley, and various ferns. Metal lathes on the elevated boards help keep the footing secure even when the surface is wet, which is most of the time because of the shelter and cooling shade of the tree canopy.

The trail reaches the southern end of the park then doubles back to the right, climbing the valley wall. Pileated woodpeckers are common here and can easily be heard or seen taking their toll on the trees nearby. The woodpeckers are only one of a large range of bird species that live in the mixed-conifer forest, which is also home to Steller's jays, song sparrows, and black-capped chickadees.

Eventually, the loop trail reaches an old road (now closed to vehicles) along the creek. Continue down the road to find a stairway on the left that will take you to the Schmitz Park Bridge, built in 1936. Head up the stairs and cross the bridge to return to your car. The road continues under the bridge and heads downhill to the Alki Community Center, an alternate place to begin the hike.

Nearby Activities

Try a meal at the Luna Park Cafe, a neighborhood staple at 2918 SW Avalon Way, just past the end of SW Admiral Way under the West Seattle Bridge. With hearty meals and an extensive children's menu, it's easy to see why Luna Park has long been a family favorite. Call the café at 206-935-7250 or check lunaparkcafe.com for more information.

GPS TRAILHEAD COORDINATES

N47° 34.654' W122° 24.121'

From I-5 just south of downtown Seattle, take Exit 163A for West Seattle Bridge–Columbian Way. Stay to the west on the off-ramp and continue onto the West Seattle Bridge. In 1.9 miles take the Admiral Way exit, then continue 2.2 miles and turn left onto SW Stevens Street just before a bridge. Park along SW Stevens Street, and find the trailhead near the intersection with Admiral Way.

5 Seward Park

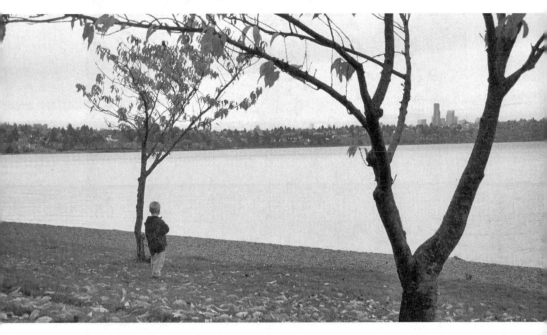

Young hiker looking toward the Seattle skyline

In Brief

Before Lake Washington was lowered by the opening of the ship canal in 1917, the peninsula now occupied by Seward Park was almost an island. Today, the park is an island of a different sort. Resisting the Seattle development that has spread around it for almost a century, Seward is now one of the last significant vestiges of old-growth forest within the city limits. A paved circular loop follows the island's lakefront shoreline and connects to a network of singletrack trails beneath the ancient trees.

Description

Seward Park was named for William Seward, who was appointed as Secretary of State by Abraham Lincoln in 1861. An outspoken critic of slavery and an ardent supporter of the Union during the Civil War, Seward became a highly visible and symbolic enemy of the Confederacy. His abuse of power as head of the government program to eliminate so-called disloyals in the North cemented his reputation among Southerners as a man to be feared and hated, and he became a supplemental target of the assassination conspiracy organized by John Wilkes Booth. On April 14, 1865, the same night Booth shot Lincoln, a

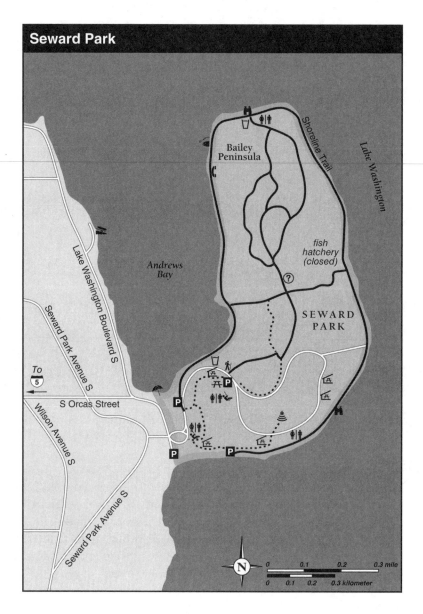

man named Lewis Powell stabbed Seward in the throat in an attempt to kill him as well. Despite suffering very serious wounds, Seward survived the attack and continued to serve as Secretary of State under Andrew Johnson.

During Johnson's administration, Seward became well known for his pivotal role in the purchase of Alaska from Russia in the spring of 1867. At the time, Alaska was generally considered a frozen wasteland and the transaction was mocked as "Seward's Folly," a monumental waste of taxpayer money.

DISTANCE & CONFIGURATION: 4.6-mile loop (2.4 miles of paved shoreline trail and 2.2 miles of interior dirt trails)	6 a.m.–10 p.m.; no fee for parking or trail access
DIFFICULTY: Easy	**WHEELCHAIR TRAVERSABLE:** Yes, on the paved Shoreline Trail
SCENERY: Views of the surrounding area and Lake Washington; old-growth forest and other picturesque plant life; lakeshore beaches	**MAP(S):** USGS *Seattle South* and *Bellevue South*
EXPOSURE: Shaded on interior trails, exposed on shoreline trail	**FACILITIES:** Toilets and water at the parking areas (some may be closed in winter)
TRAFFIC: Heavy on shoreline trail, moderate on interior trails	**DOGS:** Allowed on-leash on trails but not allowed on beach
TRAIL SURFACE: Dirt in interior, paved around perimeter	**CONTACT:** 206-684-4396; seattle.gov /parks/environment/seward.htm
HIKING TIME: 1–3 hours	**LOCATION:** 5900 Lake Washington Blvd. S, Seattle, WA 98118
ACCESS: Hikable year-round, daily,	

Today, it's hard to see how the acquisition of Alaska for the paltry sum of $7.2 million could be viewed as anything but one of the greatest bargains in US history. Seward obtained 360 million acres of land for 2 cents an acre, substantially less than Thomas Jefferson had paid for his celebrated Louisiana Purchase six decades before. Seward's $7.2 million outlay in 1867 would be the equivalent of approximately $120 million in 2015, an amount that Alaskan oil revenue alone repays approximately every five days. And this says nothing of the vast value of the other natural resources the state is famous for—including gold, which was first discovered in the Klondike in the late 1800s.

Most historians credit the ensuing Alaska gold rush with the establishment of Seattle as a major city, the last outpost of civilization for thousands of would-be prospectors on their way to the Yukon. It's safe to say that, without Alaska, Seattle would be a very different place today. For that reason, Seward's name was worthy of being attached to a 300-acre park along the western shore of Lake Washington.

Ironically, although Seward indirectly spurred Seattle's urban expansion, his namesake park is one of the few places remaining in the city that development has never reached. It's hard to imagine from looking at most parts of Seattle now, but there was a time when the entire area was covered in a thick forest—and Seward Park is one of the last remaining stands.

The 2.4-mile Shoreline Trail follows a paved road, now closed to motor vehicles, which loops around the park along the edge of Lake Washington. This route is very popular and provides views of the lake and the surrounding communities. Particularly interesting are the palatial houses visible on Mercer Island to the east; some of these estates can top the $7.2 million price tag of Seward's entire Alaska purchase. Looking northward offers a view of the I-90 Bridge and some of the tallest skyscrapers down-town, rising above the Mount Baker and Beacon Hill neighborhoods.

A fish hatchery on the eastern side of the park was constructed by the Works Progress Administration (WPA) during the New Deal to raise trout for stocking local lakes, including Lake Washington. The vision was for Seward Park to become an angler's paradise, but the reality did not quite live up to those expectations, and the fishery is now closed.

For most hikers, the primary attraction at Seward Park is its forest, which exhibits all of the required characteristics of old growth—standing snags, a layered canopy, fallen nurse logs, and some very large trees, among others. Although lacking any truly gigantic specimens, Seward Park harbors some trees that are up to 200 years old and contains one of the largest madrones in the state. Along with madrones, the lowland forest contains a mix of western red cedars, Douglas firs, western hemlocks, and big-leaf maples. The maples are notable for their ability to host epiphytes (plants that grow on other plants) such as licorice ferns, mosses, and lichens. Unfortunately, English ivy, a foreign, invasive plant that chokes out endemic species, grows here as well. Volunteer groups are working in conjunction with the park administration to eradicate the plant in an attempt to restore the natural ecosystem.

The best way to see Seward Park is to find your own way around. The spine of the park is laced with a series of dirt paths, seven separate segments (totaling 2.2 miles) linked on all sides to Shoreline Trail. By following a mix of the interior trails and Shoreline, this network can lead you to all corners of the park and its varied attractions. Thanks to the general topography and short distances involved, navigation is simple, even for first-time visitors.

Nearby Activities

Try the Columbia City Ale House for a posthike beer or meal. It's located at 4914 Rainier Ave. S. Call 206-723-5123 or visit seattlealehouses.com/columbiacity.

GPS TRAILHEAD COORDINATES
N47° 33.106' W122° 15.231'

From I-5 in downtown Seattle, take Exit 164 onto I-90 E. Immediately exit onto Rainier Avenue S, Exit 3A, and turn right onto Rainier at the bottom of the ramp. Follow Rainier Avenue S 3.0 miles through the historical downtown of Columbia City. After downtown, turn left (east) onto S. Orcas Street, which ends in 0.8 mile at Seward Park. Turn right into the park entrance, and park in one of the lower lots if you plan to walk the paved shoreline trail. Continue to the upper parking lot if you plan to hike the interior trails or if the lower lots are full.

6 Washington Park Arboretum and Foster Island

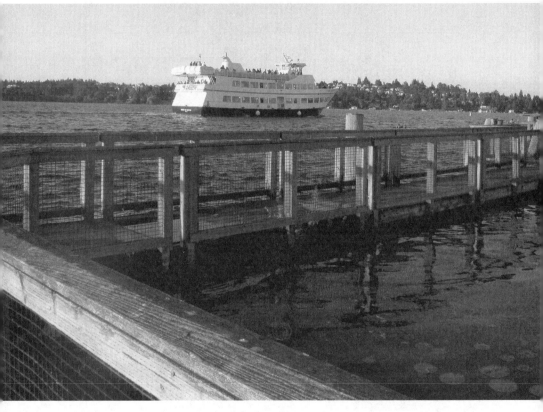

Lake Washington from Foster Island

In Brief

A few Seattle parks provide a glimpse of the way it used to be by harboring the last stands of the thick forest that once covered the region. The Washington Park Arboretum is a similar sanctuary, instead featuring exotic plant life from around the world. Rather than a trip back in time, the arboretum allows visitors to take a walk to all corners of the Earth via a peaceful system of trails through its carefully manicured gardens and groves.

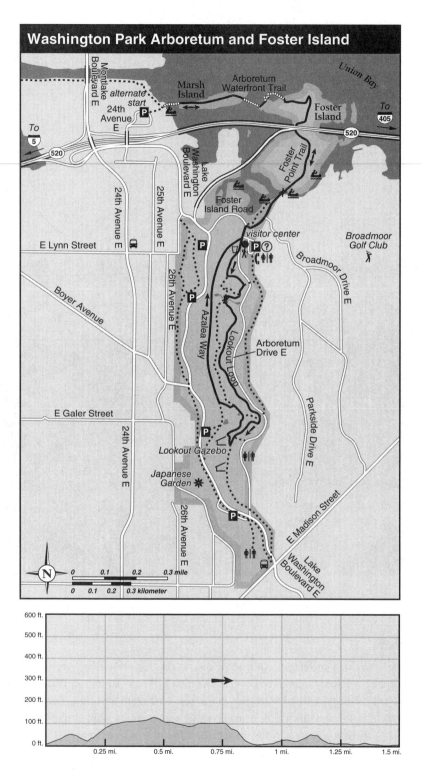

Washington Park Arboretum and Foster Island

DISTANCE & CONFIGURATION: 3.5-mile balloon (1.5-mile loop in Arboretum, plus optional 2.0-mile out-and-back on Foster Point Trail and Arboretum Waterfront Trail)	**ACCESS:** Hikable year-round, daily, sunrise–sunset; no fee for parking or trail access
DIFFICULTY: Easy	**WHEELCHAIR TRAVERSABLE:** Yes, on Azalea Way Trail
SCENERY: Incredible display of plant life from around the world, island shoreline trails, territorial views across Union Bay, bird-watching and other wildlife watching	**MAP(S):** USGS *Seattle North*
	FACILITIES: Toilets and water at the visitor center
EXPOSURE: Mostly shaded	**DOGS:** Allowed on-leash in arboretum and on Foster Point Trail but not allowed on Arboretum Waterfront Trail
TRAFFIC: Heavy	**CONTACT:** 206-543-8800; depts .washington.edu/uwbg/gardens /wpa.shtml
TRAIL SURFACE: Dirt, gravel, small amount of boardwalk	**LOCATION:** 2300 Arboretum Dr. E, Seattle, WA 98112
HIKING TIME: 1–3 hours	

Description

Any hike at the Washington Park Arboretum should begin at the visitor center, where plenty of good information on the park is available through a collection of maps, pamphlets, and handouts. An attached store sells general-interest books on botany, nature, and wildlife, and its helpful staff can assist by answering any questions. The center also occasionally hosts gala events and receptions in the great hall and under the trellis on the patio. For anyone seeking a more personal educational experience, the visitor center offers free guided walks; call 206-543-8800 for more information.

The arboretum claims to have more than 40,000 plants from 4,600 different species, 139 listed as endangered. Chances are, if something can grow in the climate and soil at Washington Park, a sample will be on display. Many are grouped into named collections, including lindens, camellias, magnolias, Asiatic maples, larches, and numerous others. Several specific exhibits highlight individual classes or geographic areas, such as a rhododendron grove and the New Zealand high country.

Multiple species are identified with signs, listing both common and scientific names. Trees range from the very familiar *Pseudotsuga menziesii,* or Douglas fir, icon of the Pacific Northwest, to the extremely rare *Franklinia alatamaha,* or Franklinia, originally from the state of Georgia and thought to be extinct in the wild since about 1800.

The arboretum is carefully landscaped with ponds, a gazebo, and plenty of places to stop and reflect. A mix of scents and fragrances fills the air. Although the park is particularly popular during the spring bloom, the wide range of species means that something is at its peak virtually every month of the year.

Laid out linearly along a north–south axis, the arboretum is generally bounded on the east by Arboretum Drive E and on the west by Lake Washington Boulevard E, though

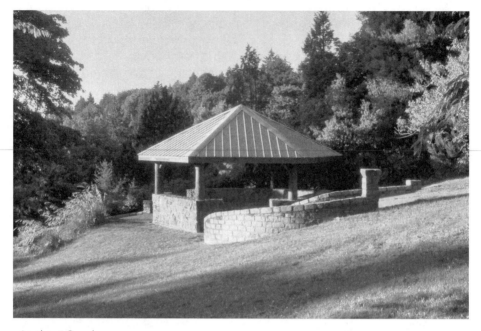

Lookout Gazebo

some sections spill over the road on either side. In between, a maze of connecting trails wind their way through the heart of the park, allowing visitors to explore the various groves and gardens.

This kind of design does not lend itself well to a single recommended route, however. The best way to see the majority of the arboretum's displays is to form an elongated loop by traveling south on the trails generally paralleling Arboretum Drive E, then returning on Azalea Way, a broad, grassy path that forms the spine of the park. Side trips to individual areas of particular interest can easily be added to this general framework to suit personal tastes.

FOSTER ISLAND TRAILS

A second hiking option, leading to Foster Island and Marsh Island, is a combination of the Foster Point Trail and the Arboretum Waterfront Trail. This route leads northeast from the visitor center parking lot. Although passing through what is technically part of the arboretum, this route explores the marshlands along Lake Washington's western shore and has an entirely different look and feel than the carefully arranged plant collections in the park's main section.

The Foster Point Trail begins as a dirt-and-gravel road and soon reaches a bridge that crosses a lake inlet to reach Foster Island. Pass through the arboretum's last identified grove of trees and then duck underneath WA 520 through a tunnel, with the traffic humming overhead. Enter a grassy area on the far side, then turn left onto the Arboretum Waterfront Trail where the trail narrows into the reeds.

A wooden observation platform is on the right, looking out over the Montlake ship canal, Union Bay, and Webster Point at the tip of the Laurelhurst neighborhood across the water. The University of Washington, with its distinctive winged stadium rising unmistakably above the lake, occupies most of the land to the left. At any time of year, a steady parade of boats will be passing by. If the Huskies are in action, an entire armada of loyal supporters unfailingly anchors in the bay.

However, the chief sightseeing attraction here is not the cityscape but the natural environment. Foster Island is an excellent bird-watching site, with flocks of ducks and other waterfowl swimming on the lake and congregating among the reeds.

The trail continues on an extensive boardwalk system of wood, metal, and concrete, occasionally reaching over the water. The lake is very shallow in this area, and it is possible to see the bottom in several places. The boardwalk eventually ends on Marsh Island, where the trail returns to dirt and enters a tangled thicket of mud and stunted trees. Additional opportunities abound for observing the island's wildlife, including beavers, whose teeth marks are visible on some of the stumps.

At the far end of Marsh Island, the trail crosses back to the mainland on a bridge and reaches its western terminus in a parking lot, a total of about 1 mile from the arboretum's visitor center and a good alternate starting point. From here, it is possible to complete a loop back to where you began by walking along Lake Washington Boulevard E. This busy road is not well suited for foot traffic, though; the safer and more scenic option is to return the way you came.

Nearby Activities

The Washington Park Arboretum also maintains an excellent 3.5-acre Japanese garden, which includes a traditional teahouse. The garden, located at 1075 Lake Washington Blvd. E, is adjacent to the southern end of the arboretum's main grounds and charges an admission fee. For more information, call 206-684-4725 or visit the website at seattle.gov /parks/parkspaces/japanesegarden.htm.

GPS TRAILHEAD COORDINATES
N47° 38.382' W122° 17.668'

From I-5 north of downtown Seattle, take Exit 168B, and go east on WA 520. In 0.5 mile take the first exit off WA 520, Montlake Boulevard. Go straight across Montlake Boulevard onto Lake Washington Boulevard E. In 0.6 mile, turn left onto Foster Island Road, then immediately turn right onto Arboretum Drive E. The parking area at the visitor center is immediately on the left.

7 Woodland Park and Green Lake Park

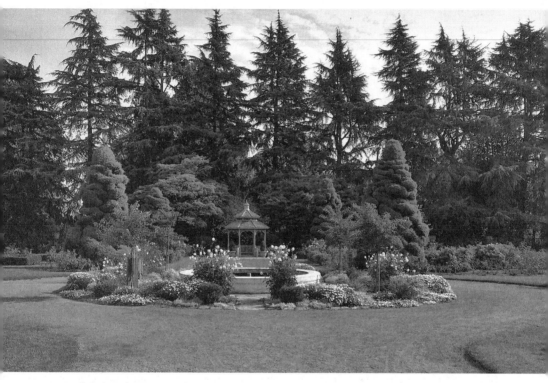

Woodland Park Rose Garden gazebo

In Brief

No one will mistake Woodland Park or Green Lake Park for wilderness, but their central location and convenient access from so many neighborhoods make this outdoor complex the signature recreation area for many Seattle residents.

Description

It is estimated that as many as 10,000 people visit Green Lake Park daily during the summer. And if you show up in midafternoon, you might think they all arrived just before you did. Woodland Park does not see quite the same crowds, but it is still sure to be busy, with its playing fields occupied and in use.

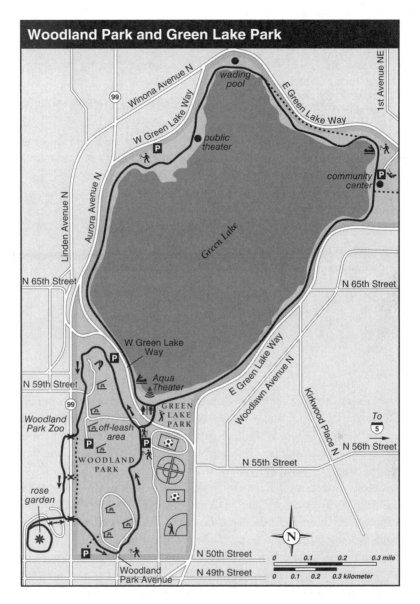

Woodland Park and Green Lake Park

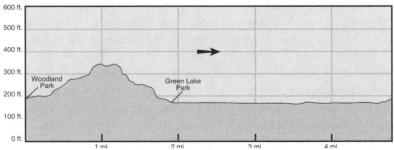

DISTANCE & CONFIGURATION:
1.3-mile loop around the perimeter; 3.0-mile Green Lake multiuse loop (many more trails in the park interior; side-trip options around Woodland Park Zoo and the rose garden)

DIFFICULTY: Easy

SCENERY: Wildlife (millions of rabbits), Woodland Zoo animals; views of Green Lake and Seattle neighborhoods

EXPOSURE: Wooded park with many shady areas

TRAFFIC: Popular on sunny days

TRAIL SURFACE: Mixture of gravel, dirt, and pavement

HIKING TIME: 1–2 hours, or longer with side trips

ACCESS: Hikable year-round, daily, 4 a.m.–11:30 p.m.; rose garden, daily, 7 a.m.–sunset; no fee for parking or trail access

WHEELCHAIR TRAVERSABLE: Yes, on the paved Green Lake Trail

MAP(S): None needed, though trails meander throughout the park; USGS *Seattle North*

FACILITIES: Toilets across the street at Green Lake; water near tennis courts

DOGS: Allowed on-leash

CONTACT: 206-684-4075; www.seattle .gov/parks/park_detail.asp?id=292 and www.seattle.gov/parks/park_detail .asp?id=307

LOCATION: Seattle

If it's solitude you seek, your best bet is to arrive at the break of dawn—or head somewhere else. However, a rewarding walk can be found here if you're willing to share the trail; special attractions like the zoo and the rose garden add a unique flavor. Woodland is also a good place to bring your pet, as a special off-leash play area allows dogs to run free in a controlled space, a relative rarity for Seattle.

Woodland Park virtually defines a multiuse facility. Tennis courts, a skate park, soccer fields, softball fields, and a running track are all immediately accessible, and walkers, runners, and cyclists utilize the area. Farther reaches of the park offer more unusual playfields, including a series of horseshoe pits and a lawn-bowling pitch.

Start your hike on the northern side of the tennis courts by heading up the park road and then veering to the right, next to the off-leash dog run. Pick any trail, and continue up a hill through a small wooded area until another parking lot and Green Lake are visible through the trees to the north.

As you advance up the hill, watch for rabbits; scores of these small mammals in all sizes and colors can be seen throughout the park, especially in the evening hours. For most visitors, this is the most exotic wildlife they will encounter. But bald eagles have been spotted in the trees here, so keep your eyes peeled.

Emerge from the woods to find a fenced-in activity area for horseshoe tossing and a green for lawn bowling. Circling the playfields, you will soon be standing above the busy traffic on Aurora Avenue N and facing a residential area on Phinney Ridge. Cut back to the left along Aurora Avenue to pass through some nicely shaded picnic areas.

Three bridges link the eastern and western sections of the park, divided when Aurora Avenue was built in the 1930s. Cross the northernmost bridge, the first one you will reach. At the far end a high fence topped with barbed wire marks the edge of the Woodland Park Zoo.

A trail circles the perimeter of the zoo, and it's possible to extend the length of the hike by turning right here and completing a loop on a mixture of trails and sidewalks. To follow the standard route, turn left and head south along the fence. With a little imagination, the traffic below sounds like a rushing river. Commingled, the noises and the scents from the animals in the zoo can make this area seem like the true outdoors.

Pass the second bridge, continue to the third, then enter an arched tunnel on the right. Go across a parking lot, climb a small rise, then bend around to the left to find the entrance to the Woodland Park Rose Garden behind some heavy wrought-iron gates. The garden is free to the public and open year-round from 7 a.m. to dusk, although the best time to visit is surely at the height of the spring bloom.

The garden displays a vast collection of roses in all colors and sizes, interspersed with a lily pond, some hedges, and a gazebo. Many of the flowers—with names such as 'Love and Peace' and 'Fragrant Cloud'—have won awards, and several hybrids bloom in shades you never imagined. This is a great area for photography, especially for capturing close-up views.

Return the way you came, and cross back on the third bridge to the eastern side of the park into more fields and picnic areas. Continue west to the edge of a short ridge, then descend through a wooded ravine to return to the parking lot where you began. There are many interconnected trails in this section of the park to extend your exploration, if time allows.

To visit Green Lake Park, cross W. Green Lake Way N and find either of two obvious loop trails. The paved inner loop is more developed, more traveled, and posted as 2.8 miles in length. The outer loop is a dirt path that follows closer to the perimeter of the park rather than the lakeshore and is slightly longer, at 3.2 miles.

Either path will lead you around the lake and back, providing a tour of Green Lake's various attractions, including basketball courts, tennis courts, a pitch-and-putt golf course, open fields, playgrounds, two fishing piers, and a boathouse. Rowing shells, kayaks, and canoes are frequently seen on the water, and various paddle boats are available for rental in the vicinity of the main north parking lot.

A sandy beach area provides a nice location for a dip in the lake, complete with a lifeguard during the summer. The indoor Evans Swimming Pool, at the northern end of the park, is a better bet for those who are seeking a more-controlled swimming environment, as does a popular wading and splash pool about 0.25 mile farther around to the west.

Although it is more of an annoyance than a hazard for swimmers, the lake once suffered from milfoil infestation. This invasive aquatic plant apparently spread here via boat trailers, just as it has at many other freshwater lakes in the Pacific Northwest. Eurasian water milfoil (*Myriophyllum spicatum*) was first found in the Seattle area in the

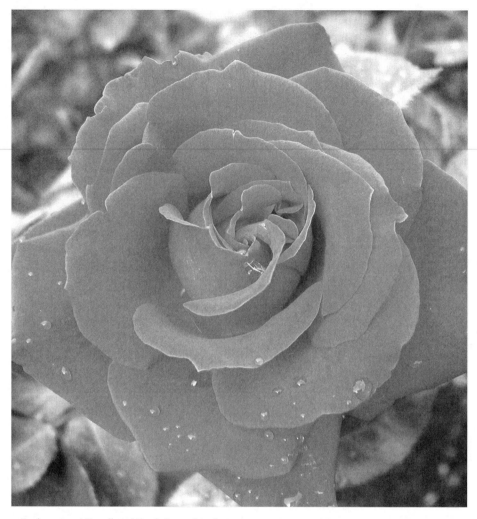

Red rose at Woodland Park Rose Garden

1960s, and has been steadily expanding its range ever since. It is now considered the most problematic plant in Washington State.

Ironically for such a pest, milfoil is quite attractive and can easily be identified by its feathery leaves and threadlike composition in areas where it reaches the surface of the lake.

Nearby Activities

The surrounding Green Lake and Wallingford neighborhoods offer countless venues for a posthike meal or drink. In particular, look along North 45th Street, a few blocks south of Woodland Park or around the northern and eastern corners of Green Lake Park. Many establishments along E. Green Lake Way N offer outdoor seating and allow for excellent people-watching. The Woodland Park Zoo also makes a great trip, especially with children. Try visiting midweek to avoid the crowds. For more information, visit zoo.org.

GPS TRAILHEAD COORDINATES

N47° 40.205' W122° 20.583'

From I-5 north of downtown Seattle, take Exit 169 for NE 50th Street, and go west 0.9 mile. Continue over a hill to a five-way intersection, and turn right onto E. Green Lake Way N. In 0.3 mile, go left at the fork in the road onto W. Green Lake Way N. Take the first left into the parking lot next to the tennis courts near the sign for Woodland Park. Additional parking is along W. Green Lake Way N and elsewhere throughout the park.

BELLEVUE AND THE EASTSIDE

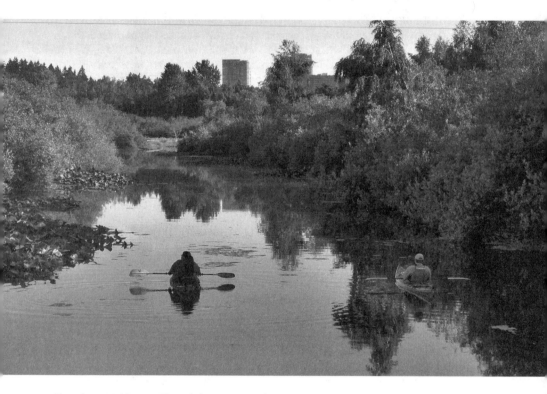

Kayakers on Mercer Slough (see page 65)

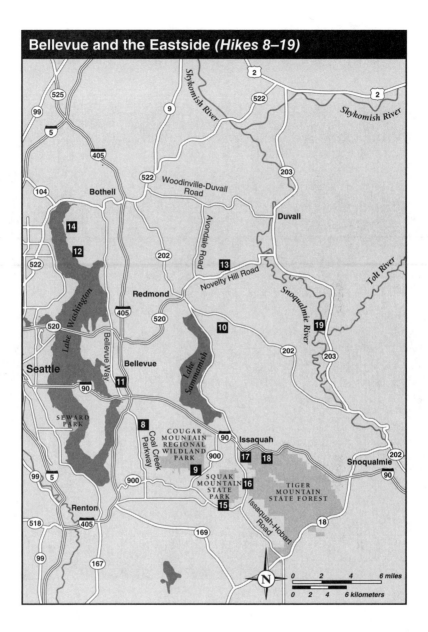

Bellevue and the Eastside *(Hikes 8–19)*

8 Coal Creek Natural Area

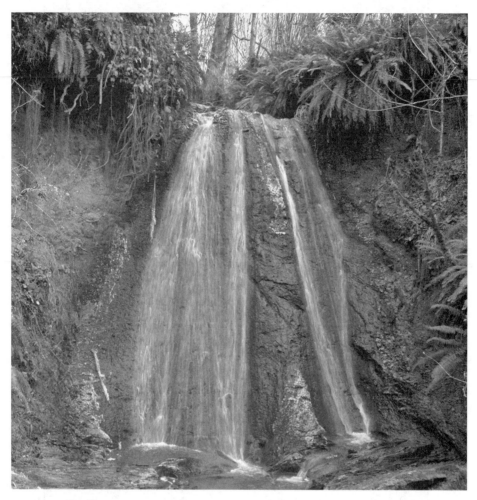

North Fork Falls

In Brief

It might be hard to believe, but this modest park helped build Seattle. Supplying coal to a rapidly expanding population across the lake, the Newcastle mine that used to operate here fueled the region's explosive growth at the end of the 19th century. Today, the park still serves the city, but as a refuge from the urban sprawl it once spawned, with a trail through a narrow creek ravine leading to two waterfalls and several excellent historical sites.

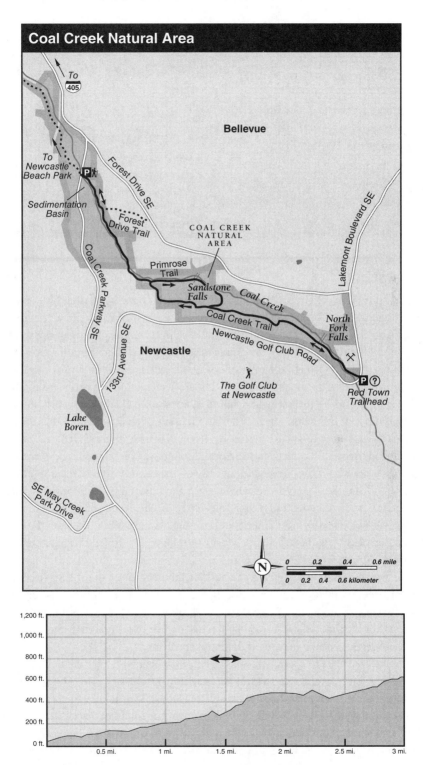

Coal Creek Natural Area

DISTANCE & CONFIGURATION: 6.0-mile out-and-back; with optional return route	**ACCESS:** Hikable year-round; no fee for parking or trail access
	WHEELCHAIR TRAVERSABLE: No
DIFFICULTY: Easy–moderate	**MAP(S):** Green Trails *Cougar Mountain/ Squak Mountain 203S*; USGS *Bellevue South*
SCENERY: Historical mines and structures; waterfalls and a creek	
EXPOSURE: Shaded	**FACILITIES:** None at trailhead
	DOGS: Allowed on-leash
TRAFFIC: Moderate	**CONTACT:** 425-452-6885; parkstrails .myparksandrecreation.com/Details .aspx?pid=463
TRAIL SURFACE: Mostly dirt; some gravel near trailhead and some boardwalk	
HIKING TIME: 2–3 hours	**LOCATION:** Bellevue

Description

The trail through Coal Creek Park is surely one of the most surprising hikes anywhere around Puget Sound. Featuring several waterfalls, a small canyon, and an environment typical of the Cascade foothills, the park straddles the boundary between the suburbs of Bellevue and the natural areas of the Issaquah Alps, a green finger pointing from the foot of Cougar Mountain through the rows of houses along Lake Washington's eastern shore.

The greater Seattle area is blessed with many excellent urban hikes, each offering a quick escape from the local neighborhood. What makes Coal Creek Park so unusual, though, is not that it is an undeveloped island in a sea of civilization but that only a century ago it was just the opposite. In the late 1800s, when virgin forest still reached all the way to the shores of Elliot Bay and today's Eastside was mostly untracked wilderness, the park was the site of the Newcastle coal mine—a substantial industrial operation that, if it were still standing, would overwhelm even the busy neighborhoods that currently surround it. As you hike the trail, watch for vestiges of the mining days, clues to the story of Newcastle coal. Yet the most compelling story in the park is undoubtedly the extent to which nature has reclaimed the land. Most of the time, it's difficult to imagine that any human development ever occurred here.

The western trailhead begins at the parking lot, near the chain-link fence protecting the Coal Creek Parkway Sedimentation Basin. Built in 1986, the basin is designed to keep the creek channel clear by capturing sediment carried by the water before it can continue downstream; it also provides habitat for fish in several man-made pools and ponds harboring a variety of trout and salmon species.

The trail narrows to a singletrack as the canyon deepens along the northern side of the creek, crossing several side streams running down from the ridge. Although the Coal Creek watershed drains only the western side of Cougar Mountain, which rarely carries a snowpack, the water is usually high enough to cover the sound of the traffic from above.

After 0.3 mile, faint Forest Drive Trail enters from the steep slope on the left. Continue past this intersection for another 0.9 mile through a mix of brush and trees until you

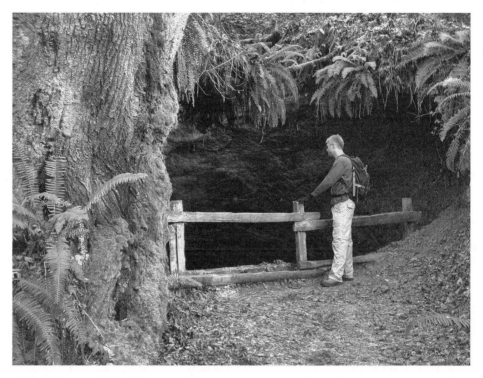

Inspecting an old coal seam

reach a signed junction with Primrose Trail, allowing you to visit Sandstone Falls and complete a short loop with the main Coal Creek Trail on the return. Strangely, the trails are not named in an intuitive way and it would make more sense if the titles were switched; Primrose Trail closely follows the creek, not Coal Creek Trail.

Follow Primrose Trail along the creek to a site with a few sandstone boulders, a relatively unusual geologic formation for this area where rocks of volcanic origin are much more common. Reach Sandstone Falls after 0.4 mile, where a side creek slides down over an exposed piece of the underlying sedimentary rock before joining the main channel. Although the 20-foot drop isn't much by high Cascade Mountain standards, it is certainly exceptional by Bellevue standards, especially during periods of peak flow.

The canyon reaches its deepest point just past the falls, and the sides begin to steepen. Watch for some remnants of the old mining operation along the southern side of the creek, including rusty iron cartwheels and a cable partially buried in the dirt.

The trail climbs out of the inner canyon to rejoin Coal Creek Trail some 0.8 mile from the previous junction. Turn left and pass below a ridge, notable for the multitude of ferns seemingly pouring down the hill from the right.

Join a dirt road through the clearing, then return to the trail on the far side at a sign for Red Town Trailhead. Just beyond the bottom of some boardwalk stairs, look for a concrete slab off to the right, the base of the old locomotive turntable. Surprisingly, the concrete looks as if it was poured yesterday, without significant weathering, yet all other evidence that a busy rail line once ran here has essentially disappeared, swallowed by the woods.

Beyond the turntable, two waterfalls mark the last 0.25 mile of the trail. Coal Creek pours over a short man-made drop of beams and planks—all that is left of a substantial wooden housing that once enclosed the entire flow—in the creek bed. Mere steps above it, North Fork Falls tumbles down a striking slab of red rock on the left, similar in height to Sandstone Falls along Primrose Trail but much more impressive, with a greater volume of water.

The trail splits nearby, creating a very short loop; be sure to explore both sides. On the north, a rich vein of coal (all that remains of an old mine shaft) is exposed and open for inspection. The opposite side features a fascinating information kiosk on the Newcastle operation from 1867 to 1929. It is almost impossible to imagine that at one time a large hotel stood nearby, locomotives steamed through, and crowds of physical laborers toiled on the very spot on which you now stand. Several old photographs tell the story, though, revealing the magnitude of the development needed to recover, process, and transport the coal.

Red Town Trailhead is just up a short hill, the turnaround point for this hike. Head back the way you came, remembering to stay on the main Coal Creek Trail at the junction for Primrose Trail to complete the central loop.

Many options are available if you wish to continue farther. Red Town is one of the most popular places for access to Cougar Mountain, just across the road from the end of Coal Creek Trail. From the western trailhead, look for a sign to Lower Coal Creek Trail on the opposite side of Coal Creek Parkway SE. The linear park continues down the canyon as far as Newcastle Beach Park via Lake Washington Trail, 2.3 miles one way.

GPS TRAILHEAD COORDINATES
N47° 33.250' W122° 9.983'

From I-405, take Exit 10 for Coal Creek Parkway. At the end of the exit, head southeast on Coal Creek Parkway. Continue on this winding road past the Factoria Mall area. In 1.4 miles from I-405, look for the trailhead parking area on the left (east) side of the road at the bottom of Coal Creek Canyon. If the lot is full, head to the Red Town Trailhead instead, located where Newcastle Golf Club Road turns into Lakemont Boulevard SE, and do the hike in reverse. To reach the Red Town Trailhead, head southeast on Coal Creek Parkway 1.2 miles, and turn left onto Forest Drive SE. In 2.1 miles turn right onto Lakemont Boulevard SE, and go 0.5 mile. The trailhead will be on your right.

9 Cougar Mountain:
WILDERNESS PEAK LOOP

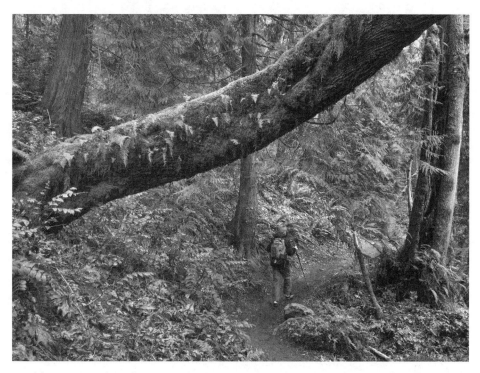

Wilderness Creek Trail

In Brief

Cougar Mountain receives many visitors, but most are concentrated at the Red Town Trailhead, far from the mountain's high point at Wilderness Peak. The Wilderness Creek Trail climbs to the park's summit via an appealing valley, passing several moderate viewpoints along the way and avoiding some of the crowds.

Description

Unlike its higher neighbors in the Issaquah Alps, Cougar Mountain has a flat, marshy area at its heart. Where both Squak and Tiger Mountains have a clearly discernible central crest, Cougar is more like a plateau, climbing on all sides to reach a broad, even middle. With this unusual topography, the true summit is difficult to discern from a wide range of similar high points among the trees.

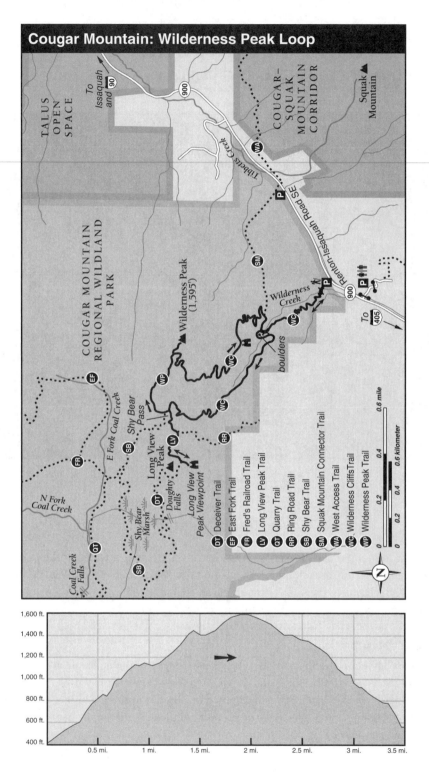

Cougar Mountain: Wilderness Peak Loop

TALUS OPEN SPACE

To Issaquah and 90

COUGAR–SQUAK MOUNTAIN CORRIDOR

Squak Mountain

COUGAR MOUNTAIN REGIONAL WILDLAND PARK

Tibbetts Creek

Wilderness Peak (1,595')

Wilderness Creek

boulders

To 405

Renton–Issaquah Road SE

Shy Bear Pass

E Fork Coal Creek

N Fork Coal Creek

Shy Bear Marsh

Long View Peak

Long View Peak Viewpoint

Doughty Falls

Coal Creek Falls

DT	Deceiver Trail
EF	East Fork Trail
FR	Fred's Railroad Trail
LV	Long View Peak Trail
QT	Quarry Trail
RR	Ring Road Trail
SB	Shy Bear Trail
SM	Squak Mountain Connector Trail
WA	West Access Trail
WC	Wilderness Cliffs Trail
WP	Wilderness Peak Trail

0   0.2   0.4   0.6 mile
0   0.2   0.4   0.6 kilometer

N

1,600 ft.
1,400 ft.
1,200 ft.
1,000 ft.
800 ft.
600 ft.
400 ft.

0.5 mi.   1 mi.   1.5 mi.   2 mi.   2.5 mi.   3 mi.   3.5 mi.

DISTANCE & CONFIGURATION: 3.5-mile loop; 0.6-mile optional side trip	**MAP(S):** Green Trails *Cougar Mountain/Squak Mountain 203S*; USGS *Bellevue South*
DIFFICULTY: Moderate	
SCENERY: Several modest viewpoints and cascading Wilderness Creek	**FACILITIES:** Toilet at trailhead; no drinking water
EXPOSURE: Mostly shaded	**DOGS:** Allowed on-leash
TRAFFIC: High	**CONTACT:** 206-205-5275; tinyurl.com /cougarmtnpark
TRAIL SURFACE: Dirt	
HIKING TIME: 2–3 hours	**LOCATION:** Issaquah
ACCESS: Hikable year-round, daily, 8 a.m.–sunset; no fee for parking or trail access	**COMMENTS:** This trailhead is prone to frequent car break-ins, so be sure to leave your valuables at home. It's also busy, so arrive early to get a parking spot.
WHEELCHAIR TRAVERSABLE: No	

Aided both by its drive-up approach and its name, which recalls the mountain's history as a military installation, Anti-Aircraft Peak attracts a lot of attention. However, at 1,483 feet it is only the second-highest point on Cougar Mountain, more than 100 feet lower than 1,595-foot Wilderness Peak, about a mile away to the south.

The hike to Wilderness Peak starts from the northwest end of the small parking lot, signed as E6 Wilderness Creek Trail. Note that the letter E indicates that this trail is in the eastern section of the park, a naming convention used throughout Cougar Mountain; other trails can also be preceded by N, W, or S, for the remaining compass directions, or C, for trails in the center.

Just past the trailhead, a footbridge crosses Wilderness Creek as it splashes down among mossy boulders and logs. The trail then climbs on the southern side of the creek through some short switchbacks, generally with the water flowing within earshot as it heads up the ridge.

Cross back over the creek on a second bridge after about 0.5 mile to reach the first junction, and stay to your left; the right-hand option, signed as Wilderness Creek Trail, serves as the end of the loop on the descent.

Some glacial erratics, not surprisingly known as The Boulders, soon appear on the right. The big rocks continue intermittently up the slope, inviting speculation on both the massive forces required to deposit them here and the power of erosion that may eventually grind them to dust.

Cross the creek several more times as the trail ascends to a flatter marshy area. Carefully laid wooden planks wind between some more erratics, keeping hikers above the mud and away from both stinging nettles and thorny devil's club, with some particularly nasty specimens reaching more than 10 feet high. Past the marsh, the trail starts climbing again through a forest of tall Douglas firs and eventually reaches an important intersection at Shy Bear Pass, elevation approximately 1,350 feet, where several S and E trails converge.

The signed trail to Long View Peak heads left, allowing a 0.8-mile out-and-back side trip to a nearby viewpoint. The overlook is far short of spectacular, and typical for Cougar Mountain, with intervening trees and a relatively narrow angle of view; nonetheless, it makes an interesting diversion. To reach the viewpoint, stay on the S4 Long View Peak Trail past a junction with S5 Ring Road Trail, then turn left onto an unsigned spur where S3 Deceiver Trail branches to the right. The spur goes up and over a small rise to reach the view, which looks out over a slice of South Seattle and Puget Sound.

Return to Shy Bear Pass and follow the signed E4 Wilderness Peak Trail on a gentle uphill singletrack to where it crests after about 0.3 mile. Descend slightly and go past the right turn onto E5 Wilderness Cliffs Trail. The high point is only another 0.1 mile, where the trail dead-ends at a bench in a circular grove of tall trees. Lacking a view or even a single exposed rock, Wilderness Peak hardly passes for a summit, by most definitions of the word. But the spot beneath the trees is pleasant and peaceful, like a quiet chapel in the woods.

Return to the previous intersection and turn left to start descending Wilderness Cliffs Trail. The route drops gradually at first, but soon becomes steeper and enters some switchbacks beneath the high Douglas firs. Two viewpoints look out over the May Creek Valley through gaps in the trees—the first just off to the right and the second farther down to the left—although neither provides what could be described as an all-encompassing vista. Wilderness Creek can be heard in the ravine below, too far down to be visible.

The signed Squak Mountain Connector Trail eventually branches off to the left. Stay to the right another 400 feet to return to Wilderness Creek Trail at the junction you encountered earlier, closing the loop. From here, continue down the same way you originally came up.

Nearby Activities

The kid-friendly Issaquah Salmon Hatchery provides a window into efforts to restore coho and chinook salmon to the Issaquah Creek Watershed. The return of the fish to spawn each fall is surely the yearly highlight, but there is always something of interest going on. To reach the hatchery, follow WA 900 (Renton-Issaquah Road SE) northeast from the trailhead, then turn right onto Newport Way NW in Issaquah. Take Newport Way into downtown, then turn left onto W. Sunset Way. The hatchery is located at 125 W. Sunset Way, on the right side of the road. For more information, visit the Friends of the Issaquah Salmon Hatchery website at issaquahfish.org or call 425-392-1118.

GPS TRAILHEAD COORDINATES

N47° 30.612' W122° 5.227'

From I-5 south of downtown Seattle, take Exit 164A, and go east on I-90. Take Exit 15 and turn right onto WA 900 West, which begins as 17th Avenue NW and then becomes Renton-Issaquah Road SE. About 3.2 miles from I-90 and just after SE 95th Street, you will reach the entrance to a parking lot for the Wilderness Creek Trailhead on the right.

10 Evans Creek Preserve

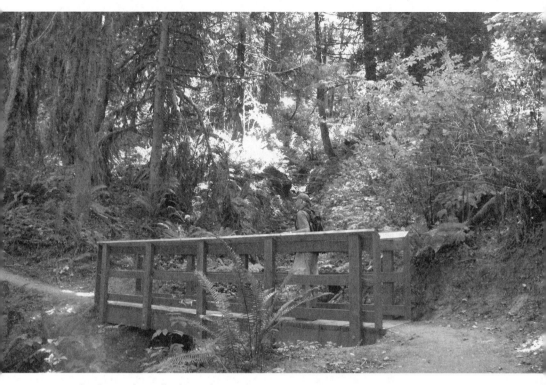

Footbridge in the Hillside Trails area

In Brief

With a mix of forest, wetlands, and meadows, Evans Creek Preserve offers an assortment of ecosystems in a semirural setting on the far outskirts of Redmond. A collection of interconnected loop trails makes it easy to wander and explore at your own pace.

Description

Thanks to the City of Sammamish Parks and Recreation Department and some generous volunteer work from the Washington Trails Association (WTA), Evans Creek Preserve opened to the public in 2011. Visitors to the preserve reap the fruits of their efforts, as the rewarding trail system is well signed, easy to navigate, and offers a host of attractions in just 179 acres.

When the preserve first opened, there was only one trailhead available (described as the alternate parking lot in the Driving Directions). A second, larger trailhead opened in

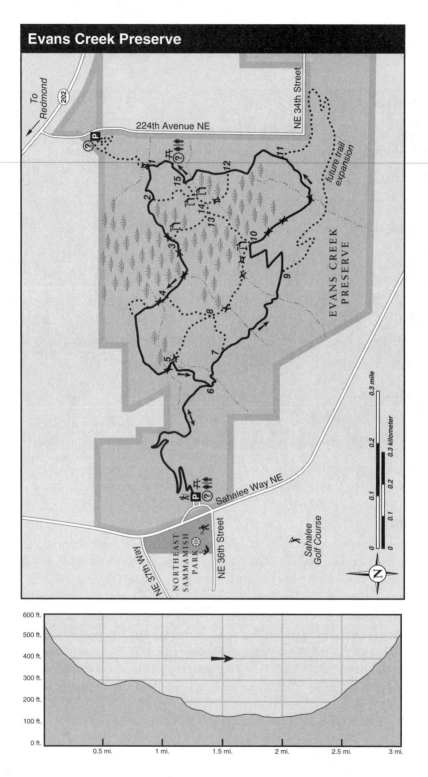

DISTANCE & CONFIGURATION: 3.0-mile loop with optional trails to make it shorter or longer	ACCESS: Hikable year-round, daily, sunrise–sunset; no fee for parking or trail access
DIFFICULTY: Easy–moderate	WHEELCHAIR TRAVERSABLE: Yes, on Meadow Trail
SCENERY: Forest, open meadows, distant mountain views, creeks, wetlands	MAP(S): At the trailheads
EXPOSURE: Over half the trails are shaded	FACILITIES: Toilet at trailhead; no drinking water
TRAFFIC: Medium	DOGS: Allowed on-leash
TRAIL SURFACE: Dirt and gravel trails with some boardwalks; ADA-accessible Meadows Trail	CONTACT: 425-295-0582; tinyurl.com /evanscreekpreserve
HIKING TIME: 1–2 hours	LOCATION: Sammamish

2014 with more amenities than the first, including toilets, bike racks, and picnic tables. The hike described here starts and ends at the newer trailhead; however, the older trailhead allows for ADA-access to the Meadow Trails, so if that is something you require, you should head to the parking lot on 224th Avenue NE.

Both trailheads provide a complete map of the preserve on an information board. This official map is the best guide to the area and displays a series of numbered trail junctions. On the trails themselves, excellent signage and short distances make finding the way simple for even the first-time visitor. No matter where you start or which way you go, it is easy to reach any section of the preserve via the multiple networked routes. This hike description follows a general counterclockwise perimeter loop that reaches every ecosystem in the preserve, but individual preferences should take you whichever way you wish to go.

From the newer parking lot, the trail starts on an impressive descent through a nice forest of ferns and mossy trees. The care and skill used by the WTA volunteers in crafting the trail here are evident, as the switchbacks are anchored with logs and stones to prevent erosion, wooden benches provide easy places to stop and relax, and the bridges are sturdy and well made.

The southwestern side of the preserve lies along the edge of a broad ravine with a surprising amount of vertical drop. Some tall trees manage to reach all the way to the top of the ravine in the canopy far above your head, making them close to 100 feet high.

After descending for 0.4 mile, reach the first trail junction, shown on the map as number 6. Take a right turn to continue on the perimeter, which should be the default choice all the way around to complete the loop. Multiple creeks run down the slope from the right to reach the wetlands and then Evans Creek itself on the valley floor below. The noise from these streams helps to mask the sound of the considerable traffic on the nearby roads. You might also hear the shouts and laughter of children through the woods; the preserve is a deservedly popular destination for families.

Another 0.5 mile leads to junction 9. As of 2016, the trail system is still a work in progress, and a future loop route through the preserve's southeastern corner from this point is still under construction.

Head downhill to the north toward junction 10 where you will exit the Hillside Trails section of the preserve and enter the central Woodland Trails area. Here the hike is much flatter since you are no longer traversing the ravine wall. Stay right to follow the perimeter and arrive at junction 11, where the future loop trail will return to the main network when complete.

Some giant stumps in the understory attest to the logging history of the former homestead that once stood on this land. As you continue north, the trees thin out until you are hiking in an open meadow. Around junctions 15, 1, and 2 lie the Meadow Trails, the easiest section for walking in the preserve. The gravel trail here is flat and wide, providing a convenient ADA-accessible loop for users entering from the alternate trailhead across Evans Creek and just up the hill to the north.

These meadows were the historical heart of the old homestead, shown by the remains of a wooden, ranch-style gate with the mysterious inscription BRAZAPPA at the top. This part of the preserve has also been the focus of most of the recent development for modern visitors. Watch for picnic tables and a toilet near junction 15 and a row of special bird feeders near junction 2.

Several marked viewpoints are located in the grass and trees, providing raised wooden platforms for observing the landscape and scenery. The views tend to be modest at best, but it is possible to see a few high peaks of the cascade front range to the east.

Moving west through junctions 3, 4, and 5, you will travel through some of the preserve's wetlands and gradually transition back from the open meadow into the forest. The wetlands are best explored through the center of the preserve near junction 13, where wooden boardwalks keep you above the giant skunk cabbage and mud below your feet.

From junction 5, another 0.5 mile of climbing via the Hillside Trails returns you to your car.

GPS TRAILHEAD COORDINATES
N47° 38.587' W122° 3.317'

From I-5 north of downtown Seattle, take Exit 168B, and go east on WA 520. In 12.1 miles exit onto Redmond Way/WA 202. Turn right (southeast) onto WA 202 (which becomes NE Redmond–Fall City Road), and go 2.5 miles; then turn right onto Sahalee Way. The parking lot is on the left in 1.0 mile. An alternate lot is located on 224th Avenue NE. To reach it, from the exit onto WA 202, travel southeast on WA 202 3.7 miles, and turn right onto 224th Avenue.

11 Mercer Slough Nature Park

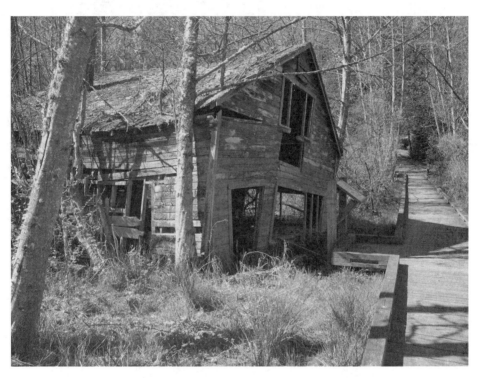

Ruined wooden structure

In Brief

This Bellevue Parks and Community Services Department gem offers easy access to a vast array of native plants and wildlife, just minutes from downtown. The vestigial wetlands provide a window into life here prior to modern development and the interesting site history and working blueberry farm ensure that everyone will find something to enjoy.

Description

Surrounded by high-rises, rampant suburbs, and two interstate highways, the Mercer Slough Nature Park is a true ecological oasis in the heart of Bellevue. Encompassing more than 320 acres of wetlands and several miles of hiking trails, the location offers a great quick escape for nature lovers of all kinds.

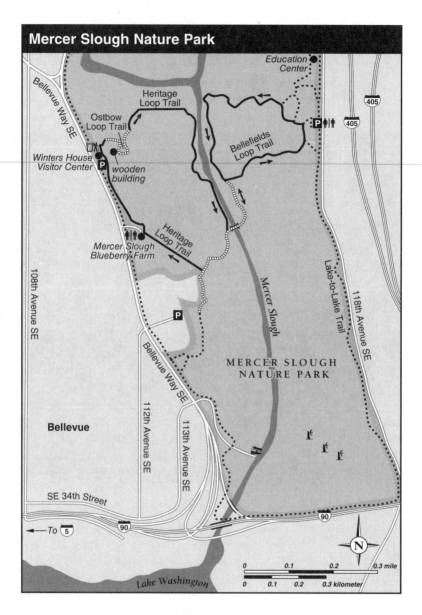

But don't be fooled; the slough's easy access does not compromise its natural setting. Mercer is the largest urban wetland in King County, and it contains an incredible range of wildlife, despite its relatively small size. Mink, otter, beaver, and even coyote call the park home, along with more than 100 species of birds, making it one of the most diverse ecosystems in the Puget Sound region.

Before beginning your hike, be sure to stop by the visitor center in the Winters House at the northern end of the parking lot. Listed on the National Register of Historic

DISTANCE & CONFIGURATION: 2.1-mile figure eight (side-trip options)	**WHEELCHAIR TRAVERSABLE:** Yes, on boardwalk and Periphery Loop
DIFFICULTY: Easy	**MAP(S):** At trailhead or pick up pamphlet in Winter House Visitor Center; USGS *Bellevue South*
SCENERY: Wetlands, slough, wildlife, blueberry farm, native flora and fauna	
EXPOSURE: Mostly open, some shady areas	**FACILITIES:** Toilets and water at visitor center
TRAFFIC: Popular on sunny days	**DOGS:** Allowed on-leash
TRAIL SURFACE: Mixture of gravel, boardwalk, dirt, and wood chip	**CONTACT:** 425-452-2565; ci.bellevue .wa.us/mercer_slough.htm
HIKING TIME: 1–2 hours	**LOCATION:** 2102 Bellevue Way SE, Bellevue, WA 98004
ACCESS: Hikable year-round, daily, sunrise–sunset; no fee for parking or trail access	

Places, the Spanish-style house was built by Frederick and Cecelia Winters in 1929 with funds earned from their on-site nursery. Initially specializing in greenhouse-raised azaleas, daffodils, and irises, the Winters attained success in bulb farming after the spread of an infectious blight led to a quarantine on imports.

The estate was purchased in 1943 by Austrian immigrants Anna and Frank Riepl; Mrs. Riepl resided in the house until 1983, when it began to fall into disrepair. Five years later, the city of Bellevue purchased the property and restored it to its current condition. In addition to serving as the park's visitor center, the Winters House is also home to the Bellevue Historical Society and serves as a gathering place for meetings, receptions, and banquets.

The hike begins on the eastern side of the parking lot; look for a display board featuring park information and an excellent map. Head north on the gravel path to the start of the Heritage Trail boardwalk. The trail is well marked, but note that on many signs decimal points are missing from the stated distances—0.3 mile looks like 3 miles, for example.

As you enter the wetlands, the ruins of an old wooden building appear on the right. The structure is falling apart and sinking into the ground, being reclaimed by the mud. Although you are only a stone's throw from Bellevue Way SE, the sounds of birds in the willows begin to overtake the dull roar of traffic.

In less than 100 yards, Ostbow Loop both starts and ends on the right. Endre Ostbow grew rhododendrons here on land purchased from the Riepls, and the side loop that now bears his name winds through many of these plants still thriving in the bog. Whether you explore this spur or not, at the second intersection follow the main trail to the left, heading north.

The boardwalk passes under a living arch of dogwood branches before bending through a cattail marsh and reaching an abrupt end. A fence separates the neatly planted

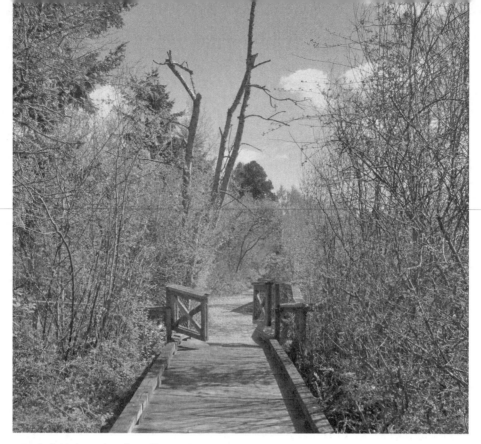

End of the boardwalk trail

rows of Mercer Slough Farm blueberry bushes on the right from the wood-chip trail and chaos of natural growth on the left. Like Ostbow's surviving rhododendrons, the blueberry farm connects the developed Bellevue of today with its agricultural roots of the past. Continue along the fence to where a riot of wild blackberry bushes lines the main channel of the slough.

Cross the footbridge over the dark, slow-moving water, watching for kayakers and canoeists paddling by. The high-rises of downtown Bellevue are visible just to the north, a reminder of the development that lays siege to this last natural refuge.

Great blue herons often fly overhead or stand in the rushes on the banks here. Despite their striking size and color, these birds can be surprisingly well camouflaged in the reeds. Other bird species you might spot include ruddy ducks, wigeons, buffleheads, hooded mergansers, and mallards. During the fall run (September–December), you may catch sight of chinook and coho salmon swimming upstream to spawn.

The boardwalk resumes on the eastern side of the bridge, reaching a T-shaped junction with the Bellefields Loop. Follow the frequently muddy, wood chip–lined trail to the right (east) into shrubs and meadows. Several interpretive displays around the loop provide valuable natural and historical information about the area.

In less than 0.25 mile, a group of benches marks a gravel path that enters from the right. Continue on the main trail to the left, past a stand of large western red cedars. These massive trees mark the original eastern shore of Lake Washington, which receded after the construction of the ship canal in 1917. Stay to the left again and cross Trail Creek, bypassing the short hill to the right leading to the Bellefields Trailhead on 118th Avenue SE.

On the far side of the stream, the trail splits, and you can veer right, over a small rise, or head left to stay along the lower path. Skunk cabbage lines both trails here; the sight of the plant's yellow flowers helps offset its thick, unpleasant odor during the spring and summer bloom. Either direction will take you to the next junction, where the trails meet again. From there, continue westward through scrub to reach the edge of the slough, passing viewpoints that offer continued chances to spot wildlife. Returning to the boardwalk, you will complete the Bellefields Loop and arrive back at the footbridge you crossed earlier.

After crossing the bridge, stay to the left and continue on the boardwalk. As you navigate the wetlands, be sure to watch for tulips in the thicket. It is amazing that these flowers can capture enough sunlight in the heavy tangle of reeds and brushes to grow. Enjoy the small miracle of these beautiful blooms if you should be lucky enough to see one.

After less than 0.2 mile, a gravel path branches to the right. Leave the boardwalk and follow this path back alongside the Mercer Slough Blueberry Farm building and then finally to the Winters House parking lot, where you began.

Note that there are many options for lengthening your hike. A paved biking and running trail circumnavigates the entire park and joins with the Lake-to-Lake Trail, which connects Lake Sammamish to Lake Washington.

Nearby Activities

Canoe and kayak lessons and rentals are available at Enatai Beach Park Boathouse, just to the south on Lake Washington; call 425-430-0111 for more information. Contact the new Mercer Slough Environmental Education Center near the Bellefields Trailhead for educational and informational programs: 425-452-2565 or bellevuewa.gov/mseec.htm.

GPS TRAILHEAD COORDINATES

N47° 35.477' W122° 11.523'

From I-5 just south of downtown Seattle, take Exit 164A, and go east on I-90. Take Exit 9 and follow the ramp as it curves to the north and becomes Bellevue Way SE. Soon you will pass a boat launch, the South Bellevue Park and Ride, and the Mercer Slough Blueberry Farm. Just past the farm, 0.6 mile from the interstate, look for the blue Winters House trailhead sign on the right and park in the adjacent lot.

12 O. O. Denny Park

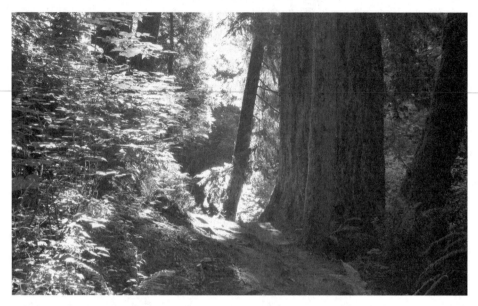

Trail winding through trees

In Brief

At O. O. Denny Park, nothing is as it seems. What looks like a small, lakefront green space in the city of Kirkland is actually a narrow slice of deep forest owned by the city of Seattle. Some of the largest trees in the city stand here, including the broken-off trunk of a 600-year-old Douglas fir, reportedly the largest tree in King County until high winds felled it in the early 1990s. An easy trail loops through the narrow creek valley.

Description

O. O. Denny Park is largely known for its beach—if it is known at all. Drawn by the open picnic area right on Lake Washington, families arrive on hot summer weekends to relax, play, and have barbecues on the grass. A large wooden shelter is often reserved for formal occasions and large gatherings, and 0.25 mile of access to the water provides good views of the opposite shore, including the enormous National Oceanic and Atmospheric Administration (NOAA) installation at Sand Point to the south.

Yet even residents of the quiet Juanita neighborhood that surrounds the park seem largely unaware of the astonishing forest that lies along the Denny Creek ravine, across the road from the lake. Even on some of the busiest days, relatively few visitors venture out on the trails and into the woods, missing out on some of the park's most outstanding features.

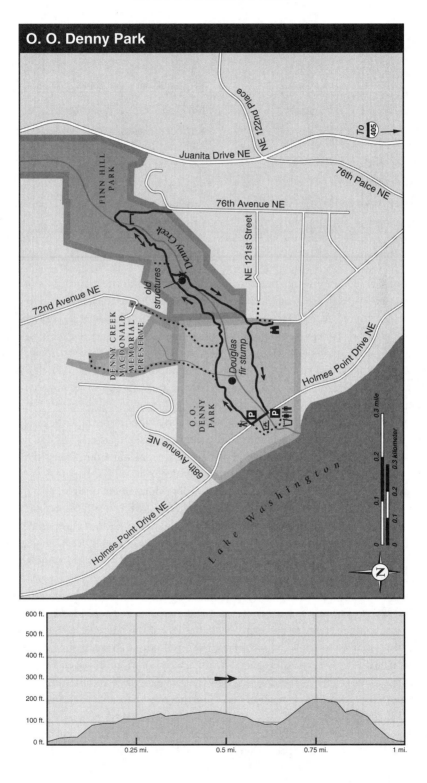

DISTANCE & CONFIGURATION: 1.0-mile loop	**ACCESS:** Hikable year-round, daily, sunrise–sunset; no fee for parking or trail access
DIFFICULTY: Easy	
SCENERY: Old-growth trees (including a 600-year-old Douglas fir), salmon-spawning creek, historical structures, views of Lake Washington	**WHEELCHAIR TRAVERSABLE:** No
	MAP(S): USGS *Bellevue North*
	FACILITIES: Toilet and water at lakefront picnic area
EXPOSURE: Shaded	
TRAFFIC: Low	**DOGS:** Allowed on-leash
TRAIL SURFACE: Dirt, gravel	**CONTACT:** 425-587-3300; tinyurl.com/oodennypark
HIKING TIME: 1–2 hours	**LOCATION:** Kirkland

The trail begins uphill into the trees from the northern side of the parking lot. Within a few hundred yards, a small network of side trails branches to the left to explore a grove of giant western red cedars. These substantial trees are just the beginning of some of the exemplary specimens representing many of the signature species of the Pacific Northwest that can be found in the park. Along with the red cedars, various Douglas firs, grand firs, black cottonwoods, and western hemlocks all stand more than 150 feet tall. Some of the trees rise more than 200 feet, placing them among the largest known samples of their kind anywhere in Seattle.

Denny Creek appears down the slope to the right, bubbling through the underbrush. The trail is frequently wet and muddy and is almost constantly shaded by the tall trees, but thoughtfully placed blocks of wood and stone set into the ground keep hikers' feet above the worst of it. The ravine is surprisingly deep, more than 100 feet to the rim, retaining the park's seclusion by keeping nearby development out of sight.

A large Douglas fir lays across the route, spanning the creek and reaching far up the bank on the far side. The trail cuts through the trunk near the roots, providing a good look at the interior of the tree and a chance to count its many rings. It is also possible to climb up around the end to inspect the tree's massive exposed root system and speculate on its demise, likely during a heavy storm.

But even that fallen tree cannot prepare you for what you will find just up the trail—the giant trunk of what was once the largest Douglas fir anywhere in King County. The word *stump* cannot adequately describe what is left of this incredible tree, which still stands more than 60 feet tall and has a base circumference that easily tops 25 feet. Even its bark is impressive, deep and rugged like an inscription from the ages, a testimony to its six centuries of survival and growth. This tree once towered far above the ravine and everything else around it, a condition that unfortunately exposed it to the wild wind that finally brought it down.

Beyond the fallen Douglas fir, an open clearing in a natural amphitheater with a few ruined buildings gives a glimpse into some local history. The park is named for Orion O.

Denny, second son of Seattle founders Arthur and Mary Denny, who once owned a country estate on the property. Named *Klahanie,* an adaptation of a Chinook tribal word meaning "the outdoors," the estate was deeded to the city as a public park in Denny's memory by his third wife around the time of World War I. This site was accessible via a gravel road on the far side of the creek, the beginning of the hike's return loop.

This trail continues up the ravine another 0.25 mile, adding an out-and-back tail to the loop. The route crosses the creek and climbs a few wooden stairs to reach a bench on the southern side of the ravine. Some short switchbacks continue up the slope, eventually ending at the side of a street in the Finn Hill community. A better option is to descend back along the creek to reach an interesting exposed clay wall in the side of the bank; an optimal turnaround point lies just around the next corner.

Return to the gravel road and cross the creek on a footbridge. Local volunteers undertook an extensive habitat-rehabilitation project here in 2002, adding boulder weirs and step pools as part of a man-made fish ladder to help with salmon recovery. Clusters of snake grass and sword ferns run along the creek, along with salmonberry, blackberry, salal, and big-leaf maples.

The wide trail climbs toward the top of the ravine, where it ends on a residential street. A view opens out to the south through the trees, encompassing Lake Washington and the eastern end of the WA 520 bridge. After enjoying the view, backtrack 20 yards to find a singletrack trail marked with a post and follow it downhill toward the creek to return to Holmes Point Drive NE, just south of where your vehicle is parked.

Nearby Activities

Kirkland's Juanita Bay Park lies just a few miles southeast of O. O. Denny Park and is particularly noted for its bird-watching opportunities. More than 150 species have been spotted at Juanita Bay, ranging from bald eagles to hairy woodpeckers. To reach Juanita Bay, turn right (south) on Juanita Drive NE from Holmes Drive NE and then right again on 98th Avenue NE for about 0.5 mile to reach the entrance. For more information or to join one of the highly recommended public tours offered by volunteers from the East Lake Washington Audubon Society, check the park's website at tinyurl.com/juanitabay.

GPS TRAILHEAD COORDINATES

N47° 42.569' W122° 14.993'

From I-405 N, take Exit 20A for NE 116th Street. Turn left onto 116th Street, which becomes NE Juanita Drive then turns north and changes its name to Juanita Drive NE. Go 3.4 miles, and turn left onto 76th Place NE, which becomes Holmes Point Drive NE. In 1.1 miles look for the trailhead parking lot on the right across the road from the O. O. Denny Park lakefront picnic area. From I-405 S, take Exit 20, and turn right onto NE 124th Street. In 1.0 mile turn left onto 100th Avenue NE, which becomes 98th Avenue NE. In 0.5 mile turn right onto NE Juanita Drive, and go 2.0 miles to 76th Place NE; follow the directions above from there.

13 Redmond Watershed Preserve

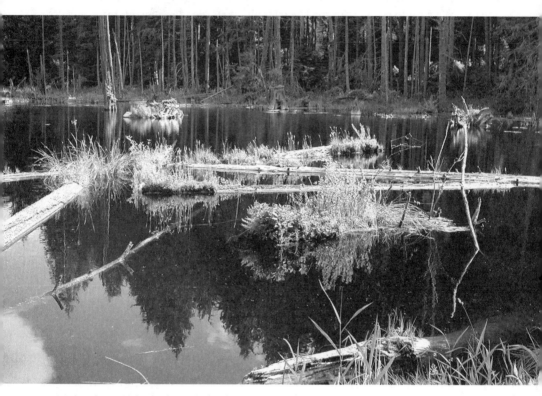

Wetlands at Redmond Watershed Preserve

In Brief

Well maintained in trails and facilities and yet well protected from encroaching development, the Redmond Watershed Preserve offers a worthwhile natural experience right on the city's doorstep. A wide network of multiple-use trails explores the reaches of the preserve, providing good hiking opportunities in a surprisingly scenic environment.

Description

The city of Redmond purchased some land from the Weyerhaeuser Corporation in 1926, hoping to use it as a source of water. At the time, the property, in what was then essentially the wilderness, must have seemed a long way outside the city. Although the

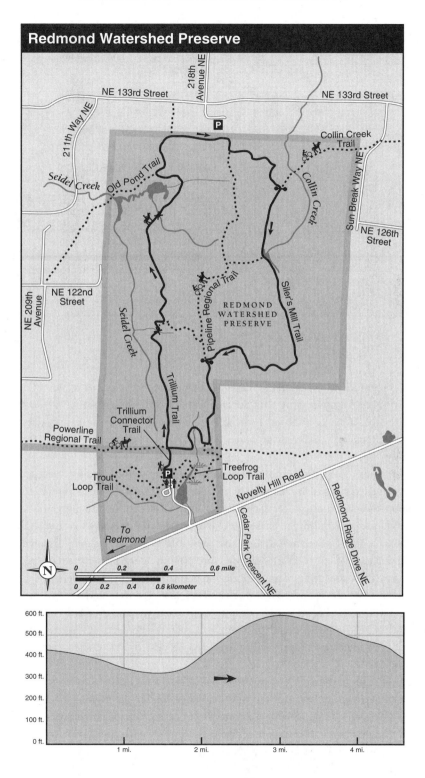

Redmond Watershed Preserve

DISTANCE & CONFIGURATION: 4.6-mile loop with side-trip options	**MAP(S):** USGS *Bellevue North*
DIFFICULTY: Easy–moderate	**FACILITIES:** Toilet at trailhead; no drinking water
SCENERY: Wetlands, plant life, well-maintained hiking trails, and optional interpretive trails	**DOGS:** Not allowed
EXPOSURE: Mostly shaded	**CONTACT:** 425-556-2311; redmond .gov/cms/one.aspx?pageId=4175
	LOCATION: Redmond
TRAFFIC: Medium–high	**COMMENTS:** Two additional short loops, both natural interpretive trails, are hiking options from the parking lot: Treefrog Loop Trail runs for 0.3 mile from the eastern side, and the 0.6-mile Trout Loop Trail starts on the western side. It is also possible to string together any number of shorter or longer trips through the preserve on any trail combination of your choosing.
TRAIL SURFACE: Mixture of dirt and gravel	
HIKING TIME: 2–3 hours	
ACCESS: Hikable year-round; no fee for parking or trail access	
WHEELCHAIR TRAVERSABLE: Yes, on interpretive trails	

site never panned out as a suitable watershed (the water was not of sufficient quality), as the city spread eastward the land became valuable for other reasons. What was once a distant piece of backwoods has now become a great outdoor-recreation site right in Redmond's backyard, and the watershed preserve has, in fact, turned into a forest and wetlands preserve instead.

Nonetheless, the setting is not entirely pristine, as open corridors for overhead power lines and a buried gas pipeline stand as reminders that the area was born to serve the urban population. But even these pieces of civilization are well integrated into the trail system: the two corridors together form the park's backbone and link the preserve to the extended Tolt Pipeline Trail, popular with mountain bikers, who follow the path on long-distance rides.

Starting in 1994, great efforts were put into upgrading the preserve's recreation facilities, enhancing everything from parking lot bathrooms to bridges, benches, and trail signs. The sign system is now so thorough and the routes so well marked you couldn't get lost if you wanted to. Yet amazingly, despite its proximity to the ever-growing suburbs of Redmond and the good natural experience available, the preserve still seems underused. The city estimates that substantially fewer people visit the watershed each year than climb Mount Si.

A grand tour of the park, linking several different trails in an extended 4.6-mile loop, presents the best hiking option. Start at the northern end of the parking lot on the signed Trillium Connector Trail, which heads into the woods on a wide gravel surface. After 0.2 mile, go straight across a four-way junction with Powerline Regional Trail to join Trillium Trail, open to hikers and equestrians but not mountain bikers.

Trillium Trail runs through a forest of second-growth Douglas firs and western hemlocks as it rolls over a few gentle ups and downs. Visible in a depression on the left is the main fork of Seidel Creek, which flows through ferns in the understory. At 0.6 mile from the junction, bypass Pipeline Connector Trail on the right and continue straight ahead, to the north. The surface underfoot changes from gravel to dirt and back again several times, but the trail remains broad and smooth. Cross two footbridges over side forks of Seidel Creek, flowing downslope from the right.

After the two creek crossings, head around to the left to reach a junction with Old Pond Trail, which leads for 0.25 mile to an exit onto 209th Avenue. The small pond itself can be seen through the trees on the left, where the three forks of Seidel Creek meet. The marshy land around the pond provides habitat for animals such as beavers, great blue herons, and other waterfowl.

Stay on Trillium Trail by following a tight turn to the right. Then curve through the northwestern corner of the park for about 0.5 mile to reach another junction. Go right on Pipeline Trail (signed as Collin Creek Trail), which runs parallel to the northern boundary of the preserve. Pass two spurs on the left that head out into the suburban neighborhood, then bend back toward the center of the park. After another 0.25 mile, you'll reach a junction with Collin Creek Trail.

Turn left onto Collin Creek Trail and walk 0.3 mile to reach a junction with the hikers-only Siler's Mill Trail on the right. Join Siler's Mill Trail and pass through a wooden gate designed to keep out horses and mountain bikers. Despite the limited access, the trail remains just as wide as the previous sections.

A pond becomes visible on the left, part of the park's most extensive wetlands ecosystem and the source of north-flowing Collin Creek. A second, substantially larger pond lies 0.25 mile behind the first, on the preserve boundary; it is neither visible nor accessible from here.

Siler's Mill Trail offers the purest hiking experience in the park, thanks to its restricted access and views of the scenic wetlands. Stay left at a junction just past the first pond to remain on the trail through the rich forest for another 1.1 miles, then pass through another wooden gate and turn left to rejoin Pipeline Trail, which is open to all users. Follow the pipeline to a major junction with Powerline Regional Trail and turn right underneath the humming wires. A final 0.7 mile returns you to Trillium Connector Trail, where a left turn carries you back to the parking lot and your vehicle.

GPS TRAILHEAD COORDINATES
N47° 41.788' W122° 3.054'

From I-5 in Seattle, take Exit 168B onto WA 520 E. Head east on WA 520 for 12.9 miles to the end in Redmond, and continue straight onto Avondale Road. After 1.0 mile, turn right onto Novelty Hill Road. Continue 2.3 miles to the park entrance on the left, across from 218th Avenue NE.

14 Saint Edward State Park

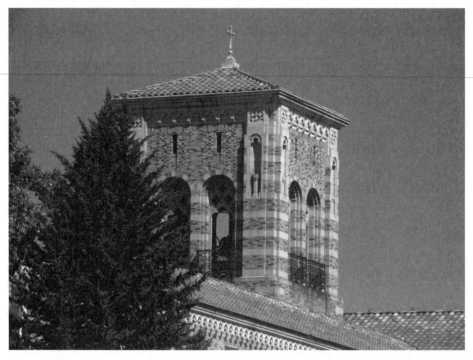

Seminary bell tower

In Brief

This former Catholic seminary sits on a high, forested bluff above the northern end of Lake Washington, providing access to one of the last stretches of undeveloped land on the waterfront via an excellent trail system.

Description

Although it hosted the raucous Washington Brewer's Festival for many years before the event moved to larger Marymoor Park in 2012, most of the time Saint Edward is quiet and calm, closer to the contemplative retreat likely envisioned when the seminary was founded by the Sulpician Order in the early 1930s. Named for Edward the Confessor, the second-to-last Anglo-Saxon king of England and founder of Westminster Abbey, the impressive facility was run by the Seattle Archdiocese until it was donated to the state of Washington in 1977 and turned into the park it is today.

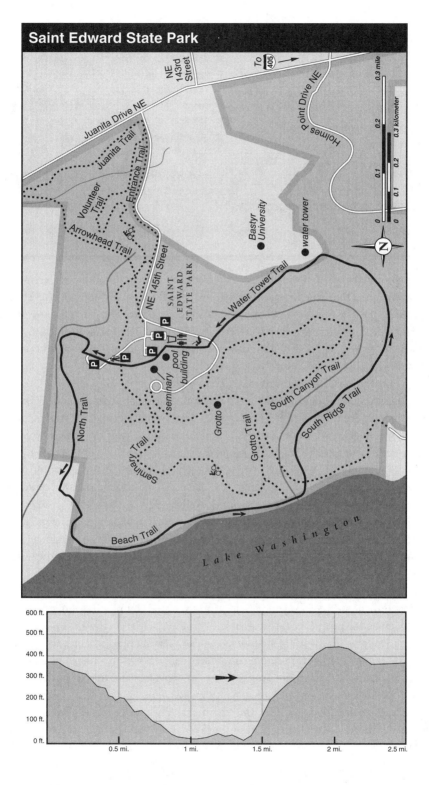

DISTANCE & CONFIGURATION: 2.5-mile loop	**WHEELCHAIR TRAVERSABLE:** No
DIFFICULTY: Moderate	**MAP(S):** USGS *Seattle North*
SCENERY: Lake Washington shoreline and area, views across the lake, a grotto	**FACILITIES:** Toilet and water available near the parking area; a great park with large play structures for small children
EXPOSURE: Mostly shaded	**DOGS:** Allowed on-leash
TRAFFIC: Moderate–heavy	**CONTACT:** 425-823-2992; parks.state.wa .us/577/Saint-Edward
TRAIL SURFACE: Dirt	**LOCATION:** 14445 Juanita Dr. NE, Kenmore, WA 98028
HIKING TIME: 1.5–2.5 hours	
ACCESS: Hikable year-round, daily, 8 a.m.–sunset; Discover Pass required for parking	

The seminary was built in a Tuscan architectural style, complete with arches and a bell tower, giving the structure a distinctly European flair. The occasional cricket or soccer game on the grass only heightens the atmosphere, extending a general sense of peace that pervades the entire property. The serenity may reach its apex at the Grotto, an outdoor sanctuary and shrine in the southwest corner of the lawn. This same tranquility is evident throughout Saint Edward's trail network as well.

A counterclockwise loop around the park perimeter is provided by linking the North, Beach, South Ridge, and Water Tower Trails, designated almost entirely as hiking only. Although Saint Edward is popular with local mountain bikers, who call it Saint Eddy, they tend to stay in the northeast corner of the park near the main entrance and have limited access to Lake Washington and the bluffs, where most of this loop occurs.

Find the trailhead by heading north from the parking lot, past the park office, some storage sheds, and another small parking area. The park's office building also houses a gymnasium (one of many fine recreation facilities available at Saint Edward), in addition to a popular indoor pool and an engaging playground for young children. Park maps can prove helpful in finding the way and are usually available at a display board near the picnic area.

North Trail (identified as Perimeter Trail) begins by ducking into the trees and then bending to the left, following a ridge downhill. A narrow ravine to the right houses a small creek that tumbles toward the lake.

The descent steepens as you get closer to the water, employing some easy switchbacks to lessen the drop. The forest is a mix of typical Pacific Northwest lowland species, including Douglas firs, western hemlocks, and big-leaf maples, with a carpet of sword ferns and other ground cover underneath. Watch for tricky roots underfoot that can trip the unwary. Gaps in the canopy provide views of the water and the houses of Lake City on the opposite side, a little more than a mile away.

After dropping about 100 feet, the North Trail ends on the lakeshore at a junction with the Beach Trail. Turn left and head south along the bank, where several distinctive red-barked Pacific madrones hang out over the water. Boats frequently pass by in summer, along with float planes from the Kenmore Air Harbor, 2 miles north at the mouth of the Sammamish River.

A thick tangle of plants prohibits easy access to the water until you reach a beach-front clearing with a swimming area along some rocks, where kayakers and stand-up paddleboarders frequently stop to rest. The wide Seminary Trail enters the clearing from the left; this is the only beach access available to mountain bikers. For hikers seeking a shorter loop, it is possible to return to the main lawn by heading directly up the hill. Just past two lavatories, the Grotto Trail branches off the Seminary Trail to the right, providing another path to the top. At 0.4 mile long, the narrow Grotto Trail is closed to mountain bikes and may be a more rewarding hike than the Seminary Trail.

To resume the Perimeter Loop, continue on the Beach Trail. Bypass the first left to the South Canyon Trail and stay right to join the South Ridge Trail, which quickly climbs above the lake. This trail is surprisingly demanding, running through a series of short ups and downs while ascending a high crest between the South Canyon on the left and a shallower ravine to the right.

Emerge from the woods below a water tower overlooking Bastyr University, a leading center for study of the natural-health sciences. Bastyr is headquartered at the Saint Thomas Seminary, which was added to the Saint Edward Seminary in 1959 and purchased by Bastyr from the Seattle Archdiocese in 2005. The Water Tower Trail starts here, heading immediately left from the wooden gate at the end of the South Ridge Trail and running through the trees along the Bastyr parking lot and access road.

Plateau Trail enters from the right and is open to mountain bikers who may share the broad Water Tower Trail with you the rest of the way. Only about 0.25 mile remains until you exit the forest next to the playground and cross the grass to return to your vehicle.

GPS TRAILHEAD COORDINATES
N47° 43.99' W122° 15.327'

From I-405 N, take Exit 20A for NE 116th Street. Turn left onto 116th Street, which becomes NE Juanita Drive then turns north and changes its name to Juanita Drive NE. Go 5.3 miles, and watch for the park entrance on the left (west) side of Juanita Drive NE, which is also the entrance to Bastyr University. After entering the park, stay to the right and park in the main parking lot near the swimming-pool building and the seminary. From I-405 S, take Exit 20, and turn right onto NE 124th Street. In 1.0 mile turn left onto 100th Avenue NE, which becomes 98th Avenue NE. In 0.5 mile turn right onto NE Juanita Drive, and go 4.0 miles to the park entrance; follow the directions above from there.

15 Squak Mountain State Park:
DOUBLE PEAK LOOP

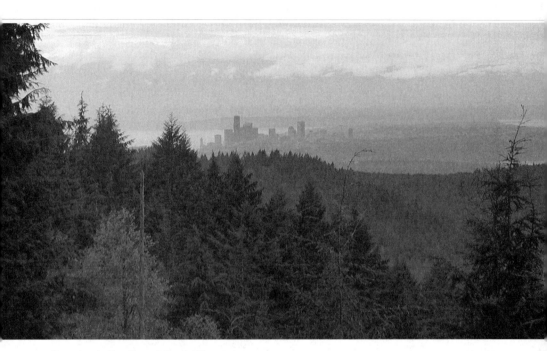

Seattle skyline from Squak Mountain

In Brief

The Double Peak Loop hike quickly escapes the lower section of Squak Mountain State Park (which is open to horses) to explore a dense forest and the historical ruins of the Bullitt family settlement, passing two good viewpoints that rival any in the Issaquah region along the way. Plus, you just might have the trail to yourself.

Description

Cougar and Tiger Mountains draw most of the attention in the Issaquah Alps, leaving central Squak Mountain relatively underused. Whether hikers stay away because of Squak's limited size, its reputation as an equestrian center, or for some other reason, their loss can be your gain.

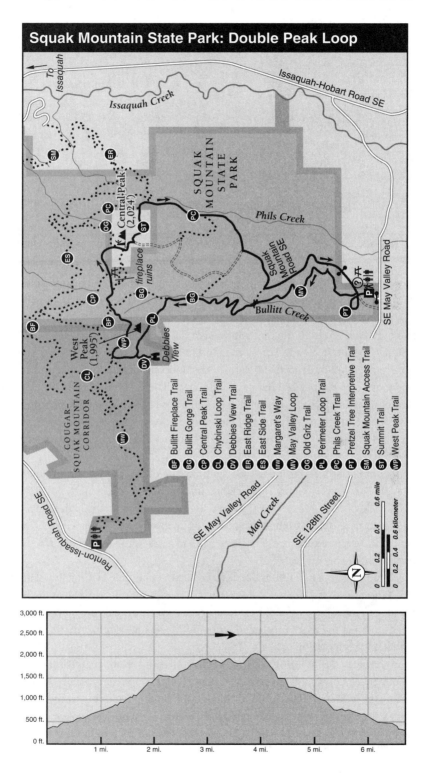

Squak Mountain State Park: Double Peak Loop

To Issaquah

Issaquah-Hobart Road SE

Issaquah Creek

SQUAK MOUNTAIN STATE PARK

Phils Creek

Central Peak (2,024')

fireplace ruins

Squak Mountain Road SE

Bullitt Creek

SE May Valley Road

West Peak (1,995')

Debbies View

COUGAR–SQUAK MOUNTAIN CORRIDOR

Renton-Issaquah Road SE

Renton-Issaquah Road SE

SE May Valley Road

May Creek

SE 128th Street

BF Bullitt Fireplace Trail
BG Bullitt Gorge Trail
CP Central Peak Trail
CL Chybinski Loop Trail
DV Debbies View Trail
ER East Ridge Trail
ES East Side Trail
MW Margaret's Way
MV May Valley Loop
OG Old Griz Trail
PL Perimeter Loop Trail
PC Phils Creek Trail
PT Pretzel Tree Interpretive Trail
SM Squak Mountain Access Trail
ST Summit Trail
WP West Peak Trail

0.6 mile
0.2   0.4   0.6 kilometer
0.2   0.4
0   0.4   0.6 kilometer
0

3,000 ft.
2,500 ft.
2,000 ft.
1,500 ft.
1,000 ft.
500 ft.
0 ft.
1 mi.   2 mi.   3 mi.   4 mi.   5 mi.   6 mi.

DISTANCE & CONFIGURATION: 6.7-mile loop	daily, 6:30 a.m.–sunset; winter: daily, 8 a.m.–sunset; Discover Pass required for parking
DIFFICULTY: Moderate	**WHEELCHAIR TRAVERSABLE:** No
SCENERY: Historical Bullitt family fire-place and homesite; views south toward Mount Rainier and northwest to the Seattle skyline	**MAP(S):** Green Trails *Cougar Mountain/ Squak Mountain 203S*; USGS *Bellevue South* and *Maple Valley*
EXPOSURE: Mostly shaded	**FACILITIES:** Toilet at trailhead; no drinking water
TRAFFIC: Low–medium	**DOGS:** Allowed on-leash
TRAIL SURFACE: Dirt	**CONTACT:** 425-455-7010; parks.state .wa.us/588/Squak-Mountain
HIKING TIME: 3–6 hours	
ACCESS: Hikable year-round, summer:	**LOCATION:** Issaquah

However, Squak Mountain's trail network is complex and can be confusing, so the best place to start this hike is at the kiosk on the eastern side of the parking lot, where free copies of a park map are available.

The trail itself starts on the opposite side of the parking lot and quickly reaches the gravel Squak Mountain Road. Across the road, a gate through a double split rail fence leads to Pretzel Tree Interpretive Trail, a short loop through a lush lowland forest of ferns and moss-covered big-leaf maples. Children will love this quick side trip, complete with interpretive displays that detail the story of a field mouse that learns about the forest and its wildlife denizens, including a crow and a beaver. They can also count the rings on several fallen logs and search for the unusual Pretzel Tree with two entwined trunks, for which the trail is named.

After completing Pretzel Tree Trail, continue uphill on the Squak Mountain Road for about 20 yards and look for a trail heading into the woods on the left, possibly signed as the May Valley Loop. Follow this trail for a long 0.25 mile or so through a carpet of triangular oak ferns until it reaches an unsigned junction with Bullitt Gorge Trail, also known as Mad Mountain Beaver Way. Turn left and head uphill on a soft surface of mud, both natural and horse-made.

If it is running, seasonal Bullitt Creek soon becomes audible in a shallow gully to the left, which the trail approaches and then crosses on a footbridge at 800 feet of elevation. Various side branches head off into the underbrush along the creek, and another leads out to the right to meet the road, creating the possibility of some confusion. Be sure to continue uphill on the main Bullitt Gorge Trail.

Climb another 0.5 mile through some giant stumps, many charred and peppered with woodpecker holes and resembling the old volcanic plugs typically found in the southern Cascade Mountains. Another junction marks the beginning of the hikers-only trail at 1,300 feet, which narrows and heads left, marked by a brown SQUAK MOUNTAIN STATE PARK NATURAL AREA sign. (Equestrians have to turn right on the wider trail, crossing Bullitt Creek.)

The primitive trail climbs steeply at first, then levels out to reach a T-junction at 1,500 feet—which is very easy to miss, so watch carefully. At the junction, the main trail continues to the right and a less-defined trail cuts to the left. Take this unsigned left turn onto Perimeter Loop Trail, which bends around the southern side of Squak Mountain on a gradual climb and then shifts back to the north.

The trail comes to its high point at about 1,750 feet and then starts to descend. At the crest, look for a path heading downhill to the left, signed as Debbies View, which leads 100 yards to a small clearing with an excellent overlook. The viewpoint provides a wide-ranging perspective over nearby neighborhoods and hills all the way to Mount Rainier. This is the best vista available anywhere on Squak's slopes, making the viewpoint a great place to stop and spend some time, especially since it faces south and gets plenty of sun.

Perimeter Loop Trail ends at a T-junction with Chybinski Loop Trail. However, the correct route to follow is on a sharp turn to the right at the same intersection, identified with a sign to West Peak and West Peak Trail. This indistinct trail, which climbs to the western summit at an elevation of just less than 2,000 feet, is steep and usually muddy.

The top of West Peak is in a grove of tall trees with no view to speak of. Just on the far side, a rapidly deteriorating cabin marks a now-abandoned communication installation. Look for the continuation of West Peak Trail (on the southeast corner of the structure), where it heads downhill through a pleasant forest of cedars and Douglas firs. The footing is soft and forgiving, thanks to a blanket of fallen needles and decaying wood.

Descend into a narrow saddle, then climb steeply back up the other side to reach a T-junction with a trail on the right. Take the fork to the left and arrive at yet another T-junction with the broad but unsigned Bullitt Fireplace Trail. Turn right and the trail narrows and climbs 150 feet to arrive at the stone chimney that marks the ruins of the original homestead that once stood here. A picnic table on the old concrete floor provides a good place to stop and rest.

The Bullitt family donated the original parcel of land that created the public park at Squak Mountain, one of the many ways the Bullitts have made their mark on the Puget Sound region over the years. The prominent clan includes Dorothy S. Bullitt, the founder of King Broadcasting; Stim Bullitt, a real estate developer whose Harbor Properties helped revitalize downtown Seattle; Harriet Bullitt, the founder of *Pacific Northwest* magazine; and Dorothy C. Bullitt, an attorney and author who helped write *Addicted to Danger,* the best-selling memoir of noted Seattle mountaineer and adventurer Jim Wickwire.

Continue east from the Bullitt fireplace and follow a short descent until the trail ends at an intersection. Take the signed Central Peak Trail uphill to the right for 0.25 mile, pass through a steel gate, and emerge at 2,024 feet, beneath the towers of the Squak Mountain Microwave Installation on the summit. An unexpected view of downtown Seattle is available through a narrow gap in the trees to the northwest, a line of sight that is the likely reason for the working radio facility.

Around the far side of the buildings, start downhill on the gravel Squak Mountain Road for a few hundred feet and turn left on the signed Summit Trail. Pass through a gate and begin a quick descent into the woods, which continue for 0.4 mile to a junction with

Phils Creek Trail. Turn right and reach another intersection with East Ridge Trail, only 0.1 mile farther along. Stay on Phils Creek Trail, once again, to the right.

The next section of trail apparently receives minimal use and may be overgrown and lined with stinging nettles, so hiking in long pants might be a good idea. Cross through a gate to return to the lower mountain, where horses are allowed, and continue downhill on Phils Creek Trail until it reaches Squak Mountain Road. Follow the road downhill back to the parking lot.

Nearby Activities

The Issaquah Depot Museum, one of two Issaquah historical museums, provides a good look into how the early fortunes of the town went hand in hand with the development of the railroad. To reach the museum, head east on SE May Valley Road and then turn left onto Issaquah-Hobart Road, which becomes Front Street in Issaquah. In the heart of downtown, turn right onto E. Sunset Way and then left onto First Avenue NE, and look for the museum next to the train tracks on the right at 78 First Avenue NE. The museum has limited hours, so check the website at issaquahhistory.org/museums/issaquah-depot or call 425-392-3500.

GPS TRAILHEAD COORDINATES

N47° 28.906' W122° 3.236'

From I-90, take Exit 15 and head south on WA 900 W, which begins as 17th Avenue NW then becomes Renton-Issaquah Road SE. After driving 4.2 miles, turn left onto SE May Valley Road. Continue another 2.5 miles to the Squak Mountain State Park parking area on the left just past the gated Squak Mountain Road.

16 Tiger Mountain:
CHIRICO TRAIL

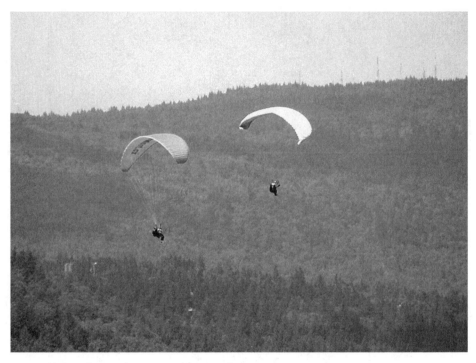

Paragliders descending toward Issaquah

In Brief

The Chirico Trail provides the shortest and easiest hike to two of the finest vistas anywhere in the Issaquah Alps, including spectacular Poo Poo Point. If the wind is right, you may share the trail with paragliders, who launch from the top and fill the sky with their colorful sails, an unforgettable sight.

Description

Although the Issaquah Alps look like a set of Cascade Mountain foothills, they are in fact part of a separate range, born long before their more famous counterparts were ever thrust up toward the sky. In contrast with the brash, young Cascades, which still show the sharp peaks and jagged spires of adolescence, the inexorable efforts of erosion have tamed and polished the geography of the Alps over the eons. Like the Appalachian

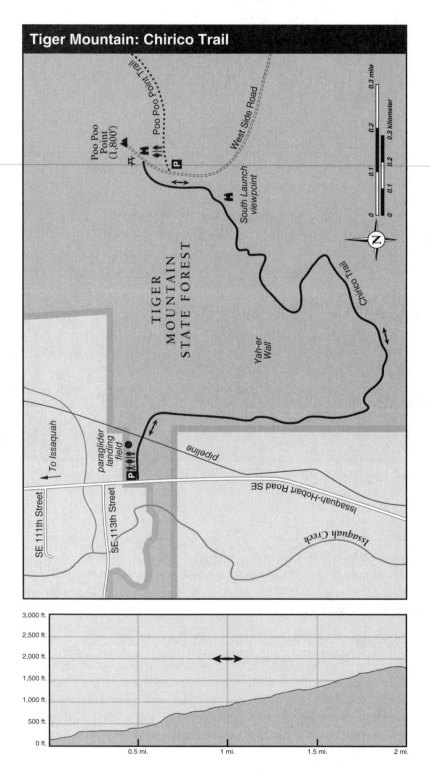

Tiger Mountain: Chirico Trail

DISTANCE & CONFIGURATION: 4.0-mile out-and-back	sunrise–sunset; Discover Pass required for parking
DIFFICULTY: Moderate	**WHEELCHAIR TRAVERSABLE:** No
SCENERY: Two separate viewpoints (one north, one south), possible paraglider watching	**MAP(S):** Green Trails *Tiger Mountain 204S*; USGS *Maple Valley*
EXPOSURE: Mostly shaded	**FACILITIES:** Toilet at trailhead; no drinking water
TRAFFIC: Crowded; get an early start	**DOGS:** Allowed on-leash
TRAIL SURFACE: Dirt	**CONTACT:** 360-825-1631; dnr.wa .gov/Tiger
HIKING TIME: 2–3 hours	
ACCESS: Hikable year-round, daily,	**LOCATION:** Issaquah

Mountains of the eastern United States, the Issaquah Alps show their advanced age with low summits and gentle grades.

Sprawling Tiger Mountain is no exception, with no dominant high point and a series of indistinct bumps spaced along a lengthy ridge passing for summits. At the extreme western end, however, an unusually steep drop-off at Poo Poo Point provides good views and a great place to launch a paraglider. Unfortunately, access to the area was difficult for many years, requiring either an endless drive on the gated West Side Road or the carrying of bulky equipment up one of the long approach trails from the north.

Chirico Trail changed all that, providing a back entrance to Poo Poo Point. The trail owes its existence to local paragliders who petitioned the Washington Department of Natural Resources to develop an access trail straight up from the valley to the west. Issaquah paragliding guide and instructor Marc Chirico spearheaded the effort, bringing together scores of contributors and volunteers to realize his vision; the trail was named in his honor.

The trailhead reveals the area's paragliding roots. The hike starts on the far side of a flat, grassy meadow, which is the traditional landing field, complete with a circular bull's-eye in the center for a target. A stream frequently referred to as Hang Glider Creek runs along the field's northern edge.

Climbing more than 1,500 feet in less than 2 miles, Chirico Trail is one of the steepest on Tiger Mountain. It begins by heading south, traversing the foot of the Yah-er Wall for the first 0.5 mile while gaining 500 feet. The trail is like a climber's use trail, with exposed roots and rocks, not surprising since its original intended users were paragliders seeking to reach the top as quickly as possible. The forest is pleasant, scenic, and damp, with heavy moss draping the trees and mud collecting underfoot. Stone stairs have been added in many places, making it easier when wet.

Near the 700-foot mark, the trail runs through a switchback and then turns right (east), escaping the sound of the traffic from the valley below. Soon after, the forest begins to thin, and occasional viewpoints open to the south through the scrubby trees as you continue to mount the ridge.

A grassy clearing just off to the right marks the beginning of the South Launch Viewpoint. Continue on the trail uphill to reach the top of the clearing, where the best views can be found. Watch out for a series of informal paths, mostly cutting switchbacks or heading out into the grass, skirting the edge of the trees.

The South Launch sits at about 1,600 feet and provides a great vista over the landscape to the south, from the community of Mirrormont all the way to Mount Rainier. The lack of trees makes the view panoramic and uninterrupted.

The trail heads back into the spongy forest on the eastern side, to the left of two doubletrack jeep roads. After another 0.25 mile you will emerge at Poo Poo Point, home to a second clearing that is the North Launch Viewpoint, elevation 1,800 feet. The view here is even more spectacular than it is on the other side, encompassing the eastern face of Squak Mountain, the Sammamish Plateau, downtown Bellevue, and even the top of the Space Needle through a saddle high on Cougar Mountain to the west. Look for a display board, which provides a helpful reference identifying the landmarks below.

When the wind is rising suitably out of the valley, typically in the afternoon, scores of paragliders use Poo Poo Point to soar into the sky. Many are able to rise far above the take-off site before eventually descending to the landing field at the bottom.

Unfortunately, the descent for most hikers will be much less exhilarating, requiring a hike back down the way you came. It is also possible to head down Poo Poo Point Trail, if you have prepared a shuttle at one of Tiger Mountain's busy northern trailheads.

Nearby Activities

Stan's Bar-B-Q at 58 Front St. N is a local favorite, showcasing Stan's signature Kansas City flavor. To get there, follow Issaquah-Hobart Road into downtown Issaquah until it becomes Front Street. Stan's is on the right, just past the Sunset Way intersection. For more information, visit stansbarbq.com or call 425-392-4551.

GPS TRAILHEAD COORDINATES
N47° 30.022' W122° 1.298'

From I-90, take Exit 17 and head south on Front Street in Issaquah. After passing through Issaquah, Front Street curves and becomes Issaquah-Hobart Road. In 3.0 miles from the interstate, the parking lot is on the left (east) side of Issaquah-Hobart Road, just past SE 111th Street. The trailhead is on the far side of the grassy paraglider-landing field.

17 Tiger Mountain:
POO POO POINT TRAIL

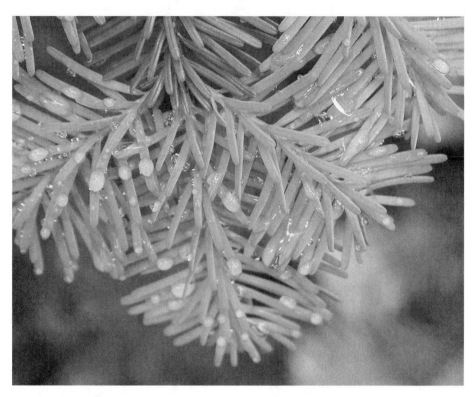

Water on needles

In Brief

Poo Poo Point is much nicer than it sounds. Perched on the western end of Tiger Mountain, it provides one of the best views anywhere in the Issaquah Alps, even though it is more than 1,000 feet below the true summit. Poo Poo Point Trail climbs to the viewpoint through some of the best forest anywhere on West Tiger Mountain and avoids some of the crowds that congregate on the mountain's northern side.

Description

Tiger Mountain's best feature might also be its worst: More trails mean more options, but confusing routes and the occasional lost hiker frequently come along with them—the

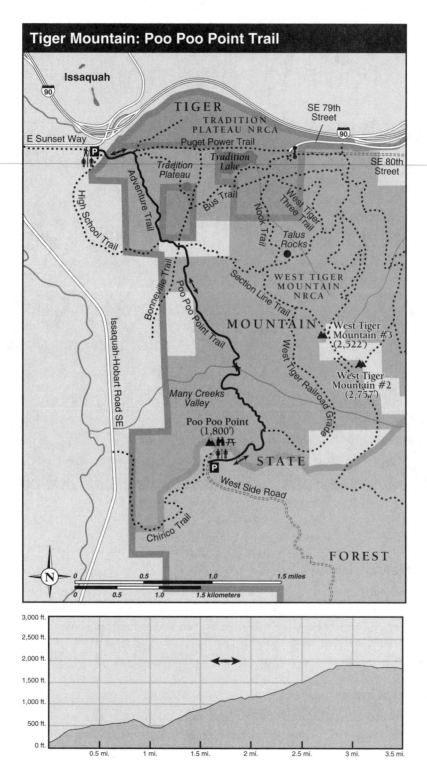

Tiger Mountain: Poo Poo Point Trail

DISTANCE & CONFIGURATION: 7.0-mile out-and-back	sunrise–sunset; Discover Pass required for parking
DIFFICULTY: Difficult	**WHEELCHAIR TRAVERSABLE:** No
SCENERY: Summit views, possible paraglider watching	**MAP(S):** Green Trails *Tiger Mountain 204S*; USGS *Bellevue South*
EXPOSURE: Mostly shaded	**FACILITIES:** Toilet at trailhead; no drinking water
TRAFFIC: Medium	**DOGS:** Allowed on-leash
TRAIL SURFACE: Dirt and gravel trails	**CONTACT:** 360-825-1631; dnr.wa .gov/Tiger
HIKING TIME: 4–6 hours	
ACCESS: Hikable year-round, daily,	**LOCATION:** Issaquah

downside to the maze of good trails available on Tiger's slopes. Hiking anywhere in the area generally requires careful consultation of the directions and the map, and Poo Poo Point Trail is no exception. However, that rarely dissuades the crowds who enjoy the easy drive from Seattle, less than 30 miles away on I-90.

Starting the hike to Poo Poo Point from the Sunset Way trailhead avoids a lot of the people who flock to the better-developed High Point Trailhead a few miles to the east. Although the early section of the hike can be confusing, lighter traffic makes it worthwhile—and this approach is no harder to follow than any of the others, some of which require navigating through the center of the complicated Tradition Plateau.

The trail starts steeply up the hillside from the east end of the parking lot, presenting one of the most demanding sections of the entire hike in the first 0.25 mile. Follow the dirt path up the slope and turn left at an unsigned four-way junction, where the trail first meets a set of power lines, running in from the right. After the turn, you will be directly above the eastbound lanes of I-90, visible through the trees.

Take the next right at another unsigned junction, climbing some steps and then following a ridgeline as it heads uphill to the east. The trail emerges under the power lines again at the top of the hill, some 300 feet above the trailhead where you started.

From here, the route is easier to find, heading left directly under the power lines on a gravel road. Known as Puget Power Line Trail, the road leads through a dense field of Scotch broom. The bright, eye-catching yellow flowers of this plant, common in the Pacific Northwest, belie its status as an invasive weed species native to Europe and Africa and originally imported as an ornamental. Puget Power Line Trail links many of the most popular routes on Tiger Mountain, so you are likely to see other hikers.

The 0.4 mile to the next junction is flat and easy. Head through a wooden split rail gate on the right, signed for Wetlands Trail and Adventure Trail. Almost immediately, the trail forks underneath the power lines; stay right, following a sign to the Adventure Trail. The brush soon gives way to trees at the edge of the forest.

Adventure Trail is a dirt singletrack, negotiating a number of quick ups and downs and short turns through cedar forest while gradually climbing to a high point at around

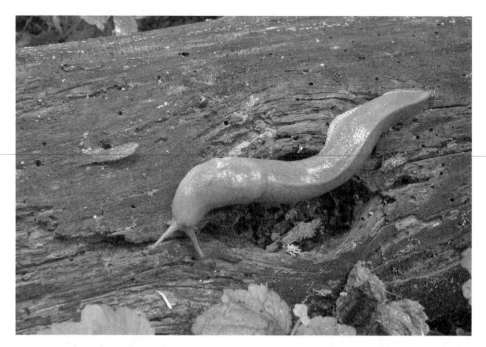

Banana slug along the trail

650 feet. It descends again on the far side to reach a T-junction at a wooden gate with the unmarked High School Trail, which has a wide, gravel surface.

Pass through the gate and turn left, starting a very gradual ascent through some stately birches. After crossing a creek, emerge from the trees to reach another set of power lines and Bonneville Trail. You have now traveled about 1.5 miles total from the trailhead and about 0.2 mile from the end of the Adventure Trail.

Stay left and head uphill under the power lines on the gravel Bonneville Trail for only about 20 yards. Watch carefully on the right for a sign to Section Line Trail and Poo Poo Point Trail, just before you reach the first metal tower.

Follow the worn trail as it crosses under the power lines and through a row of trees to reach a second clearing, where a gas pipeline runs underground. Stay right at a signed fork for Poo Poo Point Trail.

Starting at about 550 feet, this trail does most of the heavy lifting on the hike, reaching almost 2,000 feet at its highest point. Thankfully, the next junction is 2.8 miles farther up the mountain, leaving hikers free to stop worrying about navigation and to enjoy the beauty of the natural surroundings. Even though Poo Poo Point Trail is open to equestrians, both horse and human visitors tend to be much rarer here than farther down.

The trail climbs steadily over the next mile into the Many Creeks Valley. The valley is blessed with some of the nicest forest anywhere on Tiger Mountain, including some particularly large cedars that have successfully managed to avoid the ax and the saw over the years. When sunlight filters through the canopy, the woods here can feel like deep wilderness far from civilization.

Cross three separate creeks (for whom the valley is no doubt named), going over the last at around 1,200 feet of elevation on a substantial wooden footbridge with handrails. After the bridge, the trail steepens through a series of switchbacks. Mature trees tower overhead, with many decaying logs hosting thick ferns and moss underneath.

The climb abruptly levels off at a final junction, where West Tiger Railroad Grade Trail and One View Trail intersect Poo Poo Point Trail. Take a hard right, signed as Poo Poo Point Trail.

The trail has a net elevation loss over the last 0.5 mile, dropping from its high point, with an altitude of more than 1,900 feet at the junction, to about 1,800 at Poo Poo Point, but there are several short climbs and drops as the route curls around the northern side of the mountain on a flat, wide surface. The trail finally emerges at a gravel parking lot with a toilet, the end of the West Side Road.

The overlook is just up the short rise to the right, rewarding the long approach with a spectacular view to the northwest, rivaled by only a handful of others anywhere in the Issaquah Alps. Be sure to allow plenty of time to enjoy the setting and possibly observe the colorful paragliders who frequently use Poo Poo Point as a launch site in the afternoon, when rising thermals are at their best. A picnic table above the parking lot makes a great place to relax and refuel before heading back down.

The directions should be easier on the descent, although it is still necessary to pay attention to the many turns. It is also possible to head down Chirico Trail to the west, if you have left a shuttle vehicle at the second trailhead along the Issaquah-Hobart Road.

Nearby Activities

For a good northwestern microbrewed beer, head to the Issaquah Brewhouse at 35 W. Sunset Way. Follow Sunset Way west from the trailhead into downtown Issaquah to find the brewery on the left-hand side, just past the Front Street intersection. The brewhouse serves mostly handcrafted Rogue Ales, including unusual treats like chocolate stout, which can even be used to make hearty ice cream floats. For more information, check the brewery's website at rogue.com or call 425-557-1911.

GPS TRAILHEAD COORDINATES
N47° 31.796' W122° 1.519'

From I-90, take Exit 18 and head south on E. Sunset Way. The gravel parking lot is located on the left side of Sunset Way in 0.9 mile.

18 Tiger Mountain:
WEST TIGER THREE LOOP

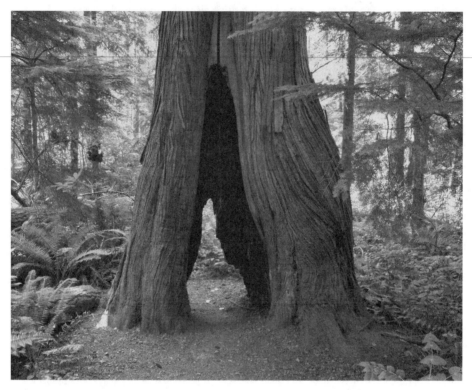

Tree on Around the Lake Trail

In Brief

Although Number Three is the lowest of West Tiger Mountain's triple summits, the view from the top is as good as from any of them. This fun loop takes a direct line to the popular peak, then descends a secluded route through the mountain's lush forests to explore some interesting natural features at Talus Rocks and Tradition Lake.

Description

With more than 80 miles of trails spread over 13,500 acres of land, Tiger Mountain attracts outdoor enthusiasts of all kinds. It is also large and complicated enough that it is possible for visitors to get lost, so it's a good idea to bring a map.

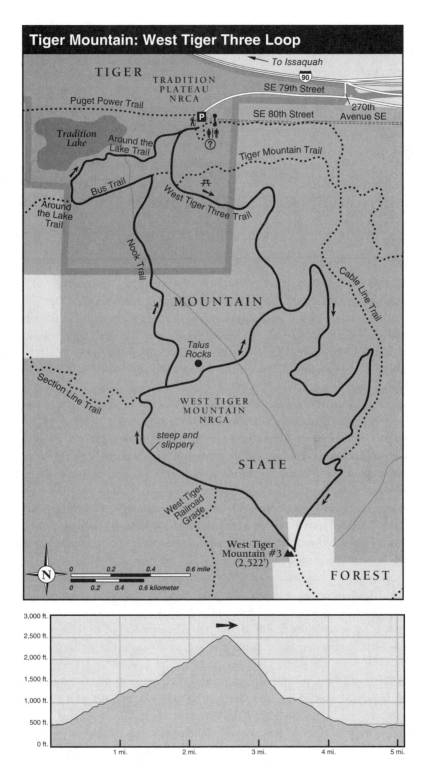

DISTANCE & CONFIGURATION: 5.1-mile loop	**ACCESS:** Hikable year-round, daily, sunrise–sunset; Discover Pass required for parking
DIFFICULTY: Moderate–difficult	
SCENERY: Tradition Lake, summit views, huge boulders and caves at the Talus Rocks area, a section of limited-use trail on popular Tiger Mountain	**WHEELCHAIR TRAVERSABLE:** No
	MAP(S): Green Trails *Tiger Mountain 204S*; USGS *Fall City*
EXPOSURE: Mostly shaded	**FACILITIES:** Toilet at trailhead; no drinking water
TRAFFIC: High on the way up, moderate on the way down	**DOGS:** Allowed on-leash
TRAIL SURFACE: Mostly dirt, a few sections of gravel	**CONTACT:** 360-825-1631; dnr.wa.gov /Tiger
HIKING TIME: 3–4 hours	**LOCATION:** Issaquah

While mountain bikers are mostly restricted to the trails and logging roads in the working forest of East Tiger, hikers tend to stay in the 4,500-acre Natural Resources Conservation Area on West Tiger. Most come to the busy High Point Trailhead, bringing families, dogs, and anyone else they can find along with them. High Point provides access to a multitude of trails laid out on the nearby Tradition Plateau, where the linking of countless small segments allows for the creation of many easy loops. The climbs to any of West Tiger's numbered peaks attract plenty of traffic as well, especially to West Tiger Three, the closest summit to the trailhead. However, it is possible to escape some of the crowds on this hike with an alternate route on the descent.

The start of the hike can be confusing, with a small maze of trails running between an educational shelter, a picnic area, a latrine, and an informational kiosk on the southern side of the parking lot. The true trailhead can be found by following various signs to the trails below the power lines at the western end.

At a four-way intersection, head south through a wooden split rail fence, signed as West Tiger Three Trail, and start hiking on a gravel surface lined with wooden planks. Moments later, head off the gravel to the left and pass through another gate to follow a muddy dirt track wide enough to be a reclaimed road, also signed for West Tiger Three Trail.

Stay straight at an intersection with Tiger Mountain Trail (TMT) to continue on West Tiger Three Trail, which soon begins to climb in earnest. The footing becomes rougher, with many rounded stones set in the ground.

About 0.8 mile from the trailhead, the trail crosses a creek and intersects with the Connector Trail, branching to the right. Stay left, continuing to climb through a bright-green forest of ferns and moss. The forest is perpetually damp here, keeping the track muddy at all times. Even though the Issaquah Alps do not scrape as much rain from the clouds as the higher Cascades farther east, the western side of Tiger gets plenty of year-round precipitation, which falls almost exclusively as rain at this elevation.

Head sharply to the right just above 1,300 feet to mount a short ridge. West Tiger Cable Line Trail comes up the steep slope from the left and runs with the main trail for a short distance before exiting again on the right. Cable Line Trail runs straight up to the summit, forgoing switchbacks and crossing West Tiger Three Trail many times. It is possible to follow the unmaintained Cable Line, although it is considerably rougher and steeper than the main trail.

In the next mile, the trail swings through a series of switchbacks and enters a glade of tall evergreens. Tiger Mountain was once extensively logged for its western red cedars, so few remain on the lower-elevation slopes. Although this section has also been harvested in the past, it nonetheless gives a better idea of what the mountain's original forests once looked like. Enjoy the easier grade through the trees, the last significant break before the ascent resumes on the far side of the flats.

Cross a junction with West Tiger Railroad Grade Trail and continue uphill, following a sign to West Tiger Three. After several more intersections with the Cable Line, the trail emerges from the trees on an open ridge with views out to the northeast, including I-90, Mount Si, and the nearby radio towers of West Tiger Two.

The summit lies just beyond at 2,522 feet, a clearing with a broad view over Tiger Mountain State Forest. To the south, Mount Rainier rises above the trees on the West Tiger Two ridgeline, and Squak and Cougar Mountains can be seen in front of downtown Seattle and the Olympic Mountains to the west. For the ambitious, a trail continues from the far side of the clearing to climb the forested ridge to the other two West Tiger summits, each a few hundred feet higher.

To start the descent, head downhill on the unsigned Cable Line Trail, the widest route leaving the summit to the north, just west of West Tiger Three Trail. After only about 50 yards on the rocky surface, the singletrack Section Line Trail drops off to the left. The start of the trail is neither signed nor obvious, so be sure to look carefully. If there is snow on the ground, the trail can be particularly hard to find and follow at the top, so a better option may be to descend the way you came until you reach the junction with West Tiger Railroad Grade, then head west (a left turn when traveling downhill) 0.5 mile until you reach the signed junction with Section Line Trail.

The path drops steeply on a narrow, tricky, and slippery surface of roots, mud, and fallen needles, but the quiet of the forest more than makes up for it. Although the Section Line Trail is unmaintained, there is minimal undergrowth in the area, making the route easy to travel. The sounds of birds singing are the rule here, rather than the loud voices and dog barking typical at the summit.

After a drop of about 500 feet in 0.4 mile, reach a junction with the wide West Tiger Railroad Grade Trail, which provides another way to reach this point (as described above). Continue straight down the hill, signed as Section Line Trail, losing another 800 feet in a steep drop over the next 0.5 mile.

Take a sharp turn to the right on a trail signed for Talus Rocks Trail and Nook Trail, leaving Section Line Trail. This connector runs only about 0.1 mile before meeting Nook Trail.

A quick side trip to the right, signed as Talus Rocks Loop Trail, is well worth the minimal effort required. The loop's name does little to illuminate its destination; *talus* typically refers to a pile of small, loose rocks at the base of a cliff or steep slope, but this trail actually runs through a series of giant glacial erratic boulders. The rocks are covered in ferns and moss, with some shallow caves, alcoves, and overhangs underneath, all suitable for exploration. The trail itself travels an inventive route, climbing over some of the boulders and squeezing through small gaps between others.

Return to the previous junction and head downhill on the signed Nook Trail, which follows a gradual descent about 0.8 mile before ending at a T-junction with Bus Trail. Head left on the wide, gravel Bus Trail, likely joining other hikers there.

A flat 0.25 mile leads to the trail's namesake, an old, rusted-out bus frame lying on its side in the woods to the right and looking like a forgotten war-zone relic. Just past the bus, continue on the gravel trail (signed as Connector Trail) as it bends around to the right. After another 500 feet, turn right, on the signed Around the Lake Trail.

The waters of Tradition Lake are visible through the trees, although it is difficult to actually reach the shore. Access used to be easier, but it was restricted in the early 1990s to protect nesting birds in the wetlands from being disturbed by frequent human traffic. Around the Lake Trail is dead flat and circles around the lake heading east about 0.5 mile before returning you to the High Point Trailhead, where you began.

Nearby Activities

The Gilman Town Hall Museum provides a good look into pioneer life in Issaquah, dating back to when the settlement was known as Gilman. The restored building looks as if it was lifted straight off a Western movie set, and the original concrete jailhouse out back is complete with iron bars on the windows. To reach the museum, head west on I-90 to Exit 18 and follow E. Sunset Way into Issaquah. The museum is at 165 SE Andrews St., one block south of Sunset Way, between First and Second Avenues. For more information, contact the Issaquah Historical Society on the Web at issaquahhistory.org or call 425-392-3500.

GPS TRAILHEAD COORDINATES
N47° 31.767' W121° 59.676'

From I-90, take Exit 20 for High Point, and head south on 270th Avenue SE. Immediately turn right onto SE 79th Street and continue past the end of the paved road through a gate (closes at sunset). The West Tiger Mountain High Point Way trailhead parking area is on the left about 0.9 mile from the interstate.

19 Tolt River– John MacDonald Park

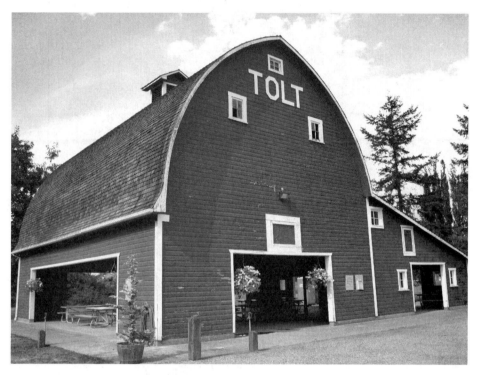

Tolt Barn covered picnic area

In Brief

An unheralded King County property in the Snoqualmie Valley, Tolt River–John Mac-Donald Park has good river access in a scenic setting. Hikers can climb to a high view-point or explore along the river on two moderate and pleasant trails.

Description

John MacDonald, the visionary behind the King County park that now bears his name, organized the development of recreational facilities at the confluence of the Tolt and Sno-qualmie Rivers in 1976 as a bicentennial project. MacDonald was the chief of the Seattle Council of Boy Scouts at the time and hoped to build campsites in the spirit of another Boy Scout facility—West Seattle's Camp Long. The fruits of his efforts are still being enjoyed

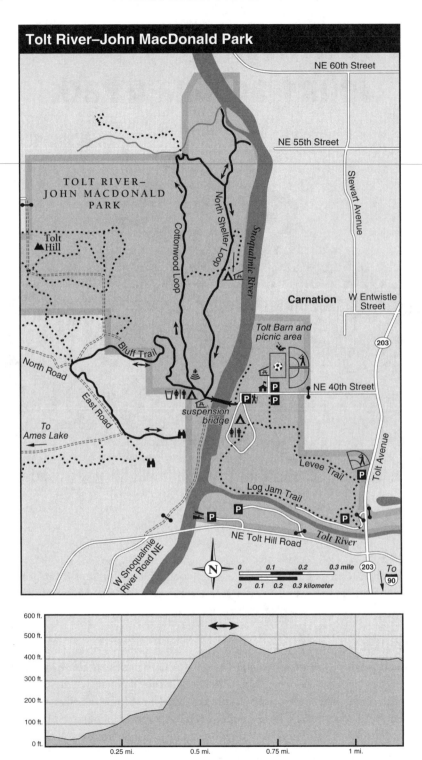

Tolt River–John MacDonald Park

DISTANCE & CONFIGURATION: 2.3-mile out-and-back on Bluff Trail; 2.0-mile North Shelter Trail and Cottonwood Loop	**HIKING TIME:** 2–4 hours
	ACCESS: Hikable year-round, May–Labor Day: daily, sunrise–10 p.m.; Labor Day– April: daily, sunrise–sunset; no fee for parking or trail access
DIFFICULTY: Easy on North Shelter Trail and Cottonwood Loop, moderate on Bluff Trail	
	WHEELCHAIR TRAVERSABLE: Yes, on suspension bridge and Levee Trail
SCENERY: High bluff viewpoint over the Snoqualmie River Valley, quiet stretch of beach along the Snoqualmie riverbank	**MAP(S):** USGS *Carnation*
	FACILITIES: Toilets, campground, cab- ins, picnic areas, and water at trailhead
EXPOSURE: Mostly shaded	**DOGS:** Allowed on-leash
TRAFFIC: Medium (note that bikes may be seen on the trails)	**CONTACT:** 206-477-6149; tinyurl.com /toltmcd
TRAIL SURFACE: Mixture of dirt and gravel	**LOCATION:** 31020 NE 40th St., Carnation, WA 98014

today, as the park provides a number of good camping spots. Other pieces of inspired devel-opment include a restored picturesque red barn that now serves as a picnic shelter and an elegant suspension footbridge that links the park's eastern and western sides.

Naturally, the park is popular with campers. But mountain bikers also like to ride a network of trails on the high bluff to the west, where it is possible to connect with trails originating at Ames Lake, about a mile away. And hikers can follow a good loop through the forest and along the river, or join the bikers on the bluff with an out-and-back trail to an impressive viewpoint.

For the loop hike, start across the suspension footbridge over the Snoqualmie River. Anglers frequently fish the waters directly below from either shore, and swimmers collect on the beach just upstream to the left, where a sandy, alluvial bank at the Tolt confluence provides good access to the shallow and easy rapids. Once across to the western side of the river, head up a gentle slope through a grass park with yurts and other camping struc-tures and stay to the right. Look for a singletrack heading into the trees, the start of a clockwise hike on the Cottonwood Loop Trail.

The trail climbs for a short distance and then contours around to the north through a forest of alders, maples, cottonwoods, ferns, and a lot of stinging nettles. Neither the river nor any of the development around the city of Carnation can be seen, providing a wel-come sense of remoteness. This stretch of trail might be the least used anywhere in the park; campers tend to stick to North Shelter Trail along the riverbank, and most moun-tain bikers prefer to stay on the bluff far above to the left. The relative seclusion here makes this a good place to spot the deer that frequent the area.

Continue 0.75 mile through the trees and then descend some switchbacks to reach a junction where a poorly defined trail leads across a creek to the left, marked with a wooden post. Stay to the right, still heading downhill, and come to an abandoned dirt

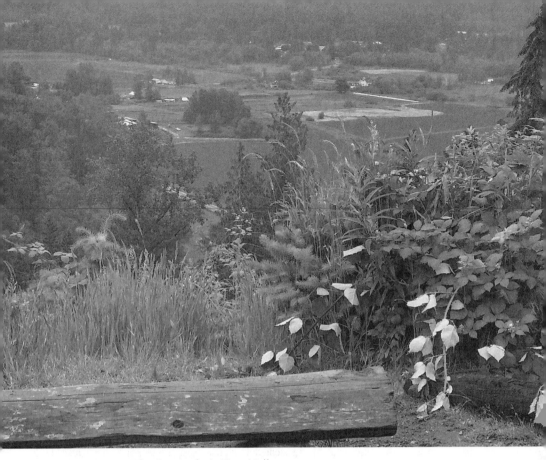

Viewpoint over the Snoqualmie River Valley

road. If you are attempting this loop in the opposite direction, this junction can be tricky to find because it is unsigned and difficult to spot.

Turn left on the road, which soon fades to a true trail, and approach the edge of the Snoqualmie River to reach a fork. Both paths are worth exploring—the overgrown left branch runs along the bank until it dead-ends in a clearing with a PRIVATE PROPERTY sign stuck to a fence at the northern end of the park boundary; the right fork leads out onto a sandy and pebbly beach on the water's edge, one of the best places to enjoy the river, although a bend to the south keeps most of the park out of sight. A gravel island is exposed just downstream at low water, when it is also possible to make your way along the bank in either direction.

Return to the trail, heading back the way you came. Follow the road southward, parallel to the river, to reach a grassy clearing, site of the North Shelter Campground. There is room for multiple tents here, centered on the shelter structure itself, and the spot makes a great place to spend a night or two in the woods. From the campground, the road follows the river back upstream to the suspension footbridge where you began. Along the way, multiple short out-and-back footpaths lead to the sandy riverbank on the left, providing access to the water. The total distance around the loop is about 2 miles.

The hike to the viewpoint on the bluff also starts from the western side of the suspension footbridge. Follow the gravel surface from the end of the bridge up the hill, to the left of the previously described loop. The wide trail bends to the right past some wooden camping shelters and narrows considerably, changing to dirt. For the next 0.5 mile, climb steeply through several turns up the side of the ridge. This is the only access to the upper part of the park, so expect to share the route with mountain bikers going in either direction.

A yellow sign on the left marks a transition to private property. Thanks to a generous easement from Port Blakely Tree Farms, the area beyond is open to public access for recreational use.

At the top of the bluff, known as Tolt Hill, a mess of poorly marked jeep roads and informal trails winds through the trees. Although the area covers only a few hundred acres, it is easy to lose your way in the complicated maze of options. Luckily, the viewpoint is easy to find.

Crest the ridge of the bluff, and you'll reach a major, five-way intersection of roads and trails. Although not indicated on any sign, the road you have been following is North Road; the one you want to take is East Road, around a sharp turn to the left. After about 100 yards uphill on East Road, watch carefully for a junction with a singletrack on the left side. If you prefer to hike on a trail, turn left and follow this narrow trail, which meanders through the forest and parallels the road; otherwise, continue uphill on the road. The trail eventually rejoins the East Road, where you'll turn left. Continue to the next road intersection and turn left on a spur road, which dead-ends at an overlook.

This high overlook stands 300 feet straight above the river. Sweeping vistas are available to the east and southeast, from the farms and development around Carnation to the Cascade Mountains' front range and the distinctive rocky western face of Mount Si, about 15 miles away.

Return the way you came, a round-trip of about 2.3 miles. To extend your hike another 2 miles, there is an additional loop available on the east side of the suspension bridge near the main campground. This loop follows the banks of the Snoqualmie and Tolt Rivers on the Log Jam Trail before returning across the meadows on the paved Levee Trail. When the river level is high, the Log Jam Trail might be under water.

GPS TRAILHEAD COORDINATES
N47° 38.650' W121° 55.455'

From I-90, take Exit 22 (Preston-Fall City), and head east on SE 82nd St. In 0.1 mile at the T-intersection, turn right onto Preston–Fall City Road SE and proceed on this winding road toward Fall City for 4.5 miles. At the edge of Fall City, stay right and cross over the Snoqualmie River on WA 202/SE Fall City–Snoqualmie Road. Immediately on the far side of the river, enter a roundabout and exit northbound onto WA 203/Fall City–Carnation Road SE. Continue 5.7 miles on this road to Carnation and turn left on NE 40th Street. Drive 0.4 mile straight down 40th to the parking lot and trailhead.

I-90 AND THE SNOQUALMIE PASS AREA

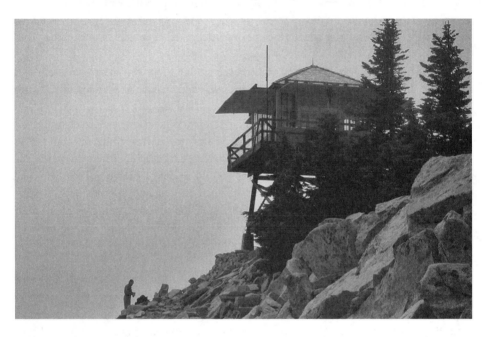

Granite Mountain Lookout

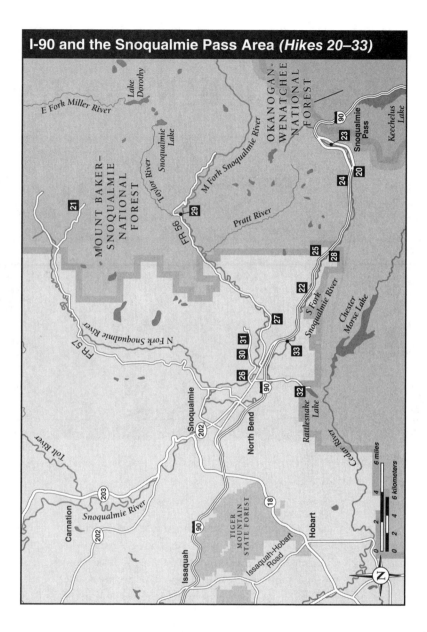

I-90 and the Snoqualmie Pass Area *(Hikes 20–33)*

20 Annette Lake and Asahel Curtis Nature Trail

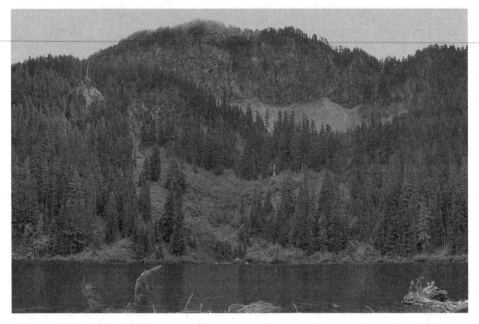

Annette Lake and Abiel Peak

In Brief

Annette, the only significant lake on the southern side of the Snoqualmie Valley, is an easier destination than many similar lakes in the well-known Alpine Lakes Wilderness to the north. Filling a subalpine bowl beneath several 5,000-foot peaks, Annette is accessed via a pleasant trail through some old-growth forest. The nearby Asahel Curtis Nature Trail and a wilderness scramble up Silver Peak expand the available hiking options.

Description

The Annette Lake Trailhead shares a parking lot with Asahel Curtis Nature Trail, worth exploring as a quick side trip or even a short and easy destination by itself. The nature trail forms a loop of 0.75 mile through some of the best old-growth forest anywhere around Snoqualmie Pass, in a representative forest typical of western Washington and Oregon. The trail stays above some swampy ground on a boardwalk while interpretive signs help identify various features of the ecosystem, from root wad to canopy and

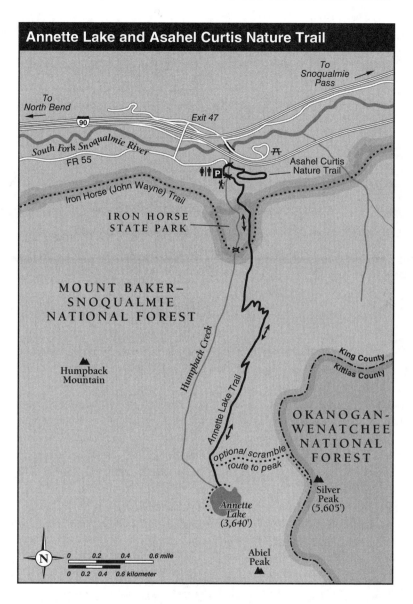

Annette Lake and Asahel Curtis Nature Trail

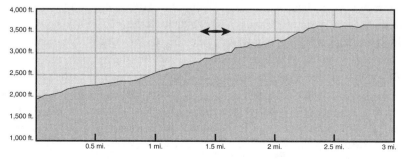

DISTANCE & CONFIGURATION:
6.0-mile out-and-back to Annette Lake;
0.75-mile loop for Asahel Curtis
Nature Trail

DIFFICULTY: Easy on nature trail, moderate to Annette Lake, difficult scramble
to Silver Peak

SCENERY: Scenic Annette Lake, old-
growth forest, educational nature-trail
loop, an optional bushwhack-and-boulder
route to Silver Peak for experienced
scramblers

EXPOSURE: Shaded

TRAFFIC: High

TRAIL SURFACE: Dirt with rocks and
roots to lake, dirt and boardwalk on
nature trail

HIKING TIME: 4–6 hours for Annette
Lake; add 30–45 minutes for the Nature
Trail, and 3–4 hours for Silver Peak

ACCESS: Hikable late spring–fall,
depending on snowpack; NW Forest Pass
required for parking

WHEELCHAIR TRAVERSABLE: No

MAP(S): Green Trails *Snoqualmie Pass
207*; USGS *Lost Lake* and *Snoqualmie Pass*

FACILITIES: Toilet at trailhead; no
drinking water

DOGS: Allowed off-leash

CONTACT: 425-888-1421; www.fs.usda
.gov/recarea/mbs/recreation
/recarea/?recid=17966

LOCATION: North Bend

everything in between. The most impressive trees here are western hemlock, Douglas fir, and western red cedar; other species, such as Pacific silver fir, noble fir, and western white pine, are present as well.

Asahel Curtis, for whom the nature trail is named, was a founding member of The Mountaineers and an accomplished climber who served as chief guide at Mount Rainier National Park in 1917. His achievements include summiting Rainier many times and completing the first documented ascent of Mount Shuksan in 1906 with W. Montelius Price. But Curtis is probably best known for his photographs documenting the natural landscape of the Pacific Northwest, including the early years of Mount Rainier National Park just as it was first reached by road. His work was often overshadowed, however, by that of his more famous brother Edward, who ran a photography studio out of Seattle and whose controversial images of the fading cultures of American Indians are now preserved in the Library of Congress as one of the most important historical records of the era. Edward Curtis's portrait of Chief Joseph of the Nez Percé is now famous, and the renowned photographer once filmed the snake dance of the Arizona Hopi in a rare, early motion picture.

Annette Lake Trail leaves the parking lot to head nearly due south, climbing steadily from a starting elevation of 1,900 feet. Enter a dense forest of alders and cross Humpback Creek on a bridge, with a pretty waterfall flowing down through some boulders on the right. The trail remains on the eastern side of the creek for the rest of its run up the valley.

Reach an old, unmaintained forest road within 0.5 mile, cross to the right, and follow a sign for Annette Lake. Soon thereafter, pass underneath some power lines in a clearing and then emerge on the gravel Iron Horse State Park rail-trail near 2,400 feet. Look for another sign to Annette Lake Trail about 20 yards to the right and reenter the trees; you'll be heading uphill.

Some of the old-growth starts to become apparent after another 0.25 mile. Although this patch of forest is less impressive than the area showcased along Asahel Curtis Nature Trail, there are still plenty of significantly large and ancient trees. An inventively designed section of the trail actually runs along the top of a giant downed log, complete with flat steps laboriously carved and leveled out of the rounded surface.

Running through a mix of switchbacks and flatter sections, the trail climbs steadily while angling up the valley's eastern wall. Near 3,500 feet, you'll cross some steep brush fields with open views to the right. Humpback Creek runs far below, and the rocky, exposed Humpback Peak is visible above at 5,174 feet. With another 100 feet of climbing, the trail reaches a high point, crosses some talus slopes, then begins a gradual descent with a few muddy ups and downs to enter the bowl that holds the lake, which is less than another 0.5 mile away.

Annette Lake, sitting at 3,640 feet, is surrounded by trees on all sides and bounded by Silver Peak (5,605') to the east, the long ridge of Humpback Peak to the west, and the high basalt walls of Abiel Peak (5,365') to the south. A small seasonal waterfall pours into the lake on the far eastern shore, collecting runoff from the western slopes of Silver. On the near side, the lake outflow empties into the Humpback Creek Valley. This is not the source of the creek itself, which originates in a drainage gap 0.25 mile away. Expect to share the tranquil and picturesque lake with other users, and possibly even fly-fishermen who cast their lines out of boats and others in float tubes on the water.

Some campsites are available; check signs at the lake and at the trailhead for more information. It is possible to continue farther around the lake by bushwhacking along the water's edge, but the thick brush and steep walls soon make this endeavor prohibitively difficult, and there are certainly no good campsites to be found there.

Dedicated scramblers will invariably be drawn to the upper slopes of Silver Peak, which is usually climbed from Pacific Crest Trail on the mountain's opposite side but can also be reached from here. Backtrack slightly along the trail from the lake and then pick a way uphill through the woods due east, aiming for the nearest visible clearing. With a little effort, you can reach the start of the long boulder field that climbs to the northern ridge and then the summit. Should you choose this adventurous side trip, you'll be rewarded with commanding views of the Snoqualmie Pass region.

GPS TRAILHEAD COORDINATES
N47° 23.572' W121° 28.48'

From I-90, take Exit 47 for Denny Creek–Asahel Curtis, and head south. At the T-intersection in 0.1 mile, turn left onto Forest Route 55/Asahel Curtis Road and drive 0.3 mile to the parking lot entrance on the right.

21 Bare Mountain

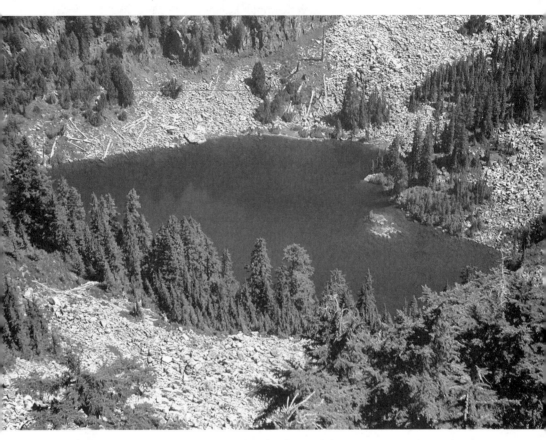

One of the Paradise Lakes on the north side of Bare Mountain

In Brief

Covering more than 400,000 acres between Snoqualmie Pass and Stevens Pass, the Alpine Lakes Wilderness attracts some 150,000 visitors each year. On a typical summer weekend when the hordes are camped at the Enchantment Lakes, Bare Mountain presents a great alternate escape. Tucked into a little-used corner of the wilderness area, this former fire-lookout site provides great high Cascade views, including three glaciated volcanoes.

Description

According to the U.S. Forest Service, more than half the population of Washington State lives within an hour's drive of the Alpine Lakes Wilderness. With its proximity to several

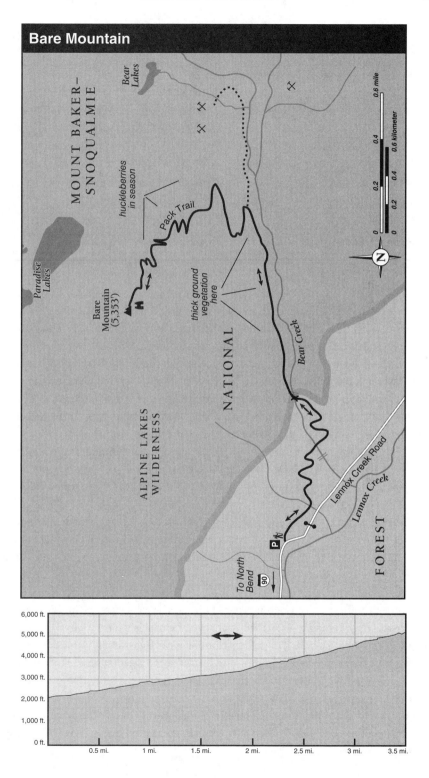

Bare Mountain

MOUNT BAKER–SNOQUALMIE

Bear Lakes

huckleberries in season

Pack Trail

Paradise Lakes

Bare Mountain (5,353')

thick ground vegetation here

NATIONAL

ALPINE LAKES WILDERNESS

Bear Creek

Lennox Creek Road

Lennox Creek

FOREST

To North Bend

90

0.6 mile

0.6 kilometer

DISTANCE & CONFIGURATION: 7.0-mile out-and-back	ACCESS: Hikable late spring–early fall; NW Forest Pass required for parking; self-issue wilderness permits at trailhead
DIFFICULTY: Difficult (3,250' elevation gain)	
	WHEELCHAIR TRAVERSABLE: No
SCENERY: Forested trails, old-growth forest, creek cascades, swimming hole, historical mines, views from summit	MAP(S): Green Trails *Mount Si 174* and *Skykomish 175*; USGS *Mount Phelps* and *Grotto*
EXPOSURE: Last two-thirds is exposed	FACILITIES: None
TRAFFIC: Low	DOGS: Allowed on-leash
TRAIL SURFACE: Dirt; watch for deep holes hidden by vegetation	CONTACT: 425-888-1421; www.fs.usda.gov/recarea/mbs/recarea/?recid=17970
HIKING TIME: 5–6 hours	LOCATION: North Bend

urban centers and the undeniable attraction of its magnificent high country, many of the most popular sections of the wilderness unfortunately no longer provide much isolation.

Bare Mountain, on the other hand, lies at the extreme western edge of the Alpine Lakes and is protected by a long gravel road through the North Fork Snoqualmie River Valley. Although the drive is accessible to any vehicle during good weather, the tedious, time-consuming approach deters many potential visitors from making the trip. Take advantage of their reluctance and see what this challenging and rewarding hike has to offer, including solitude, wild huckleberries, and top-of-the-world views.

A board on the northern side of the road marks the beginning of the hike, signed BARE MOUNTAIN TRAIL 1037. Look for a host of relevant information, including an area map, wilderness regulations, and notes from the rangers. Wilderness permits are free and can be self-issued here.

The trail departs from behind the information board and immediately comes to the first of several creek crossings. These creeks drain the southern side of Prospectors Ridge and may run dry in the summer. Underfoot, the surface is lined with smooth, round rocks, more typical of a desert wash from the Southwest's Canyon Country than a trail in the western Cascades.

The path follows an old mining road, built to service several claims farther up the Bear Creek Valley. Owing to its original purpose, the trail is wide with a moderate grade, easing the long uphill grind. The steady climb is a constant reminder of the daily hardships faced by the region's early settlers and the lure of riches that brought them here.

After around 0.75 mile, Bear Creek appears, flowing steeply down on the right. Note the different spellings of the creek and the mountain, which may be a testament to the illiteracy of the miners but is more likely the result of two separate derivations. Unlike many of the hikes along the I-90 corridor, there is no traffic noise here, only the sound of the rushing water.

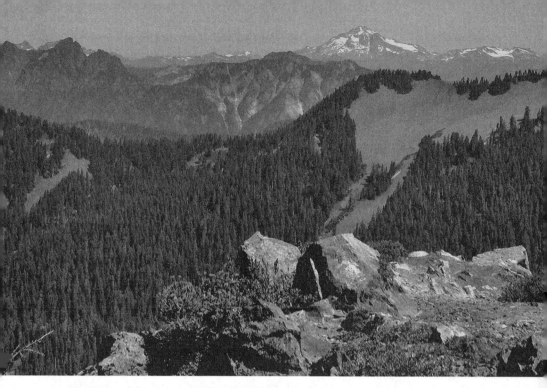

Glacier Peak from the summit of Bare Mountain

The trail crosses the creek below a long slab waterfall, reminiscent of the exposed granite faces of Kings Canyon or Yosemite. Various bolted and decaying timbers are all that remain of a ruined bridge that once spanned the water as part of the miner's road. Pick your way across the creek on a series of stepping-stones and logs. A crystal-clear pool among the rocks allows for an icy dip on a hot day, probably best saved for the descent. Note that this section may be dangerous during periods of high water, requiring a tricky wade, so proceed carefully.

Near the one-mile mark, the route crosses the creek again over a more recent and permanent bridge and then passes the official Alpine Lakes Wilderness boundary. On the far side, the trail surface changes to packed dirt and may be periodically muddy in areas even during the driest parts of the year due to the shade of several giant old-growth trees.

The ancient trees provide the last significant cover from the sun along the way, so appreciate it while it lasts. As the trail continues to climb eastward along Bear Creek, the path emerges into a vast field of bracken ferns crowding in from either side. Much of the thick growth reaches to chest or shoulder height, and the limited foot traffic on this hike does little to regularly beat it back.

Be careful through this section, as the ferns often hide the ground and the tread is highly uneven. Rocks, holes, and even streams can be hazardous and difficult to see. If the plants are wet, your legs soon will be, so hiking sticks, gaiters, and zip-off pants legs are recommended. Keep your eyes peeled for hummingbirds that can occasionally be spotted flitting through the bushes.

Near the head of the valley, the main trail makes a hairpin turn to the left and a spur continues through even thicker growth to the right. This side path dead-ends after another 0.5 mile at one of the old mines below the cliffs on the opposite side of Bear Creek, although the entrance can be difficult to find. Do not enter the dangerous shaft if you decide to explore among the rocks.

The junction with the side trail is beyond the halfway point of the 4.3-mile horizontal distance but only 1,300 vertical feet above the trailhead, with another 1,900 remaining to the summit. Needless to say, the bulk of the climbing occurs in the next part of the hike.

Start the long haul up a series of more than 50 switchbacks that leads to the top. For comparison, consider that the 14,494-foot summit of Mount Whitney in California can be reached via its famous 100 switchbacks. Look for wild huckleberry bushes as you near the crest of the ridge. A few small streams flow down the slope and could prove useful water sources if properly treated.

Persevere through several false summits and finally scramble up the last few switchbacks to the rocky peak at 5,353 feet. It's easy to see why a fire lookout stood here until it was torn down in 1973—the view stretches far and wide to all points on the compass. The only evidence remaining of the lookout is a few twisted pieces of wood and metal, but the view is as good as ever.

On a clear day, the high-rises of Seattle are just visible out to the west, dwarfed by the Olympic Mountains on the far side of Puget Sound. The familiar profiles of both the Brothers and Mount Constance are easily recognizable, some 80 miles away. Mount Baker and Glacier Peak poke above the northern Cascades, and Mount Rainier and the high crags of Summit Chief Mountain and Chimney Rock dominate the skyline to the south.

When you have had your fill of the commanding view, head back down the way you came. Use care on the descent, as the first few steps are slightly exposed and it may appear that a slip could plunge you into one of the Paradise Lakes that sparkle 1,300 feet below the northern side of the ridge. The section through the ferns is also trickier downhill, as your greater speed will make the hidden rocks and holes that much more treacherous.

GPS TRAILHEAD COORDINATES
N47° 38.378' W121° 31.710'

From I-90, take Exit 31, and at the roundabout turn north under I-90 on Bendigo Boulevard S/WA 202 toward North Bend. In 0.7 mile turn right on North Bend Way, and two blocks later turn left onto Ballarat Avenue N. Stay on this winding road 4.8 miles (it changes names several times), and turn onto the unsigned Forest Route 57 heading uphill on the left. This road begins paved, then soon turns to gravel and winds past many gated spur roads along the North Fork Snoqualmie River Valley. At 14.6 miles, there is an intersection where the left branch quickly crosses Lennox Creek. Make this left then another quick right on Lennox Creek Road/FR 57. Proceed 3.2 miles to the well-signed Bare Mountain Trailhead.

22 Dirty Harry's Peak and Balcony Trail

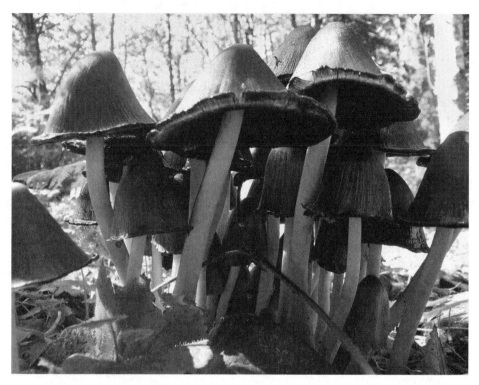

Mushrooms along the trail

In Brief

Dirty Harry's Peak is a lesser-known destination along the popular I-90 corridor, attracting significantly less traffic than its more prominent neighbors. Nonetheless, it makes a worthwhile outing, offering two good hiking options: the balcony, an easy-to-reach ledge that looks out to the south, and the more distant and challenging summit, with wide views to the north.

Description

It's almost impossible to talk about Dirty Harry's Peak without making the obvious reference to Clint Eastwood's signature role as fictional San Francisco detective Harry Callahan. But the mountain is actually named for an independent logger who once worked its

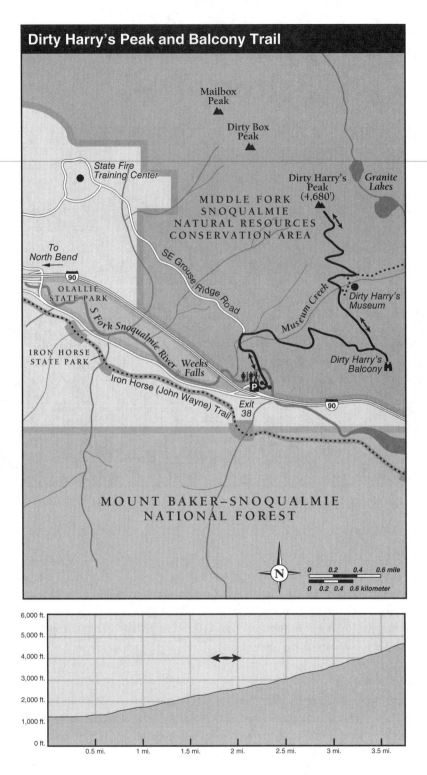

Dirty Harry's Peak and Balcony Trail

DISTANCE & CONFIGURATION: 7.5-mile out-and-back to peak, with an optional 0.3-mile round-trip side trip to the balcony	**HIKING TIME:** 5–8 hours
	ACCESS: Hikable summer–fall; Discover Pass required for parking
DIFFICULTY: Difficult	**WHEELCHAIR TRAVERSABLE:** No
SCENERY: Forested trails, old logging artifacts, views from the balcony and summit	**MAP(S):** Green Trails *Mount Si 206S*; USGS *Chester Morse Lake* and *Bandera*
EXPOSURE: Shaded most of the way, but some final sections to summit are exposed	**FACILITIES:** Toilets; bring water
	DOGS: Allowed on-leash
TRAFFIC: Light–moderate	**CONTACT:** 206-375-3558; dnr.wa.gov /MiddleForkSnoqualmie
TRAIL SURFACE: Dirt trails; rocky and slippery in many places	**LOCATION:** North Bend

slopes, a job perhaps as gritty as investigating murders in the City by the Bay but hardly as glamorous. The real-life Harry Gault is now gone, but the current hiking route still follows the main road he built up the side of the mountain. Try it for a rewarding day hike—if you feel lucky, punk.

From your car, hike through the gate and up the Fire Training Center Road. You can also follow a trail behind the information board on the north side of the parking lot, but this merely cuts off the first curve and puts you back on the road. At about 0.5 mile above the gate, look carefully for a trail leading into the woods on the right, elevation approximately 1,400 feet. This poorly marked junction may be indicated by a small sign with a hiker icon. You can also look for a moss-covered concrete block buried in the undergrowth.

Start climbing on this trail on a steady uphill slope into the forest. The surface is rocky and many of the stones underfoot can be slippery or loose, so proceed with caution, especially when it is wet. The footing becomes even more hazardous on the descent and sometimes sections of the route carry a flowing stream, most commonly during spring thaw.

Stumps in the woods on either side attest to Harry's relentless labor here in the past. The trees at the lower elevations were surely the first to be harvested since the access quickly gets more difficult at higher elevations. After about 0.5 mile, cross a small creek flowing down from the left. The wood bridge is rapidly crumbling, but the creek is little more than a ditch and easy enough for hikers to negotiate even if the bridge is totally unusable.

At times the trail is obviously an old road, complete with parallel rutted tracks, but other times it looks more like a true footpath. As it continues uphill, follow a gradual turn to the left 0.5 mile beyond the bridge and then bend back to the right near 2,000 feet. Along the way, keep your eyes peeled for random pieces of metal and other debris left behind by Harry's industrial operations.

About 1.3 miles from the trailhead, look for a cairn and a collection of artifacts just after a broad turn to the left at an elevation of approximately 2,450 feet. This marks the turnoff to the balcony, so be sure to watch for it carefully.

Turn right on the spur trail and follow this boot-beaten track uphill for another 0.25 mile to where it dead-ends at the rocky viewpoint. The traffic on I-90 rumbles through the Snoqualmie Valley directly below while McClellan Butte rises on the far side, its rocky peak by far the most prominent visible landmark. Iron Horse Trail runs parallel to the highway farther up the opposite side, marked by the chain of utility poles that follows the historical railroad right-of-way.

After visiting Dirty Harry's Balcony, you can return down the way you came or continue on the main trail to the summit, 2 more miles and a climb of 2,200 feet.

To continue uphill, follow the road on its relentless ascent and soon reach a traverse with views across the valley. One mile above the balcony, at an elevation of 3,000 feet, Museum Creek runs across the trail and drops steeply off to the left over a hidden slab-slide waterfall. During high-flow periods, the creek overruns its usual course and this rocky section of the trail turns into a free-running creek itself, making the footing particularly tricky and requiring some careful rock-hopping and route finding.

The creek is named for Dirty Harry's Museum, a collection of old logging gear abandoned in the woods somewhere above the trail. The centerpiece of the museum is the deteriorating shell of an old logging truck now permanently parked on the mountainside and rusting into oblivion, a fascinating relic of the past.

However, the vegetation grows thicker every year and the museum becomes harder and harder to find. Although it's difficult to imagine the challenge in locating a large truck in a relatively limited space, most hikers end up disappointed and merely waste time searching up and down the slope. But if you are a would-be Indiana Jones with some extra time and motivation, perhaps the hidden site will reveal its secrets.

A short distance past the creek, follow a steep switchback to the right on a section of true singletrack and then climb to an important junction at approximately 3,300 feet. Here the main trail starts to descend slightly into a swampy area, but the correct route is the left turn that continues uphill on the rocks.

Another critical intersection comes up moments later, requiring a second left turn; keeping straight would take you on a traverse beneath a large talus field. The correct trail is essentially a switchback and will once again keep you heading uphill on a rocky surface. Be sure to find this sharp turn, as many hikers keep going straight and never reach Dirty Harry's Peak, ending up on an adjacent high point instead.

However, above this junction the route is easy to follow to the summit, even as the trail narrows and looks less and less like the road it used to be. Proceed through several switchbacks as views begin to open out to the east.

The summit ridge is well below the timberline, so unfortunately there are no panoramic views, and it can be hard to even tell exactly where the highest point (4,680') is. Look for a collection of boulders with an open sight line to the northeast over the edge of a high cliff. The westernmost of the two Granite Lakes lies straight below, while the rocky double peak of Russian Butte rises prominently on the far side of the Granite Creek Valley.

It is worth exploring the far western end of the ridge, which dead-ends at a steep drop-off and a view across a long notch. The next peak over is commonly known as Dirty Box Peak, since it lies between Dirty Harry's Peak and Mailbox Peak to the west. Dirty Box is the highest of the three at 4,926 feet, but it is labeled only with its elevation on the USGS map since the name is unofficial.

After exploring the summit area, descend the way you came.

GPS TRAILHEAD COORDINATES

N47° 25.87' W121° 37.949'

From I-90 E, take Exit 38 and turn right onto SE Homestead Valley Road. Drive 1.8 miles and go left under I-90 toward the State Fire Training Center. Park outside the gate in the Olallie State Park Far Side trailhead parking lot. From I-90 W, take Exit 38, and turn right into the parking lot.

23 Franklin Falls and Old Snoqualmie Pass Wagon Road

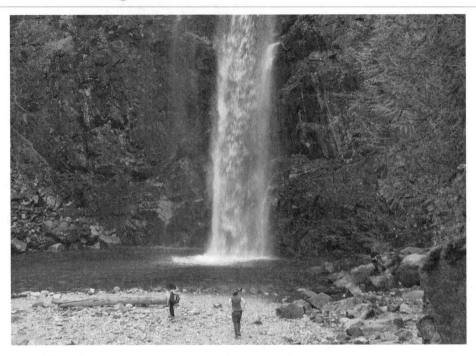

Franklin Falls

In Brief

The trail to Franklin Falls combines history and natural beauty along a compact and easily accessible loop. A visit to the falls makes for a particularly enjoyable half-day's outing for anyone who wants to explore the Snoqualmie Pass region but isn't looking for a demanding mountain hike.

Description

It sounds like a joke or the effects of some terrible flood: a scenic waterfall in the middle of I-90—not off to the side somewhere or even visible from the pavement but right in the center—with traffic driving by on either side. Yet this improbable juxtaposition of natural

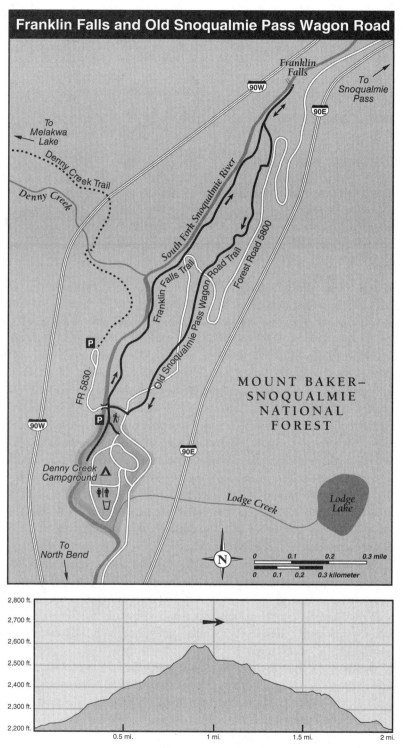

DISTANCE & CONFIGURATION: 2.0-mile loop	**ACCESS:** Hikable late spring–fall; NW Forest Pass required for parking
DIFFICULTY: Easy	**WHEELCHAIR TRAVERSABLE:** No
SCENERY: Franklin Falls and the picturesque South Fork Snoqualmie River Gorge, old-growth forest, a walk along a historical wagon route	**MAP(S):** Green Trails *Snoqualmie Pass 207*; USGS *Snoqualmie Pass*
EXPOSURE: Shaded	**FACILITIES:** No facilities at trailhead; Denny Creek Campground has toilets and water
TRAFFIC: Get an early start to beat crowds and get parking.	**DOGS:** Allowed on-leash
TRAIL SURFACE: Dirt (well-maintained with steps and bridges)	**CONTACT:** 425-888-1421; www.fs.usda .gov/recarea/mbs/recreation /recarea/?recid=17980
HIKING TIME: 1–2 hours	**LOCATION:** North Bend

and man-made elements is found just west of Snoqualmie Pass, where the two directions of I-90 are split. More than 25,000 people pass within 0.25 mile of Franklin Falls every day, and most would never guess that it is there. Amazingly, an old-growth forest still hangs on in the area as well, seemingly oblivious to the cars and trucks humming overhead.

Long before there was an I-90, however, human traffic passed much closer to the falls on the Old Snoqualmie Wagon Road, developed by pioneers heading west toward Seattle. Without the miracles of modern engineering that elevate the current roadway, the horse-drawn wagons had to stay at the bottom of the valley on their arduous journey through the mountains. The road often amounted to little more than two wheel-worn ruts in the mud. Nonetheless, it was the primary route across the Central Washington Cascades.

Unlike the cars on the interstate, today's hikers tend to travel at a pace similar to that of the pioneers, which makes the former site of the Wagon Road a great place to explore the natural beauty and history of the area on foot.

At the Franklin Falls Trailhead, the correct trail is signed as FRANKLIN FALLS TRAIL NO. 1036. The return for the 2-mile loop is on the other side of the junction where Forest Route 5830 branches off FR 58.

The hike starts out heading northeast along the South Fork Snoqualmie River. The water is clear with a greenish tinge, and runs fast through a mix of gray and reddish rocks. There are plenty of good places to stop and dip your toes in the rushing water, including a polished-rock chute in an exposed slab that could double as a water slide a short distance upstream. There is even a small sandy beach on the bank and a pool at the bottom when the river is low.

The trail is wide and easy to follow, with some private rustic cabins visible on either side of the river. Old-growth stands of western red cedar, western hemlock, and Douglas fir appear in the forest to the right, displaying some truly outstanding giant specimens. An epic cedar with a circumference easily 20 feet or more stands watch at the bottom of a set of wooden stairs.

The stairs ascend the bank as the river quickly drops away into a narrow gorge on the left, guarded by a wooden safety fence on the rim. More seemingly good swimming holes appear below, but they are unreachable at the bottom of the sheer rock walls. Various tributary streams flow into the river, including Denny Creek on the far side (although it is difficult to spot through the trees).

In just under a mile, a trail joins from the right at a junction, the start of the Old Snoqualmie Wagon Road and the return route on the second half of the loop. Stay straight ahead along the fence for another 0.1 mile to reach the splendor of Franklin Falls, where the river pours over a 70-foot cliff into a natural amphitheater of black and reddish rocks, misting everything nearby and making the trail muddy and slippery. The westbound lanes of I-90 cross overhead on a bridge to the left, clearly visible above. When the river is low, it is possible to explore the riverbed by walking on the rocks.

Return to the previous junction and turn onto the Old Wagon Road. Surprisingly, although the falls tend to attract considerable crowds, many hikers return the way they came, ignoring the simple loop option. The 1-mile descent back to the trailhead is pleasant and comfortable, with a spongy and forgiving surface of decaying wood underfoot that is easy on the joints. The perspective on the forest is different as well, with the river mostly out of sight.

Hard evidence of the old road is well hidden, and only the most diligent or lucky observer is likely to find anything specific to mark the pioneers' passing. It is difficult enough to even imagine covered wagons making it through the mud and trees of the forest. Not so well hidden, however, is the modern, paved FR 58, which must be crossed several times along the way. At each intersection, look for an inconspicuous wooden post on the opposite side to show the continuation of the trail, usually within 10 yards to the left or right.

The end of the Old Wagon Road returns you to the junction of FR 58 and FR 5830, as mentioned earlier, where it is a short walk across the parking lot back to your vehicle.

Nearby Activities

From the parking area, you can hike to two good waterfalls on Denny Creek Trail, which starts from the end of FR 5830: Keekwulee Falls is about 2 miles up the trail, and Snowshoe Falls is another 0.25 mile beyond.

GPS TRAILHEAD COORDINATES

N47° 24.79' W121° 26.535'

From I-90, take Exit 47 for Denny Creek–Asahel Curtis, and head north. At the T-intersection in 0.1 mile, turn right onto Forest Route 9034. In 0.3 mile, turn left onto FR 58 toward Denny Creek. In 2.3 miles, turn left onto FR 5830 toward the Denny Creek and Melakwa Lake Trail. Just before the bridge over the river, you'll find the trailhead for Franklin Falls Trail on the right. Park anywhere along FR 5830 near the trailhead, or drive to the end of FR 5830 for additional parking spots.

24 Granite Mountain Lookout Tower

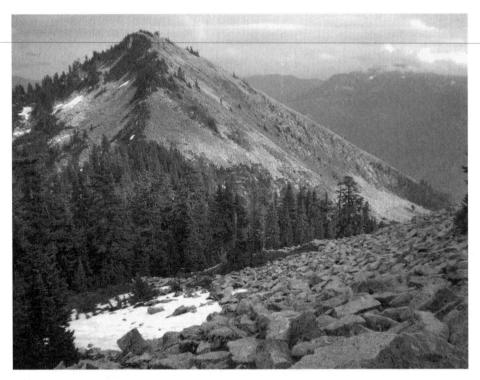

West Granite Mountain

In Brief

This tough but rewarding hike leads to one of the highest peaks west of Snoqualmie Pass and includes some 2,000 feet of climbing in the alpine zone; the trek is capped by a long boulder hop up the final ridge. The summit lookout tower provides a commanding view of the surrounding area and much of the central Washington Cascades, with four high volcanoes framing the unforgettable scene.

Description

Most of the summits along I-90 can provide excellent views, and Granite Mountain is no exception. However, there is a reason Granite was selected as a fire-lookout site when so many others were not. Even among the exemplary collection of peaks between North

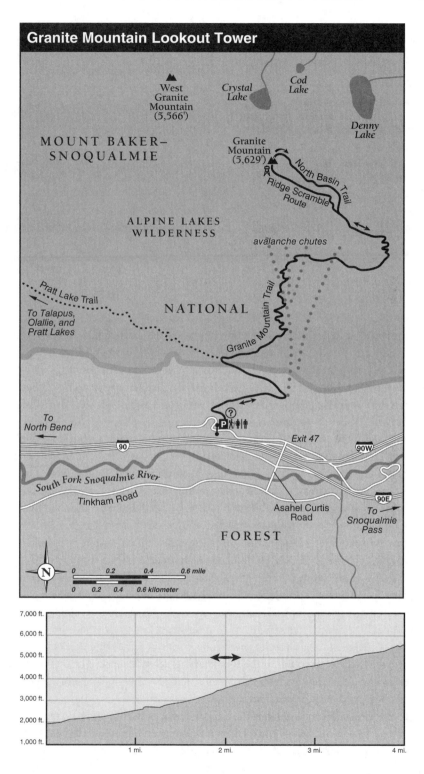

Granite Mountain Lookout Tower

DISTANCE & CONFIGURATION: 8.0-mile out-and-back, with summit loop option	spring); NW Forest Pass required for parking; self-issue wilderness permit at trailhead
DIFFICULTY: Difficult	**WHEELCHAIR TRAVERSABLE:** No
SCENERY: Active lookout tower on summit with distant views, optional scramble route along a boulder-strewn ridge	**MAP(S):** Green Trails *Snoqualmie Pass 207*; USGS *Snoqualmie Pass*
EXPOSURE: Shaded on lower half, exposed on upper half	**FACILITIES:** Toilet at trailhead, no drinking water
TRAFFIC: Moderate–high	**DOGS:** Allowed on-leash
TRAIL SURFACE: Dirt	**CONTACT:** 425-888-1421; www.fs.usda.gov/recarea/mbs/recarea/?recid=17986
HIKING TIME: 5–7 hours	
ACCESS: Hikable late spring–fall (avalanche chutes can be dangerous in	**LOCATION:** North Bend

Bend and Snoqualmie Pass, Granite stands out, reaching just a little bit higher, with a grander view to match. The price of admission is the demanding haul up the mountain's long south slope, a trip that's guaranteed to exact its toll in sweat and lactic acid.

Granite Mountain shares a trailhead with several other destinations, listed with specific mileages and trail numbers on a prominent sign at the northern side of the parking lot, where trail reports and other useful information are also displayed. All the hikes start on Pratt Lake Trail 1007 before branching off to their separate endpoints. Note that the hike to the Granite Mountain Lookout is listed as 4 miles one-way, but it certainly feels farther, given the tough character of the climb.

The trail begins on a rocky uphill, rising quickly above the trailhead at 1,880 feet. A series of seasonal streams flows down the mountainside and crosses underfoot as the route contours eastward, reaches a major switchback at 2,200 feet, and then bends back to the left beneath a forest of tall Douglas firs.

After about a mile, a sign marks Granite Mountain Trail, where it branches to the right from Pratt Lake Trail. The climb becomes noticeably steeper and reaches the bottom of a series of avalanche chutes near 3,000 feet. These chutes are hazardous in winter and spring and are often a problem early in the hiking season if a heavy snowpack lingers on the mountain's upper slopes. If you have any doubts at all about crossing this section, your best bet is to return to the trailhead. You're always better safe than sorry.

Skirt the edge of the avalanche chutes on a series of tight switchbacks before finally crossing over to the eastern side at the top, near the 2.5-mile mark. The open gullies provide good views of the Snoqualmie Valley below and are often full of colorful wildflowers and puffy beargrass in the spring and summer.

Large rocks start to appear along the trail, evidence of the mountain's namesake underlying granite. As you climb above 4,000 feet and enter the alpine zone, the steepness relents and the landscape continues to open up. This section can be cruelly deceptive—even though it seems the top must be just above the next rise, there is still a long way to go. The area is also exposed to the weather, which could mean anything from cold wind and rain to a burning sun, depending on seasonal conditions.

At around 5,000 feet, some social trails branch to the left and lead to the foot of a long ridge of granite boulders that reaches to the summit, still 600 feet above. The main trail continues into an open alpine bowl and crosses toward the mountain's scenic, quiet northern side before climbing through stunted trees to the lookout tower. Many hikers take the most direct route to the top, enjoying the fun and easy scramble through the massive rocks. In some years, snow remains on the official trail well into July, making the boulders an even more attractive option. It is also possible to make a short loop by climbing one route and descending the other, getting a feel for both.

At 5,629 feet, Granite Mountain is high enough that it is possible to feel some minor effects of the altitude over the last few hundred feet of climbing. The thin air will be most apparent to anyone coming up from sea level, which means essentially all hikers from the Puget Sound lowlands.

The sturdy wooden lookout is perched on the southern end of the summit crest, capping a jumble of lichen-encrusted rocks. The lichen adds a mix of green and black to the gray and white slabs, and even throws in a splash of pink. Unfortunately, the lookout is kept locked and is not available for public rental, as it is still in use by the U.S. Forest Service. Fire spotting is mostly done by helicopters these days, but rangers and volunteers are sometimes stationed in the tower.

If someone is on duty and it is possible to get inside, the interesting fire-finder compass in the center of the structure is worth investigating. Surrounding peaks up to a radius of about 9 miles are labeled and can be lined up with a set of crosshairs to provide bearing and elevation data, traditionally used to report the locations of potential wildfires. The compass is also useful for identifying many geographic landmarks visible from the lookout.

On a clear day, no one will have any trouble picking out Mount Rainier and Mount Adams to the south and Mount Baker and Glacier Peak to the north; all are unmistakable. Although not quite as scenic as the mountain peaks, I-90 also requires no guide for identification, as it winds through the valley far below. All around, a sea of peaks, valleys, lakes, and rivers invites quiet contemplation.

GPS TRAILHEAD COORDINATES
N47° 23.863' W121° 29.221'

From I-90, take Exit 47 for Denny Creek–Asahel Curtis, and head north. In 0.1 mile at the T-intersection, turn left onto Forest Route 9034. Drive 0.4 mile to the parking lot and trailhead.

25 Ira Spring Trail to Mason Lake, Mount Defiance, and Bandera Mountain

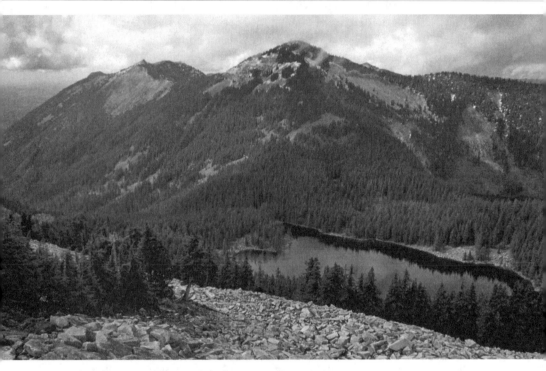

Mount Defiance and Mason Lake from Bandera

In Brief

With multiple worthwhile destinations, this hike is really three trails in one—two difficult options climb the high peaks of either Mount Defiance or Bandera Mountain, while a moderate option leads to peaceful Mason Lake in between. No matter which one you choose, vibrant wildflowers, alpine wilderness, and great views will be your reward.

Description

The formerly sketchy Bandera Mountain–Mason Lake Trail saw major renovation in 2003 and was renamed Ira Spring Trail a year later in memory of the famous outdoor advocate

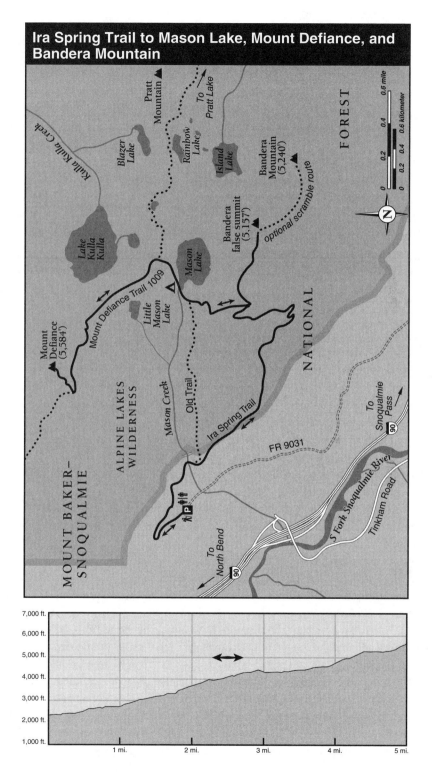

DISTANCE & CONFIGURATION: 6.5-mile out-and-back to Mason Lake; 10.0-mile out-and-back to Mount Defiance; 6.5-mile out-and-back to Bandera Mountain false summit	abandoned gravel-road approach and boulder hopping on Bandera
	HIKING TIME: Half day to Mason Lake, all day for either summit
DIFFICULTY: Moderate to Mason Lake, difficult to either summit	**ACCESS:** Hikable late spring–early fall; NW Forest Pass required for parking; self-issue wilderness permit at trailhead
SCENERY: Mountain lake; a waterfall; two mountains to ascend, including a scramble route on a boulder ridge; and many great viewpoints along the way	**WHEELCHAIR TRAVERSABLE:** No
	MAP(S): Green Trails *Bandera 206*; USGS *Bandera*
EXPOSURE: Shaded on lower portions and around Mason Lake	**FACILITIES:** Toilet at trailhead; no drinking water
TRAFFIC: High to Mason Lake, less on summit routes	**DOGS:** Allowed on-leash
	CONTACT: 425-888-1421; www.fs.usda .gov/recarea/mbs/recarea/?recid=17992
TRAIL SURFACE: Dirt, with an	**LOCATION:** North Bend

and photographer, who had just died from cancer at the age of 84. The tribute was especially fitting, both because the Spring Family Trust was established to support just this type of project and because the trail leads to a Pacific Northwest landscape with deep evergreen forests, grand mountain scenery, and sparkling alpine lakes that Spring would have loved to capture on film.

If there is any drawback to the Ira Spring Trail, it's that, despite the considerable improvements, it still can't be described as easy. Mason Lake is the least demanding destination but nonetheless requires a tough climb of 2,000 feet over 3.3 miles. Add 1,200 feet and another 1.75 miles to reach the summit of Mount Defiance, or a little more than a mile to get to the top of Bandera. Still, each destination is well worth the exertion.

Note that the Alpine Lakes Wilderness was expanded in December 2014, adding this entire area, so a self-issued permit is required at the trailhead no matter where you decide to go.

Whichever destination you choose, the first several miles of the route are the same for all three and involve climbing a high, south-facing ridge. The trail starts near 2,300 feet on an abandoned gravel road that quickly bends to the east and enters a forest of alders. Several creeks—including Mason Creek, with a particularly large and impressive waterfall worth stopping to photograph—flow down the slope from the left and pass under the roadbed. The water bounces down through a series of boulders and logs in a cascade of crashing foam and mist, with the top too far up to be seen through the trees.

The trail climbs steadily as it continues to head eastward, ascending on a long traverse. The trees gradually thin, providing views of the I-90 corridor and McClellan Butte directly across the valley, and are replaced by some lichen-encrusted boulders. Eventually the old road ends, but the trail branches off uphill to the left and continues through several avalanche gaps before reaching its first switchback, near 3,500 feet. Evidence of an old forest fire can be seen in some charred stumps scattered across the mountainside, sticking up out of the beargrass, huckleberry bushes, and wildflowers.

Several more switchbacks run back and forth across the fire-scarred slope and through some substantial piles of rock, where the trail displays some of the best handiwork of the tireless volunteers who labored to create it. The effort required to lay a flat dirt trail through a wide boulder field is nothing short of monumental, and the sandy surface provides great drainage, even in the rain and snow.

At 4,100 feet, you'll finally reach the signed split to Bandera Mountain on the right. The trail to Bandera above the junction is much rougher than Ira Spring Trail, not far removed from a scramble through bear grass and exposed rocks. It is much steeper as well, running virtually straight uphill. However, it seems like the entire Snoqualmie Valley is at your feet and the wide-ranging views make it easy to forget the physical challenge. The south-facing slope gets plenty of sunlight, nurturing huckleberries, Indian paintbrush, purple lupine, and a host of other colorful wildflowers while keeping the ground generally dry.

Skirt some low trees and continue up the rocky ridge toward the crest. Occasional cairns show the way, but the boot-polished boulders are generally equally good indicators of the correct route, which is never hard to follow.

A small clearing marks the end of the hike at about 5,200 feet, just before it would be necessary to descend into a notch. The true summit is actually another 0.5 mile away, but it is only marginally higher, at 5,241 feet, and the crossing is little more than a bushwhack. Few hikers make the journey to the summit. And why should they? The view from the false summit is hard to beat, taking in a vast stretch of land that on a clear day includes everything from the peaks around Snoqualmie Pass to downtown Seattle and Mount Rainier. Mason Lake shimmers directly below to the north, along with Island Lake and several others. Lake Kulla Kulla sits below some exposed slabs on the northern buttress of Mount Defiance, whose distinctive pyramidal summit is the highest point anywhere to the west other than in the Olympic range.

Mason Lake and Mount Defiance can be reached by continuing on Ira Spring Trail from the junction at 4,100 feet. Follow the path until it reaches a saddle and then descend through an evergreen forest on the opposite side.

Cross the Mason Creek outflow to find the lake itself, sitting in an alpine bowl directly below the Bandera ridge. The trail wraps around through the trees on the northern shore, where a clearing among the boulders provides a good campsite and many places to sit and relax. There are plenty of opportunities to explore on your own as well, if this is your final destination.

To continue to Mount Defiance, follow the extension of the trail through the jumbled rocks and back into the forest. A sign reading MAIN TRAIL tacked high on a tree may help show the way, although it is easy to miss. The trail soon leads to a more obvious T-junction, with a sign for Mount Defiance Trail 1009 to the left, and a trail to Island Lake and distant Pratt Lake to the right. The dry and sandy tread hiked earlier will likely seem very far away, as mud puddles big enough to be called ponds can collect on the trail when it is wet.

Take the left fork and begin climbing once again on a shallow ridge, with glimpses of Lake Kulla Kulla visible through the stately trees to the right. As the trail continues to ascend, it feels almost like an organic part of the forest, winding in and out of the moss-covered trunks until finally emerging into an avalanche gap at 5,100 feet, about 900 feet above Mason Lake.

Cross the chute and continue west on an open, wildflower-studded slope with spectacular views similar to those on summit ridge on Bandera (although the trail here is mercifully flat). After a long but glorious 0.25 mile, look for a narrow trail switchbacking straight up to the right just short of where you would reenter the trees. This steep and rocky path is the final stretch to the summit, where the ridge ends in a pile of boulders at 5,584 feet.

The view from the top of Defiance is just as panoramic as the one from nearby Bandera, with an even better vantage for observing the southwest corner of the Alpine Lakes Wilderness and the high summits of Kaleetan Peak, Mount Roosevelt, and Preacher Mountain across the Pratt River Valley to the northeast.

GPS TRAILHEAD COORDINATES
N47° 25.477' W121° 35.003'

From I-90, take Exit 45 and head north on Forest Route 9030, which bends left to parallel the interstate. At a junction in 0.9 mile, stay left (straight) on FR 9031/Mason Lake Road, and continue 2.9 more miles to the road's end at the Mason Lake Trail–Ira Spring Trail parking lot and trailhead.

26 Little Si

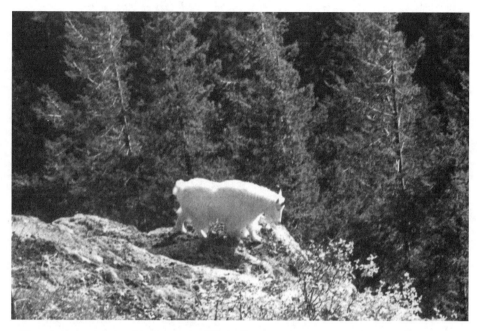

Mountain goat below the summit of Little Si

In Brief

Long overshadowed both literally and figuratively by its big brother next door, Little Si is a worthwhile destination on its own and offers a good alternative when its hulking neighbor is too busy, too socked in, or too demanding. Watching rock climbers on the lower cliffs is an interesting diversion along the way.

Description

From a distance, it can be hard to even identify Little Si as a separate peak from Mount Si proper. So complete is Mount Si's dominance over the area that the insignificant-seeming bump in front seems hardly worth noticing.

A closer view reveals that this is all an illusion. The minor notch that separates the peaks is actually a deep cleft, and the tree-clad summit ridge of Little Si actually hides impressive cliff faces far more sought by climbers than any on the exposed rock of the bigger peak next door. For hikers, the manageable distance married with a moderate elevation gain presents a solid challenge, although well short of extreme.

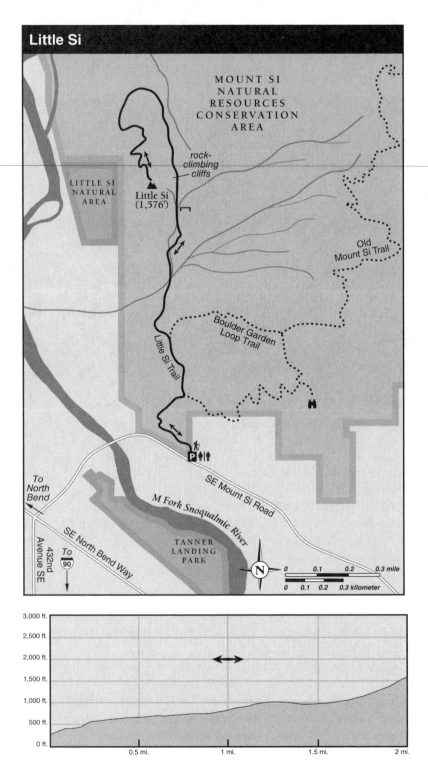

Little Si

DISTANCE & CONFIGURATION: 4.0-mile out-and-back	**ACCESS:** Hikable year-round; Discover Pass required for parking
DIFFICULTY: Moderate	**WHEELCHAIR TRAVERSABLE:** No
SCENERY: An easier alternative to Mount Si, with similar views of North Bend and the Snoqualmie River Valley	**MAP(S):** Green Trails *Mount Si NRCA 206S*; USGS *North Bend*
EXPOSURE: Mostly shaded	**FACILITIES:** Toilet at the trailhead; no water available
TRAFFIC: High	**DOGS:** Allowed on-leash
TRAIL SURFACE: Dirt with rocks and roots	**CONTACT:** 206-375-3558; dnr.wa.gov /MountSi
HIKING TIME: 2–3 hours	**LOCATION:** North Bend

Little Si's attractiveness for rock climbers plays a big role in the tight trailhead parking, especially when the rock is dry. The good news is that this means even when the lot is full the trail itself will probably be less crowded than you might think. The bad news is that more often than not there will be a considerable volume of cars to contend with.

The trailhead has space for more than 40 vehicles, but on some days you may need to arrive early to get a space.

Start up the trail from the southeast corner of the parking lot, behind the toilets. Right away, you face a tough incline on rocks and dirt. A glance back over your shoulder across the broad Snoqualmie River Valley reveals the long ridge of Rattlesnake Mountain, with pockets of radio towers marking its many peaks. The sun here can be brutal, thanks to thin growth and a south-facing slope. Luckily, a series of switchbacks soon leads into some shady trees and ferns where the trail levels out. The forest here is typical of the western Cascade foothills, with a primary mix of Douglas firs, alders, and maples.

After about half a mile, Boulder Garden Loop branches off to the right. This junction can be tricky to identify since it is unsigned and sometimes obscured by logs or other debris, but it is well worth finding. The loop trail winds past some giant rocks in a section of beautiful, mossy forest. Along the way, stay straight where Old Mount Si Trail heads uphill to the right.

The return of Boulder Garden Loop to the main Little Si Trail is clearly signed, making this second junction much easier to find than the first. A good option would be to explore the Boulder Garden on the way down, avoiding the difficulty of finding the lower intersection altogether.

To continue up Little Si, descend to a creek crossing as the trail enters the gap between the peaks. Views start to open through the trees onto the southwest face of Mount Si, with the summit of Little Si now to the left. An information board marks the first of many access points for rock climbers into the Mount Si Natural Resource Conservation Area, available for day use only.

The canyon between the two Si's is defined on its western side by a long wall of rock below the Little Si summit ridge, where climbers test their skills. Several vantage points offer the opportunity to stop and watch them tackle the challenging routes and listen to their voices carry through the trees.

A memorial bench dedicated to Doug Hansen provides a place to sit along the way. Hansen was a popular Seattle-area mountaineer who honed his skills in the high Cascades and ended up being killed along with 11 others on Mount Everest in May 1996. Under the guidance of New Zealand guide Rob Hall, Hansen successfully reached the summit, but then died in a storm on the descent, events tragically immortalized in Jon Krakauer's *Into Thin Air.*

Past the bench, the trail starts to climb again, now heavily shaded below the rock wall. Even on a hot summer day, the temperatures are surprisingly cool here, where the sun never really penetrates. After reaching an old rockslide on the left, the trail enters a beautiful fern valley, a mix of dappled greens, sunlight, and shadow. Look for some of the ferns hanging off boulders along the wall and spreading like a carpet over the forest floor.

At the northern end of the valley, the path swings hard to the left and steeply uphill. Unfortunately, the bulk of the climbing on this trail occurs in the last third of its distance as the route exits the valley and mounts the summit ridge, doubling back in the direction you've already come. Prepare for a near scramble through a few short sections.

When you finally reach the summit, you will feel like you have come a lot farther than the actual distance. Various ledges surround the high point; poke around for a while to find the one that suits you best. Don't miss the rocks slightly down the far side, which have some of the best views over North Bend and where mountain goats can occasionally be spotted. There are also several viewpoints just before the top that face Mount Si, clearly showing its much larger size. Stay back from the edge, and be careful not to knock anything off that could hit the rock climbers directly below. The return route is the way you came.

GPS TRAILHEAD COORDINATES
N47° 29.193' W121° 45.186'

From I-90, take Exit 32 and head north on 436th Avenue SE. In 0.5 mile turn left onto SE North Bend Way, and then in 0.3 mile turn right onto SE Mount Si Road. In 0.6 mile, just after crossing the river and rounding a bend to the right, look for the trailhead parking area on the left signed for Little Si.

27 Mailbox Peak

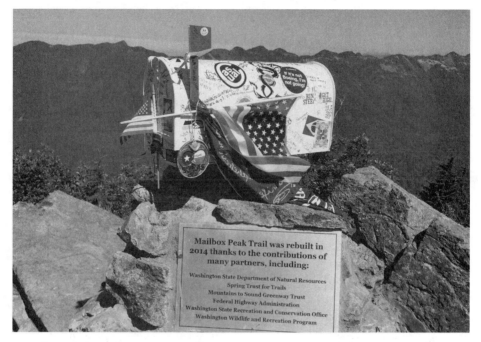

Mailbox Peak summit marker

In Brief

Once reserved for the elite club of people who knew about it, Mailbox Peak has become a flagship destination for Puget Sound hikers. Anyone completing the difficult climb to the summit will be amply rewarded with a sea of wildflowers in season and a 360-degree view of the western Cascades and Mount Rainier.

Description

Mailbox Peak was unknown to the general public for a long time, the trail and mountain traditionally unmarked on most maps. With a top elevation of less than 5,000 feet, the summit was easily overlooked by most hikers, who instead headed to several more-famous destinations along the Snoqualmie River Valley.

Locals in the know shared the peak with friends and family, eventually beating a trail up the mountain's western ridge. Mostly devoid of the smooth surface, measured grading, and other niceties typical of a well-maintained path, the steep route ascended more than 4,000 feet in about 2 miles.

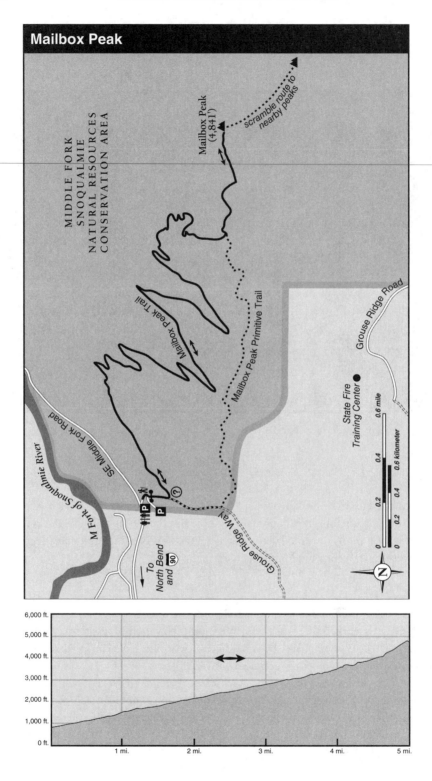

DISTANCE & CONFIGURATION: 10.0-mile out-and-back	**ACCESS:** Hikable late spring–fall, daily, sunrise–sunset; Discover Pass required for parking
DIFFICULTY: Difficult (more than a 4,000' elevation gain)	**WHEELCHAIR TRAVERSABLE:** No
SCENERY: Forested trails, wildflowers along the summit ridge, views from the summit	**MAP(S):** Green Trails *Mount Si NRCA 206S*; USGS *Chester Morse Lake*
	FACILITIES: Toilets at upper parking lot
EXPOSURE: Mostly shaded; final ridge walk and summit are exposed	**DOGS:** Allowed on-leash
TRAFFIC: High (get an early start to beat the heat and the crowds)	**CONTACT:** 206-375-3558; dnr.wa.gov /MiddleForkSnoqualmie
	LOCATION: North Bend
TRAIL SURFACE: Dirt; steep near summit	**COMMENTS:** The gate at the upper parking lot is open only 7 a.m.–7 p.m., so park at the lower lot if necessary.
HIKING TIME: 5–8 hours	

Many of the peak's hikers were mountaineers in training, who used the brutal climb as off-season preparation for high volcano ascents. Although the twin complicating factors of high altitude and glacier travel can't easily be re-created here, some extra weight carried in a backpack could help to make up the difference.

The peak's name is derived from an actual mailbox that appeared on the summit in years past, hauled up by some intrepid hiker. Since then, the original has been replaced multiple times and a wide assortment of other unlikely artifacts has come and gone, including a box for the *Olympian* newspaper, a fire hydrant, and an aluminum stepladder, but the Mailbox name has stuck.

By the mid-2000s, word had gotten around, and more and more people were coming to test themselves on the challenging route. Responding to the growing popularity of the peak and the need to protect it from being loved to death, the Washington State Department of Natural Resources (DNR) set aside the mountain and surrounding land as the Middle Fork Snoqualmie Natural Resource Conservation Area in 2011.

At the same time, the need for a better hiker experience spurred construction of a new parking lot and an easier way to the summit. With support and volunteer hours from a wide range of interested groups, including Spring Trust for Trails, Mountains to Sound Greenway Trust, and even the Federal Highway Administration, the new Mailbox Peak Trail was opened to the public in 2014. Climbing Mailbox Peak remains a challenge, but the challenge is now much more manageable.

However, this is still a difficult hike and anyone attempting it should carry adequate supplies, including clothing, food, and water. Regardless of the outside temperature, you are guaranteed to sweat, so hydration is important.

To begin the hike, go around a heavy metal gate and follow the old road (unsigned Mailbox Peak Road) through scrub brush up the hill.

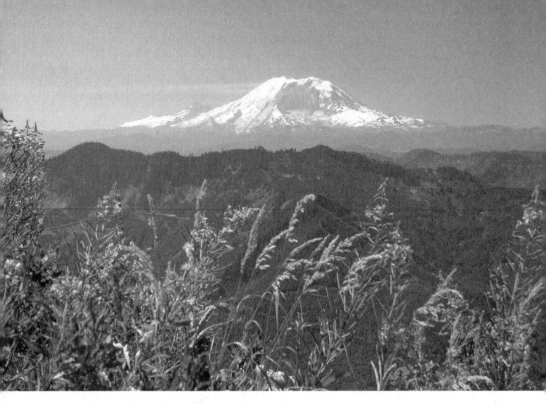

Mount Rainier through wildflowers

The trailhead is marked with an information board on the left after 0.1 mile. Anyone familiar with the old trail will be amazed by the new one, smooth and wide enough to accommodate a riding mower as it begins the steady but moderate ascent.

The trail climbs for more than 2,000 vertical feet through 3.5 miles of long switchbacks before crossing an open, rocky area with some views to the north. Be careful of giant, thorny devil's club (*Oplopanax horridus*) visible below. Devil's club has a long history as a useful medicinal plant, but because its spines can be very painful and difficult to extract from the skin, it is best avoided.

Shortly after the open area, wrap around a rock outcrop that marks the mountain's western ridgeline. A few more switchbacks bring you to a junction with the old Mailbox trail on the right, at an elevation of approximately 3,800 feet.

Here the new trail merges with the old for the rest of the trip to the summit, so the route becomes much steeper and more challenging. Watch for white diamond blazes on the trees to show the way as you scramble through loose dirt and rocks. Sections of exposed roots climb like stairs, and you may find yourself grabbing trees to pull yourself up. Patches of worn bark indicate that you are not the first to employ this strategy.

Good views begin to appear on either side as the trees give way to boulders and brush, including wild blackberries, ferns, and bear grass. Kinnikinnick covers the ground, with stunted evergreens and Indian paintbrush poking through.

At 400 feet above the junction, the trail reaches an alpine meadow perched on the crest of the final ridge. A spectacular rainbow of wildflowers populates the slope in spring and summer; the higher you go, the later the blooms. From the ridgeline, the world seems to drop steeply away to either side, especially to the right (south) where the buildings of the State Fire Training Center are virtually straight below. Although the climb is still demanding, the views near and far give your mind something else to focus on as you continue to ascend.

The trail abruptly reaches the summit at 4,841 feet, with its signature mailbox stuck in a pile of boulders. Inside, find the summit register and a collection of other random pieces of literature to keep you entertained as you relax among the bear grass.

However, your attention is best spent on the amazing view. To the north, the Middle Fork Snoqualmie River runs like a blue ribbon below the dominant crags and cliffs of Russian Butte. Mounts Si and Teneriffe are immediately to the west, with the radio towers of Rattlesnake Mountain visible across the Snoqualmie Valley. Mount Rainier and its huge Willis Wall rise to the south beyond Mount Washington and McClellan Butte. For the truly adventurous, a scrambler's trail runs toward the southeast, first descending into a saddle and then climbing up the other side to a high point (4,926') informally known as Dirty Box Peak, the name a mash-up of Dirty Harry's and Mailbox, the two peaks it stands between.

Be careful on the descent of the summit ridge. Despite the temptation, the steepness of the trail makes it difficult to go much faster on the way down than on the way up, and the roots and loose dirt make it easy to lose your footing.

Nearby Activities

Looking to test yourself on the old Mailbox trail? It's possible to complete a loop in either direction using the old and new trails together. The old trailhead is just up Mailbox Peak Road from the new one. Expect a real grind if you ascend that way—and commensurately greater satisfaction at the summit. Watch for white diamond blazes to keep you on the correct route.

GPS TRAILHEAD COORDINATES

N47° 28.058' W121° 40.494'

From I-90, take Exit 34 for 486th Avenue SE, and head north, proceeding through the Edgewick "Truck Town" area. In 0.5 mile, turn right onto SE Middle Fork Road. In 1.0 mile Middle Fork Road and Lake Dorothy Road meet at a fork. You can take either road because they meet up again in 1.2 miles. After the two roads come back together, continue 0.3 mile on Middle Fork Road to a parking area on the left and right. A road ascends from here to another parking lot, but note that cars must be out before 7 p.m.

28 McClellan Butte

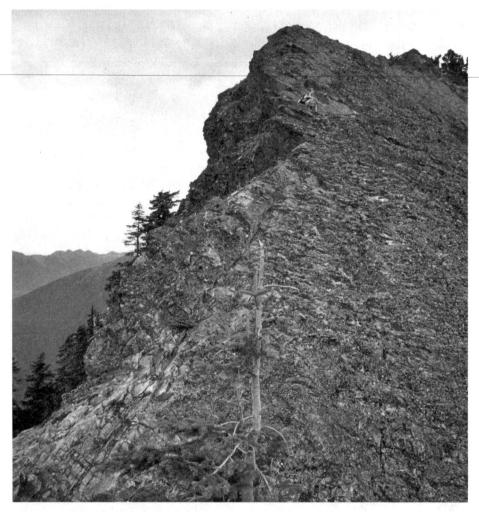

Summit scramble on McClellan Butte

In Brief

Thanks to its rocky summit and central location, 5,162-foot McClellan Butte provides one of the best views of the high peaks lining I-90 between North Bend and Snoqualmie Pass. On the final ridge, an optional scramble presents an additional challenge, suitable for experienced hikers who are comfortable using handholds and facing considerable exposure.

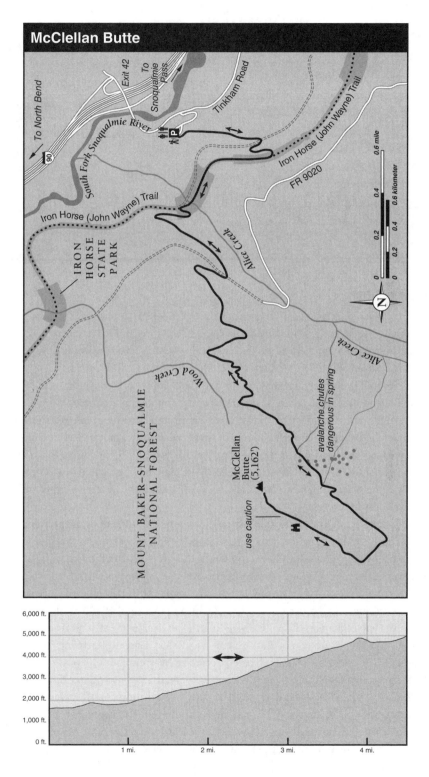

McClellan Butte

DISTANCE & CONFIGURATION: 9.0-mile out-and-back	ACCESS: Hikable summer–fall (don't cross avalanche chutes when snow-filled); NW Forest Pass required for parking
DIFFICULTY: Difficult	
SCENERY: Old-growth forest, subalpine meadows, historical rail-trail, summit scramble, views from summit	WHEELCHAIR TRAVERSABLE: No
	MAP(S): Green Trails *Mount Si NRCA 206S*; USGS *Bandera*
EXPOSURE: Mostly shaded; summit is exposed	FACILITIES: Toilet at trailhead, no drinking water
TRAFFIC: Moderate	DOGS: Allowed on-leash
TRAIL SURFACE: Dirt with a short crushed-rock rail-trail segment	CONTACT: 425-888-1421; www.fs.usda .gov/recarea/mbs/recreation /recarea/?recid=18002
HIKING TIME: 5–8 hours	LOCATION: North Bend

Description

From the approach drive, the prominent peak of McClellan Butte does not seem to be far above the highway. Don't be deceived; the route to the top gains 3,700 feet over 4.5 miles, a demanding average gradient of 820 feet per mile, ranking this hike among the most difficult in the Snoqualmie River Valley.

Yet the trail is more than just an uphill slog, since it passes through old-growth forest, subalpine meadows, and a series of avalanche chutes on its way to the top. The route also wraps around to the far side of the butte, crossing through a corner of the restricted Cedar River Watershed and presenting a unique southerly view away from the I-90 corridor.

Check the trailhead information board before beginning your hike. At an altitude of more than 4,000 feet, snow can linger in the avalanche chutes late into July and can be challenging to cross safely. Look for notes from the local rangers on this and other potential items of interest.

McClellan Butte Trail 1015 starts at an elevation of 1,600 feet at the western end of the parking lot. Almost immediately, pass under some power lines, the first of many traces of historical and modern development in this area. Within the first mile, expect to cross several more sets of power lines and gravel roads as you switchback uphill.

The second set of power lines you encounter runs through linear Iron Horse State Park. A reclaimed right-of-way from the old Chicago–Milwaukee–St. Paul–Pacific Railroad (commonly known as the Milwaukee Road), the Iron Horse stretches across most of Washington State. Snoqualmie Pass offers the easiest Cascade crossing between the Columbia River and the Canadian border, so the railway climbed the pass from the east and traveled down the Snoqualmie River Valley to Seattle just as I-90 does today.

The Milwaukee Road was converted to electricity through the Rockies in 1915 and then through the Cascades in 1917, making it the first electrified transcontinental railway in the United States. Although the tracks are long gone, the right-of-way still boasts forward-thinking technology in the form of buried fiber-optic cables underground.

McClellan Butte Trail shares 0.4 mile with John Wayne Pioneer Trail (also called Iron Horse Trail), which travels more than 100 miles through Iron Horse State Park and was named a National Millennium Legacy Trail in fall of 1999. For many, John Wayne was the physical embodiment of the spirit of the West, and this rail-trail was named after him as a tribute. Although generally pictured riding into the sunset somewhere in the desert, the Duke was actually a frequent visitor to the Pacific Northwest and enjoyed exploring the waters around the Olympic Peninsula in his boat *Wild Goose*; he eventually donated 22 acres on Sequim Bay to what is now known as the John Wayne Marina. He has fictional ties to the region as well; in the 1960 film *North to Alaska,* he portrayed Sam McCord, who visited Seattle during the gold rush era in search of his partner's girlfriend.

The shared section of the trail is well signed at both ends. As you walk the wide gravel surface, look for a marker on the right showing 2,126 miles to Chicago. Also watch for the Alice Creek camp 0.25 mile farther along (with tent platforms, picnic tables, and a toilet), one of a series of public campsites available in Iron Horse State Park. Bypass an unmarked gravel spur off to the left that leads down to Alice Creek.

Reach the second trail junction and head uphill on the hikers-only trail. The first section of the route features notched logs, water bars, bridges, and occasional steps, making the traveling easy despite the incline. Pass through some massive old-growth Douglas firs and enjoy the thick scent of cedar, which can permeate the lower forest.

Head straight across the final gravel road and begin the climb in earnest, as the trail becomes steeper and more rugged with less evidence of regular maintenance. For the next 2 miles, expect to grind up the mountain on a series of switchbacks, gradually working your way southwest. An occasional viewpoint to the left reveals I-90 below and shows how far you have come, although there is still a long way to go.

Just past the 3-mile mark, cross a series of creek beds, usually dry in summer. A glance up to the right reveals the rocky crags of the summit, which the trail skirts with a back side approach. The creek beds grow successively larger and the last few are avalanche chutes, the final one characterized by pinkish rocks. Watch for snow here, which can be dangerous to cross as you navigate the boulders and brush.

Finally, the trail bends to the right and then crests the ridge near 5,000 feet, presenting a view of Chester Morse Lake in the heart of the Cedar River Watershed. Descend for 0.25 mile to reach a subalpine bowl with views out to the west, a small meadow, and a pond. Gradually head uphill once again, passing beneath some rocky cliffs, and then emerge on the summit ridge at the end of the hikers' trail. The opposite side of the ridge drops sharply into the avalanche chutes you crossed earlier, and the northern face of Mount Rainier appears through a notch on Mount Kent to the south. The icy giant looks close enough to touch but is actually more than 40 miles away.

A rocky fin leads northeast to the true summit, 100 feet higher and laced with mountain heather. The route is a short Class 3 scramble along the right side of the ridge. But despite plenty of good holds, it is exposed, and a fall from the scramble could result in serious injury or death. If you are unsure whether this is for you, then it probably isn't.

Proceed with extreme caution and be aware of external factors, such as wet rocks or high winds, that could make the climb more dangerous.

Those continuing to the top will be rewarded with grand views on all sides and plenty of room to relax on the broad, flat boulders. Climbers or other hikers may be ascending any of the faces, so be careful not to knock anything off; you never know who is below.

The view is particularly good of the peaks just across the valley, including Mailbox, Defiance, and Bandera. Look for Mount Stuart to the northeast, poking far above the intervening ridges at 9,415 feet. Below, the tiny cars crawl past on I-90, dwarfed by the mountains.

Return the way you came, and take extra care through the scramble; going down is typically more difficult than going up.

Nearby Activities

Hiker, bikers, equestrians, cross-country skiers, and snowshoers can all take advantage of John Wayne Pioneer Trail in Iron Horse State Park to trek for virtually any distance, short or long. Multiple access points and campsites along the way allow for easy overnight travel, and attractions like the 2.3-mile Snoqualmie Tunnel add special interest. For more information, visit the Iron Horse State Park website at parks.state.wa.us/521/iron-horse.

GPS TRAILHEAD COORDINATES
N47° 24.730' W121° 35.353'

From I-90, take Exit 42 for Tinkham Road, and head south. After about 0.25 mile, go right on a short road that ascends to the official McClellan Butte Trailhead parking lot.

29 Middle Fork Snoqualmie River Trail

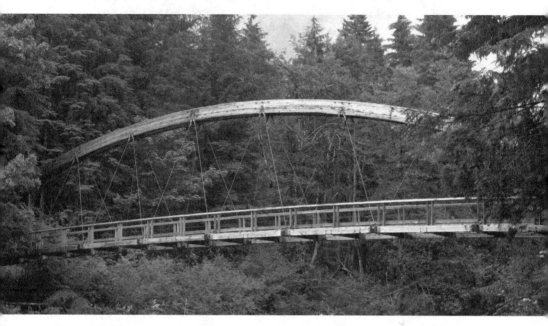

Gateway Bridge

In Brief

Middle Fork Trail reaches deep into an area that is ripe for rediscovery. After years of U.S. Forest Service neglect, the low-elevation trail has been reborn, allowing hikers to explore along the banks of the scenic Middle Fork Snoqualmie River and access much of the mountain wilderness beyond.

Description

If there is a dark side to the Alpine Lakes Wilderness, it can be found on the Middle Fork Snoqualmie River. The word *wild* describes equally well the natural environment of the mountain valley and its historical lawlessness: abandoned cars, dumped garbage, and even mobile methamphetamine labs are among the unwelcome artifacts that have appeared in the woods in the past, like a scene from *Deliverance* or *Breaking Bad.* Although these unsavory elements might have added a certain frontier authenticity to the region, not surprisingly many people decided to look elsewhere for their outdoor recreation.

149

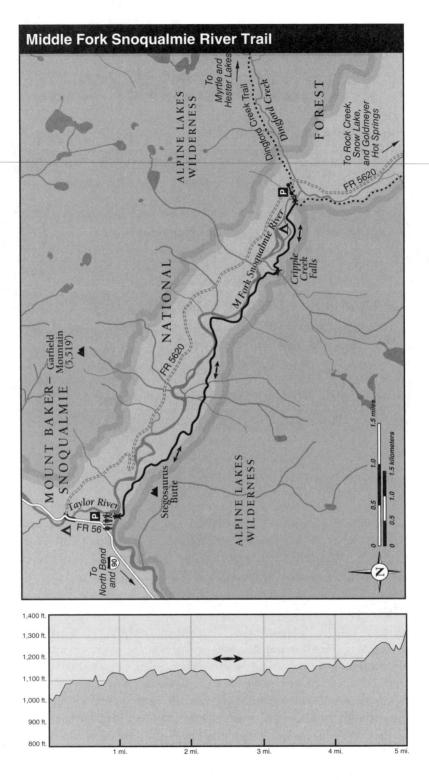

Middle Fork Snoqualmie River Trail

DISTANCE & CONFIGURATION: 6.0-mile out-and-back to river access point; 10.0-mile out-and-back to Dingford Creek	snowy in winter); NW Forest Pass required for parking
DIFFICULTY: Moderate	**WHEELCHAIR TRAVERSABLE:** No
SCENERY: Middle Fork Snoqualmie River, views of nearby peaks	**MAP(S):** Green Trails *Mount Si 174*, *Skykomish 175*, and *Snoqualmie Pass 207*; USGS *Lake Philippa*, *Snoqualmie Lake*, and *Snoqualmie Pass*
EXPOSURE: Shaded	
TRAFFIC: Medium; mountain bikers on odd-numbered days	**FACILITIES:** Toilet at trailhead; no drinking water
	DOGS: Allowed off-leash
TRAIL SURFACE: Dirt and gravel trails	**CONTACT:** 425-888-1421; www.fs.usda .gov/recarea/mbs/recarea/?recid=18006
HIKING TIME: 3–6 hours	
ACCESS: Hikable year-round (may be	**LOCATION:** North Bend

All that began to change a few years ago, when the U.S. Forest Service decided to take back the more than 100,000 acres of natural land accessible from along the river. The centerpiece of the reclamation project is the paving of the rough Middle Fork Road/ Forest Route 56. Depending on when you visit, the road could be a washboarded and rutted nightmare or a smooth, newly sealed dream.

The linear Middle Fork trail provides multiple hiking opportunities from several access points. The easiest place to begin is at the Middle Fork Trailhead (also known as the Gateway Parking Area), elevation 1,000 feet, which has already seen some significant physical development as part of the region's overall rehabilitation. The wide parking lot stands prepared to deal with the increased traffic that the road improvements are sure to bring and a drive-in campground is available on the northern side of the road near the Taylor River Confluence.

There are two trailheads at the Gateway Parking Area, but both lead to the same place, meeting 50 yards into the woods at the beautifully crafted Gateway Bridge over the Middle Fork River. The graceful bridge sports an unusual compression-arch, suspended-deck design with a single central span, and provides good views up and down the valley. On the far side, turn left and start heading upstream. The gravel singletrack soon changes to dirt as the trail runs above some walls 20 feet above the clear water. On the right side, the slope climbs steeply away to some high cliffs overhead. This is the northern side of Stegosaurus Butte, a sharp, rocky fin rising about 1,000 feet that apparently bears some resemblance to the bony plates on the back of the dinosaur for which it is named, although you will be hard-pressed to discern that from here.

The trail gradually climbs away from the river on a series of short ups and downs through a forest of mixed second-growth deciduous and coniferous trees. Big-leaf maples tower over ferns and devil's club in the underbrush, and pretty orange chanterelle mushrooms grow on some of the fallen logs and giant stumps underneath. An area of downed trees and high, upturned root wads provides a great view across the valley to

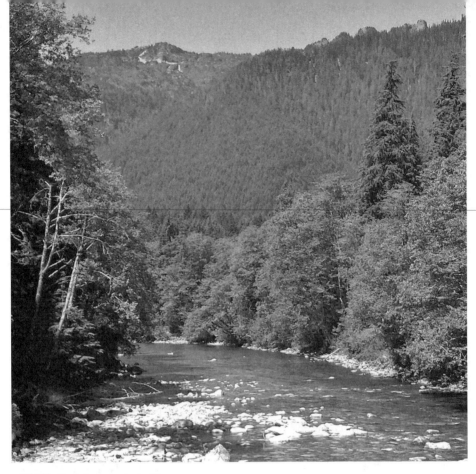

Middle Fork Snoqualmie River

the seemingly impregnable walls of Garfield Mountain (5,519') on the far side. The summit is frequently obscured by clouds billowing up the valley.

The trail flirts with the riverbank for another mile, sometimes close to the edge and other times far above it. Although the trail seems to follow an excessively circuitous route, it actually takes a reasonably direct line; the deep bends and oxbows of the river cause the frequent separation. Views of Garfield come and go through the trees.

About 3 miles from the trailhead, you'll reach a clearing on the river's edge at an elevation of approximately 1,100 feet. The small open space makes a good place to stop, rest, and enjoy the view. A wide field of white rocks sits on the riverbed on the opposite side, and some high cliffs are visible upstream, the abrupt terminus of the far northeastern ridge of Preacher Mountain (5,924') to the south. The clearing is a little past the halfway point between the Middle Fork and Dingford Creek Trailheads and can potentially make a good turnaround point for a 6-mile out-and-back from Middle Fork or a slightly shorter trip from Dingford Creek.

Pass beneath the cliffs and continue almost another mile to a bridge over a thundering falls on the right. Huge boulders and logs sit in the stream, known as Cripple Creek, fed by a cluster of alpine lakes far above in a bowl bounded by the eastern shoulder of Preacher Mountain and the northern side of Mount Roosevelt.

Another mile through the forest brings you to a spur trail on the left, heading sharply downhill to an undeveloped campsite. Soon after, look for a sign pointing to the left at a junction for Middle Fork Road and Dingford Creek Trail. The main Middle Fork Trail continues to follow the river upstream straight ahead, bound for Wildcat Creek about a mile away, Rock Creek and Snow Lake Trail another 0.5 mile beyond that, and the privately owned Goldmyer Hot Springs still another few miles distant. The hot springs mark the end of the Middle Fork Road, although the trail itself continues on to eventually reach Dutch Miller Gap below Summit Chief Mountain.

From the junction, turn left to reach a sturdy bridge over the river, then climb up the far bank to reach the end at Dingford Creek Trailhead on FR 56. Note that if you are running a shuttle and need to leave a vehicle here or you have decided to start hiking from this point, this trailhead is not well marked. Look for a turnout on the right side of the road just before the bridge over Dingford Creek Falls.

For a point-to-point hike between the trailheads, there is a small elevation advantage to starting at Dingford Creek, which is 400 feet above Middle Fork. However, the many short climbs and drops along the way are likely to eliminate any feeling of overall net elevation gain or loss in either direction.

Options abound for alternate ways to experience Middle Fork Trail and the surrounding Alpine Lakes Wilderness. From Dingford Creek, hikers can continue up Middle Fork Trail as mentioned earlier or tackle the tough climb on the northern side of the road on Dingford Creek Trail, which rises 3,000 feet to Myrtle and Hester Lakes, 5 miles distant.

It's also possible to return to the Taylor River Trailhead on FR 56 via mountain bike, an option that is likely to remain viable even if the road becomes gated and closed to motor vehicle traffic somewhere along the way. In fact, the U.S. Forest Service decided in 2003 to allow mountain bikes on Middle Fork Trail itself on odd-numbered calendar days, which makes a loop ride combining the trail and road a great option if you time your visit accordingly.

GPS TRAILHEAD COORDINATES
N47° 32.853' W121° 32.238'

From I-90, take Exit 34 for 486th Avenue SE, and head north, proceeding through the Edgewick "Truck Town" area. In 0.5 mile, turn right onto SE Middle Fork Road, which becomes Forest Route 56. Continue 11.6 miles to the signed Middle Fork Trailhead and parking area on the right. To reach the alternate Dingford Creek Trailhead, go 0.5 mile past Middle Fork Trailhead, and turn right onto FR 110, which becomes FR 5620. The road is rough beyond the Middle Fork Trailhead, so a high-clearance vehicle is recommended. In 5.3 miles the small parking area and trailhead are located on the right, just before the bridge over Dingford Creek.

30 Mount Si

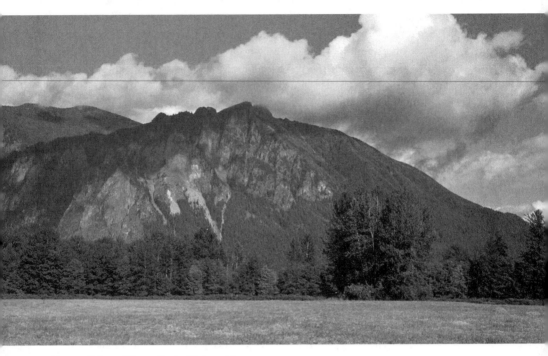

Mount Si from Three Forks Natural Area

In Brief

Just as no tourist can claim to have seen downtown Seattle without a visit to Pike Place Market, there is no such thing as a Seattle hiker who hasn't been to the top of Mount Si. Easy to reach, physically challenging, and capped by a commanding view, the mountain known simply as Si is like a city park crossed with a serious Cascade Mountain peak.

Description

Mount Si is crowned by the Haystack, a rock outcrop boosting the summit elevation by about 200 feet and providing a significant visual landmark for much of the Puget Sound region. This landmark apparently works as a beacon, summoning people from all over western Washington on weekends year-round. No matter what season they come, the hikers who are drawn here keep the giant parking lot busy for most of the day, no easy feat given that Mount Si has room for at least 150 vehicles.

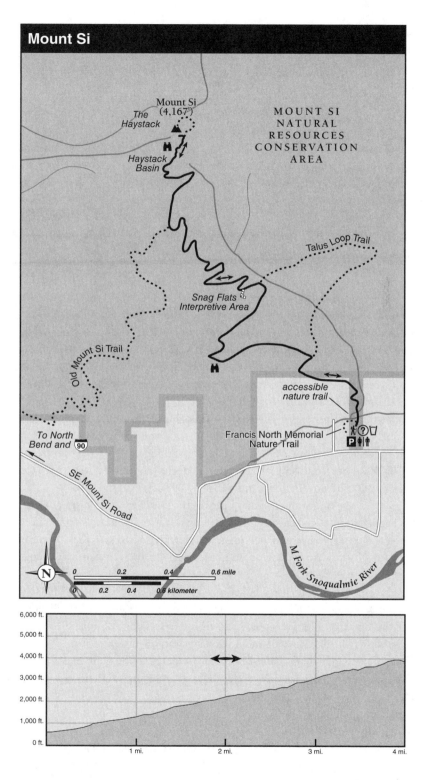

DISTANCE & CONFIGURATION: 8.0-mile out-and-back	**HIKING TIME:** 4–7 hours
DIFFICULTY: Difficult hike, optional exposed-rock scramble	**ACCESS:** Hikable year-round (may be snowy or icy in winter); Discover Pass required for parking
SCENERY: One of the best western views from the Cascade foothills to the Puget Sound lowlands, great rock scramble to summit of the Haystack	**WHEELCHAIR TRAVERSABLE:** Yes, on Francis North Trail
	MAP(S): Green Trails *Mount Si NRCA 206S*; USGS *Mount Si* and *Chester Morse Lake*
EXPOSURE: Mostly shaded; exposed in Haystack Basin and on the Haystack	**FACILITIES:** Toilet and water at trailhead
TRAFFIC: High; get an early start or hike midweek	**DOGS:** Allowed on-leash
TRAIL SURFACE: Mostly dirt, boardwalk (at Snag Flat), gravel (near trailhead)	**CONTACT:** 206-375-3558; dnr.wa.gov /MountSi
	LOCATION: North Bend

It's a safe bet that hikers do not come to Si to find solitude in the outdoors. Yet what they do find is a great hike, enjoyed by everyone from extended families with young children to mountaineers in training and hard-core trail runners chasing serious vertical gain.

The trailhead can be found past the last row of cars in the northeast corner of the parking lot, at an elevation of 500 feet. It is worth filling up with water from the public tap because there is no treated water available anywhere else along the way and the top is 4 miles up the trail—with a 3,500-foot climb.

Before the trail proper, a wheelchair-accessible loop trail, a memorial to Francis North, runs 0.2 mile off the main trail. Look for a plaque detailing North's committed efforts toward the protection of Mount Si in the Washington State Legislature in the late 1970s. Thanks to her leadership, the region was declared a Natural Resources Conservation Area in 1987 and now includes more than 20,000 acres of land.

A bench at the end of the side loop provides a last chance for rest before the climb begins. Thanks to its popularity and the continual labor of volunteers and maintenance crews, the trail is well worn and well maintained, with graded stairs and water bars as it ascends through the woods. The uphill grade is steady and constant with long switchbacks, but never too steep.

The low-elevation forest is characterized by tall second-growth Douglas firs with high canopies, giving the understory an open, airy feeling. Watch for a small wooden sign marking the first 0.5 mile, elevation 1,120 feet. These signs are posted every 0.5 mile, although they can be hard to spot and do not always show the elevation.

Short of the 1-mile mark, Talus Loop Trail branches to the right, heading uphill. The Talus Loop traverses several small creek valleys draining the southern side of the mountain and can provide an alternate route over the next mile, although adding slightly to the total distance. Along the main trail, look for a viewpoint over a cliff at a great resting spot after a long traverse to the west.

Talus Loop Trail returns to the main Mount Si Trail at a signed junction just short of Snag Flats. Appropriately named, the flats is the only significant level section of the hike,

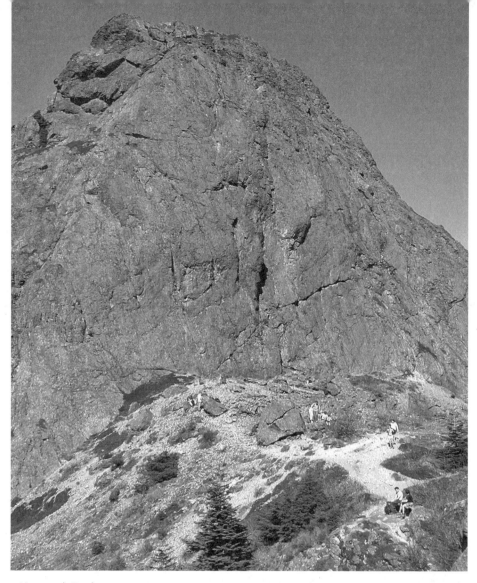

Haystack Rock

making it a good spot for a rest. A short interpretive trail explores the area's namesake snags, describing the forest and its wildlife, on a boardwalk that keeps hikers above the frequently muddy ground. Pileated woodpeckers are common here; they hammer the decaying trees in search of insects.

The climb begins again in earnest on the far side of Snag Flats, rising through a series of switchbacks over the next 1.5 miles and gradually becoming rockier near the end. By the time the 3-mile mark is reached, the trees have become noticeably thinner and shorter, stunted by the harsher climate at the higher elevation.

A viewpoint finally opens to the right after another 0.5 mile, revealing Mailbox Peak, the Snoqualmie River Valley, and Mount Rainier to the south. The trail then climbs through rocks and salal in its steepest section before emerging from the trees into a jumble of boulders.

It is not unusual to find scores of hikers relaxing here, enjoying the southern view and exposure to the sun that comes with it. The trail continues upward through the rocks, requiring an occasional moment of route finding or scrambling. Concrete added in a few spots to create stairs, and boot-polished stone to show the way, make the going easy enough for everyone.

The trail branches at a sign, showing Snoqualmie Valley Viewpoint to the left and the Haystack Scramble to the right. For most Mount Si hikers, the effective summit is the wide bowl known as Haystack Basin to the left, whose views to the west and south are nothing short of spectacular. The name Snoqualmie Valley Viewpoint does not even begin to describe the view, which stretches far beyond the Snoqualmie River Valley to include downtown Seattle, Puget Sound, the Olympic Peninsula, and much of the southern Cascades, including Mount Rainier. It is worth poking around in the rocks to find an ideal spot to relax, as there is plenty of space to accommodate everyone.

The Haystack towers above the northern end of the basin, seemingly out of reach thanks to its sheer, daunting cliffs. However, experienced scramblers can reach the top via an easy Class 3 route on the rock's eastern face, starting from the end of the hiking trail. The ascent is not for beginners or children, but it has plenty of good, obvious holds, so qualified climbers should have no difficulty reaching the top. The view from Mount Si's true summit at 4,167 feet adds a northern aspect to what can be seen from the basin, including the high summits of Mount Baker and Glacier Peak, but adjacent Mount Teneriffe at 4,788 feet blocks sight lines to the northeast and keeps the view from being truly panoramic.

Nearby Activities

Twede's Cafe, immortalized in David Lynch's TV show *Twin Peaks* as the T-Mar Cafe, where FBI Special Agent Dale Cooper came to get his cherry pie, lies on the southeast corner of the Bendigo Boulevard/WA 202 and North Bend Way intersection in the town of North Bend. The retro 1950s-style diner features 40 different burgers—and that's just for starters. Find more information at twedescafe.com or 425-831-5511.

You could also do this hike as a shuttle. Park one car at Little Si (see page 135), and add 5 miles to your hike by taking the Old Mount Si Trail to the summit, returning via Mount Si Trail.

GPS TRAILHEAD COORDINATES
N47° 29.228' W121° 43.383'

From I-90, take Exit 32 and head north on 436th Avenue SE. In 0.5 mile turn left onto SE North Bend Way, and then in 0.3 mile turn right onto SE Mount Si Road. Continue 2.4 miles on this road to a well-signed parking lot on the left for the Mount Si Trailhead.

31 Mount Teneriffe and Teneriffe Falls

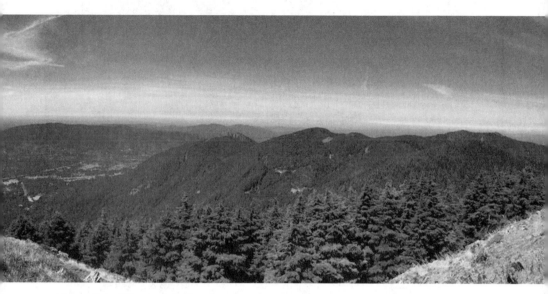

Mount Teneriffe summit view

In Brief

Rising above Mount Si's eastern shoulder, Mount Teneriffe tops its popular neighbor by several hundred feet and presents similarly grand views, stretching from the Puget Sound lowlands to the high crags of the Central Cascades. A stunning (although seasonal) waterfall along the way makes a great destination by itself.

Description

Mount Teneriffe has long escaped the notice of many Seattle hikers, despite being highly visible from the busy summit of Mount Si and having a trailhead just up the road. With Si's ever-growing popularity, the attractions of the peak next door deserve wider attention.

Starting in 2005, the Washington Department of Natural Resources (DNR) made significant upgrades to the Mount Si Natural Resources Conservation Area (NRCA), most visibly with three big parking lots at Mount Si and Little Si and extensive trail renovations. Yet there is still occasional overflow from these lots on busy summer weekends, to say nothing of the hordes frequently encountered on the trails. Further

159

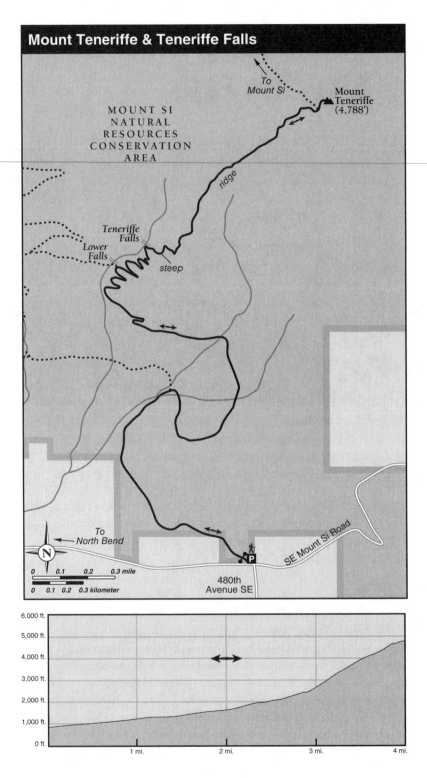

DISTANCE & CONFIGURATION: 5.6-mile out-and-back to falls; 8.0-mile out-and-back to summit	**TRAIL SURFACE:** Dirt trails, rocky in places
	HIKING TIME: 5–8 hours
DIFFICULTY: Moderate to falls; difficult to summit (4,000' elevation gain and rough trail)	**ACCESS:** Hikable late spring–early fall; Discover Pass required for parking
	WHEELCHAIR TRAVERSABLE: No
SCENERY: Waterfall (seasonal), 360-degree views from summit, forested trails	**MAP(S):** Green Trails *Mount Si NRCA 206S*; USGS *Mount Si* and *Chester Morse Lake*
	FACILITIES: None
	DOGS: Allowed on-leash
EXPOSURE: Shaded most of the way, final approach to summit is exposed	**CONTACT:** 206-375-3558; dnr.wa.gov /MountSi
TRAFFIC: Low–medium	**LOCATION:** North Bend

attempting to mitigate hiker impact, DNR now actively encourages visitors to consider heading for other nearby destinations.

As part of the upgrade effort, DNR also made some modest improvements at Mount Teneriffe (contained in the NRCA), adding new signage and replacing a section of a difficult climbers' route with some easier switchbacks. Although these improvements didn't receive much fanfare, they have considerably improved the hiker experience. Thanks to its new face-lift and the opportunity it provides to literally look down on everyone at Mount Si, Teneriffe has gained a lot of appeal.

Unfortunately, the trailhead parking for Mount Teneriffe is still cramped, and local space restrictions probably prevent it from ever getting much bigger, no matter what DNR would like. There is only room for about 10 vehicles along the road here, so it still pays to arrive early. And, as at many other trailheads, shattered glass on the ground tells a sad story about recent break-ins, so be sure to remove valuables from your car.

The trail starts at about 860 feet of elevation and begins on an old logging road behind a large locked gate. Climb through the forest on an easy uphill slope for about a mile, then look for a signed right turn onto another road at elevation 1,190 feet. The sign reads TENERIFFE FALLS TRAIL and was part of the recent DNR work. In addition to showing the way, the sign also helps cement local nomenclature; Teneriffe Falls was once informally known as Kamikaze Falls, a name shared through popular word of mouth.

After making the turn, continue uphill through the woods. A few giant stumps among the ferns in the understory reveal the logging history of the area. Ignore several side trails that branch off to the right and stay on the main road. Despite some stones, the surface is good for hiking; smooth and fast, with continued moderate climbing.

Just above 1,400 feet, the road takes a general turn to the left, contouring to the west for about half a mile. A few glimpses of the valley below begin to show through the trees, including the buildings at the Edgewick "Truck Town" area and the curved lines of I-90.

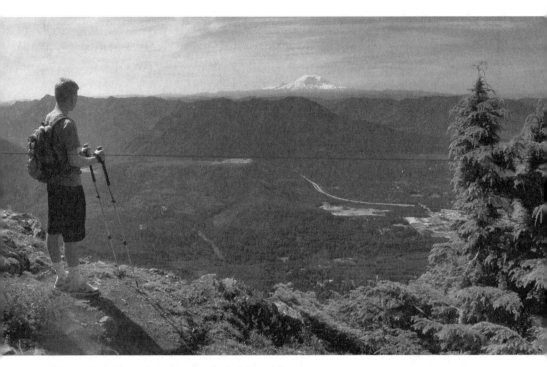

Mount Rainier and the Snoqualmie River Valley

A prominent switchback leads into a rocky section and the start of more serious climbing as the logging road fades to a singletrack trail. Cross an open rockslide section with short cliff bands visible above and a nice view of Rattlesnake Mountain across the I-90 corridor. By 2,000 feet, the top of Mount Rainier starts to poke above Mount Washington and McClellan Butte on the far side of the Snoqualmie River Valley.

Another 200 feet of climbing lead to Lower Teneriffe Falls, where the water tumbles down through a long series of stones. This section of the falls is best described as a cascade since there is no large, single pour off. Although the creek often rages through here in a mess of whitewater, some summers it may have very little flow or even dry up and disappear altogether. Its seasonal nature explains why this prominent landmark is absent from some area maps.

From here, the old climbers' route is visible, headed straight up the slope next to the creek. The new switchbacks lead to the same destination but on an easier grade just to the right.

Follow the short climb to a viewpoint on the left for Upper Teneriffe Falls, where the water pours over an exposed rock face in a true plunge drop. Mist and spray sweep through the trees, either refreshing or chilling, depending on the conditions.

This point marks the end of the improved trail and is a good turnaround spot for a moderate day hike. For those seeking more challenge and the commensurate reward of the sweeping views from the summit, trudge uphill on the continuation of the old climbers' trail. Roots, rocks, mud, gravel, and many other obstacles underfoot will hinder your progress, and expect to use trees and other nearby natural features as handholds for assistance.

After 400 feet of climbing in a deceptively short distance, emerge to an obvious saddle at 2,800 feet. To your right an exposed rock outcrop makes a nice rest area, although any view is blocked by tall trees on all sides. The trail continues uphill to the left, just as steep as the previous section.

The good news is you have now attained the long ridge that leads to the summit. The bad news is there are almost 2,000 feet of climbing remaining over the last mile, a mostly grueling ascent. The rough nature of the climbers' trail continues as you mount the rocky ridge. In some areas the steepness relents slightly but in others once again expect to use your hands for occasional support.

At about 4,300 feet, enter an area where the forest thins to a carpet of ferns. The sudden view includes the east face of Mount Si, whose crowning Haystack tops out at 4,167 feet. Surprisingly, you are now well above this famous point.

But now is no time to rest because the Teneriffe summit is within reach. A junction with a wider, better trail descending to the left shows you are moments from the top. This other trail heads west along the ridge, eventually reaching Si by a sparsely used back door.

Stay right for another 40 yards then clamber up the rocks immediately on the right to reach the Mount Teneriffe summit at 4,788 feet. On a clear day, the 360-degree view encompasses the distant high volcanoes of Mount Baker and Glacier Peak to the north and Mount Rainier dominating the skyline to the south. To the west, it is possible to make out the skyscrapers of downtown Seattle and Bellevue and the crest of the Olympic Mountains beyond. Mailbox Peak is the nearest landmark to the southeast, only 53 feet higher than where you now stand and easily identifiable by its distinctive pyramidal shape on the other side of the Middle Fork Snoqualmie River.

Away to the northeast, a sea of rugged mountains in the Central Cascades reaches to the horizon. Even with a compass and good topographic map, it would be a considerable challenge to identify them all.

Linger at this excellent vantage point as long as time allows, and then return down the way you came. Take special care in the steep sections above the falls as it is easy to lose your footing in the loose dirt and rocks.

GPS TRAILHEAD COORDINATES
N47° 29.160' W121° 42.052'

From I-90, take Exit 32 and head north on 436th Avenue SE. In 0.5 mile turn left onto SE North Bend Way, and then in 0.3 mile turn right onto SE Mount Si Road. Continue 3.5 miles on this road to a gated, gravel road on the left (1.0 mile past the Mount Si Trailhead parking lot). There is only room for about 10 cars at the Teneriffe trailhead, so arrive early.

32 Rattlesnake Ledge and Rattlesnake Mountain

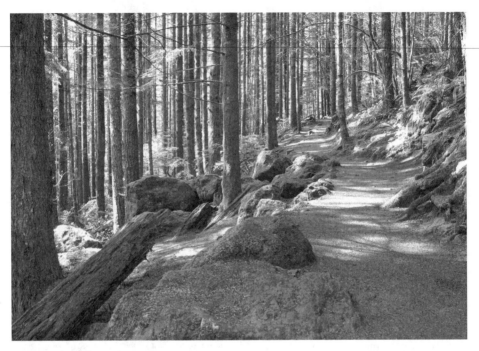

The trail climbing through trees

In Brief

Long a popular outing for its proximity to Seattle and commanding views of the Snoqualmie Valley, Rattlesnake Ledge is a well-known hiker's destination. Far less traveled, however, are the trails that continue past the ledge up onto Rattlesnake Mountain and stretch almost 10 miles along its broad summit ridge. For two excellent trip options, either climb to Rattlesnake Ledge if you have just a few hours, or head to the solitude of the East Peak and return for a full day's hike.

Description

In 1911 Seattle closed off the Cedar River Watershed to protect the city's primary source of drinking water, established 22 years earlier, in 1889. For almost a century since, careful stewardship of the pristine waters and surrounding land has seen the area largely

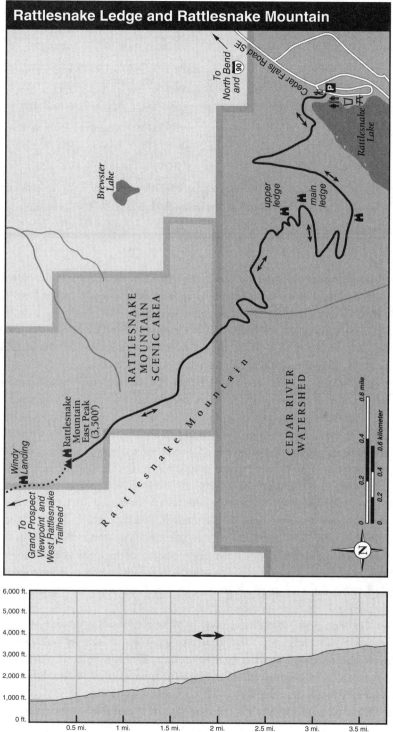

Rattlesnake Ledge and Rattlesnake Mountain

DISTANCE & CONFIGURATION: 4.0-mile out-and-back to the ledge; 8.8-mile out-and-back to East Peak	sunrise–sunset, though Rattlesnake Mountain may be snow-covered in winter; no fee for parking or trail access
DIFFICULTY: Moderate–difficult	**WHEELCHAIR TRAVERSABLE:** No
SCENERY: Forest, views	**MAP(S):** Green Trails *Rattlesnake*
EXPOSURE: Mostly shaded	*Mountain 205S*; USGS *North Bend*
TRAFFIC: High on trail to ledge; trail beyond sees fewer hikers	**FACILITIES:** Toilets near the Rattlesnake Lake parking area
TRAIL SURFACE: Dirt	**DOGS:** Allowed on-leash
HIKING TIME: 2–6 hours (depending on how far you travel from the trailhead)	**CONTACT:** 206-477-4527; dnr.wa.gov /RattlesnakeMountain
ACCESS: Hikable year-round, daily,	**LOCATION:** North Bend

undisturbed, leaving a semiwilderness right on the doorstep of the now-developed town of North Bend. The elk that occasionally wander through residents' yards are a testament to the still-untamed nature of the protected region.

The trails on Rattlesnake Mountain skirt the edge of the Cedar River Watershed and allow the public to get as close to the area as possible without special access. An education center lies along the southern side of Rattlesnake Lake on Cedar Falls Road; it provides information on the natural and human history of the region along with an overview of many of the issues surrounding water storage and use and can easily be reached via a lakeshore trail that originates at the parking lot and is open to foot traffic and bicycles.

The ample parking area is well developed and offers special lots for boat trailers and handicapped access. Many visitors come only to spend a day at the edge of the lake for a barbecue and swim, or to paddle a canoe on the water. No overnight camping is allowed, though, and the gates are closed and locked each night at 9:30.

The crowds of today are no anomaly; this area has seen regular human use for close to 10,000 years, starting when the first American Indians arrived. Establishing routes around what was then a tallgrass prairie, they came from nearby settlements in search of berries, herbs, animals, and fish. Although the source of the Rattlesnake name remains unknown, it may date back to these early inhabitants. The lake remains an important site for modern American Indians and is stocked with rainbow trout for anglers, under standard Washington State regulations.

The hikers-only trail starts as a gravel road from the southwest side of the parking lot; it's marked with a large sign. Note that although the trail is never hard to find or follow, the signage is often inconsistent and inaccurate. The information board and map by the lakeshore fail to show any of the Rattlesnake Mountain trails beyond the ledge, and distances tend to be underestimated.

Find the true trailhead a few minutes along the gravel road to the right. From this point, it is 2 miles one-way to Rattlesnake Ledge and a climb of 1,175 feet. Several signs here also give conflicting information, so look for the newest ones, which show the correct distance. Similar signs along the way correctly mark each 0.5 mile to the ledge.

The trail starts on a gradual climb through a forest of moss-covered trees and ferns, with the occasional boulder or stump along the way. The Douglas firs are particularly impressive here, some more than 100 feet tall with diameters of less than 4 feet. Their lack of low-level branches yields a pleasing display of strong vertical lines. The well-worn trail continues to gain altitude as it leads through a series of broad switchbacks up the slope.

Immediately before the 1-mile mark, a viewpoint opens out to the left, revealing views deep into the watershed protected area. Rattlesnake Lake and the education center appear to the southwest, with Mount Lindsay beyond.

A short downhill section follows, the only relief from the relentless climb. NO TRESPASSING signs hang on some of the trees on the side of the trail to mark the watershed boundary. A few more long switchbacks lead to a signed junction with a map.

The fork to the right leads to Rattlesnake Ledge, just a few steps away at an elevation of 2,080 feet. Even if you plan to head farther up the mountain, the ledge should not be missed. Considered the eastern terminus of the Issaquah Alps, the rocky ledge has a commanding view of almost 270 degrees, including the entire lower Snoqualmie Valley. Rattlesnake Lake and distant Chester Morse Lake sparkle below Cedar Butte and Mount Washington.

This is a great place to sun yourself on a rock and enjoy the view; arrive in the morning to take advantage of the southeastern-facing aspect. However, be careful of your footing, especially when hiking with children, as a deep chasm runs through the center of the ledge and cliffs drop off on all sides.

After visiting the ledge, return to the nearby junction. From here, you can descend the way you came or continue up the Rattlesnake Mountain summit ridge. The East Peak and Tower Viewpoint are another 2.4 miles distant and a climb of an additional 1,400 feet. For the truly fit or adventurous, the trail continues beyond the East Peak for another 2.7 miles to Grand Prospect viewpoint and another 4.7 miles to the west Rattlesnake Mountain Trailhead. With a shuttle, the entire ridge from the eastern trailhead at the lake to the new western trailhead makes a great long traverse of approximately 11 miles.

The climb up the ridge immediately becomes steeper, harder, and narrower, a true trail compared with the broad conduit from the lake. Underfoot, packed earth and mud give way to sections of exposed rocks and roots. Far fewer people venture this way, so with just a few steps you'll leave most of the crowd behind.

In less than 0.25 mile, a spur leads to an obvious viewpoint to the right on a precipitous outcrop. The elevation here is close to 2,200 feet, providing a view of Rattlesnake Ledge just below.

Resume the uphill slog through a long tangle of salal. On a dewy morning, passage through this section can leave you soaked from the waist down, so be prepared for wetness. Persevere through the thick growth and enjoy the occasional view out to either side of the ridge. You will notice that the forest here is much less uniform than it is down below, with sudden changes in density and types of trees. Some areas are particularly damp and dark with thick decay underneath.

Ironically, although the upper section of Rattlesnake Mountain sees far fewer visitors than the area just above the lake, it nonetheless displays greater evidence of human activity. More than once you will encounter a network of dirt roads feeding some borrow pits (small, quarry-like excavations where material such as gravel is extracted for use as fill elsewhere) scattered along the ridge. However, the correct way is marked with arrows, and a large wooden sign is at the most confusing intersection, where you need to cross a road. Look for the trail to Snoqualmie Point, another name for the western trailhead, and enter a dark forest of short pines.

Almost immediately you will cross the road a second time and then emerge at the East Peak. A bench on the left below another trail sign (which understates the distance you have just traveled from the lake) marks the spot. Make a sharp turn to the right to reach two radio towers on the 3,500-foot summit. Unfortunately, tower access is prohibited, so you will have to enjoy the view from ground level only.

There is no single point here that provides a panoramic view, so explore the area to look through various gaps in the trees. An even larger tower facility can be seen to the northwest, marking Prospect Point farther along the ridge. A broad valley opens to the west and south, leading down to a corner of Puget Sound.

The best view, out to the north, is conveniently provided by a second wooden bench. The landmark Mount Si dominates the head of the valley, with some of the more-jagged Cascade Mountain peaks looming above the other end. In between, I-90 climbs toward Snoqualmie Pass. Traffic on the highway can be seen and heard, but it seems far away, some 2,700 feet below.

Enjoy the view from the bench, a great place for a snack and a drink of water. Relax here for a while before heading back down.

Nearby Activities

To reach the western Rattlesnake Mountain Trailhead at Snoqualmie Point, take I-90 E to Exit 27. Turn right at the end of the ramp and head up the hill to where the road ends at the trailhead parking lot. If you're not up for the full mountain traverse, a good day-hike destination from here is Stan's Overlook, a round-trip of about 5.4 miles and a climb of 1,100 feet.

GPS TRAILHEAD COORDINATES

N47° 26.159' W121° 46.071'

From I-90, take Exit 32 for 436th Avenue SE, and head south. The road becomes Cedar Falls Road and winds 3.0 miles to a large sign for Rattlesnake Lake; turn right off Cedar Falls Road here. Immediately make another right into a parking lot signed RATTLESNAKE LEDGE TRAIL PARKING. If this lot is full, there are many more spaces in the southern lot next to the lake.

33 Twin Falls Natural Area and Olallie State Park

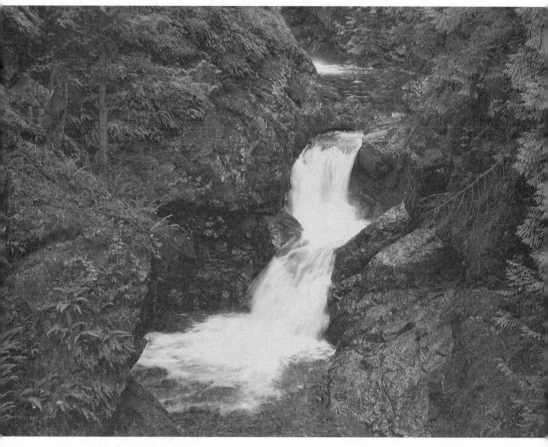

Upper Twin Falls

In Brief

Located well below 2,000 feet and just off I-90, Twin Falls makes a great year-round destination, especially when winter snows close many of the hikes farther up toward Snoqualmie Pass. This hike follows the rocky South Fork Snoqualmie River and climbs to two significant waterfalls before connecting to a larger network of trails exploring Olallie State Park.

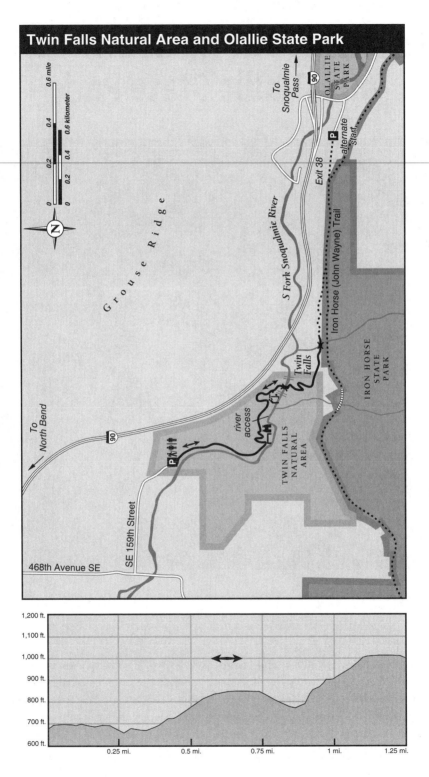

Twin Falls Natural Area and Olallie State Park

DISTANCE & CONFIGURATION: 2.5-mile out-and-back or longer

DIFFICULTY: Moderate

SCENERY: Waterfalls, old-growth trees, river viewpoints, riverside access

EXPOSURE: Shaded

TRAFFIC: Moderate–heavy; many dogs on this hike; go midweek for less traffic

TRAIL SURFACE: Dirt (gravel on Iron Horse Trail)

HIKING TIME: 2–3 hours

ACCESS: Hikable year-round, summer: daily, 6:30 a.m.–sunset; winter: daily, 8 a.m.–sunset; Discover Pass required for parking

WHEELCHAIR TRAVERSABLE: No

MAP(S): Green Trails *Mount Si NRCA 206S*; USGS *Chester Morse Lake*

FACILITIES: Toilets but no water at both trailheads

DOGS: Allowed on-leash

CONTACT: 425-455-7010; parks.state .wa.us/555/Olallie

LOCATION: North Bend

Description

Mention Seattle and the first thing people think of is rain. The city is almost universally identified as one of the wettest places anywhere in the United States, despite the persistent efforts of the Washington State Tourism Department to dispel this image; travelers are invited to the Emerald City with the lure of only 36 inches of annual rainfall, less than such so-called dry places as New York (47 inches) or Atlanta (48 inches). And don't tell the sunbathers and scantily clad club-hoppers at famous South Beach, but the joke is on them: Miami receives 59 inches a year, some 50% more than Seattle.

The difference is that, where other cities receive most of their rain in concentrated downpours, Seattle usually sees mist and drizzle that lasts for days but doesn't add up to much, leaving endlessly cloudy skies for nine months out of the year—almost 300 days, on average—but limited total rainfall accumulations. Just 30 miles east, however, the region lives up to its reputation.

The lower western slope of the Cascades is probably the second-wettest place in the state, trailing only the western side of the Olympic Peninsula. Although no match for the Hoh Rain Forest (at 140 inches per year), the Twin Falls region gets more than 90 inches, 2.5 times as much as downtown Seattle. The heavy clouds from the Gulf of Alaska that sweep over the city, keeping it gray but relatively dry, get trapped by the mountains and dump their precipitation here.

However, the rain is not evenly distributed throughout the year, falling primarily in the winter and going through wide seasonal variations. In turn, the South Fork Snoqualmie River rises and wanes as well, showing a remarkable range between the flow at low and high water.

According to the U.S. Geological Survey gauge at Edgewick, the river in this area reached an all-time record-low flow on September 28, 2001—172 gallons of water per second. The record high occurred on November 24, 1990, at 80,790 gallons per second, a volume almost 470 times greater. Although this is a comparison between extreme values, fluctuations within the year also show amazing disparities. The flow on January 31, 2003, reached 44,359 gallons per second, 141 times the 314 gallons per second recorded on September 6 that year. Even day-to-day readings can oscillate wildly; November 18, 2002, saw 1,571 gallons per second, but 14,288 the next day, and then the flow fell back over the next week to less than 1,500. All of this occurs in a drainage area of less than 65 square miles.

The character of Twin Falls is naturally dependent on the flow of the river. At high-water periods, typically in late winter and spring, expect to see a single thundering torrent. The low water of late summer and fall presents a much more peaceful display, as the falls split into several separate braids. This hike may well warrant several trips at different times of the year to appreciate the full range of experiences available.

The trail starts out winding along the bank of the river. When the flow is suitable, watch for whitewater kayakers who come here to hone their skills by "play boating" sometimes only a stone's throw from the parking lot. About 0.25 mile along, some big boulders shelter several potential swimming holes.

Licorice and sword ferns testify to the volume of rain that falls here, but the thick canopy created by the tall Douglas firs can keep the worst of it from reaching the ground, making this a better option than it would seem for hiking during the frequently questionable weather.

Climb through a few long switchbacks to arrive at a high point with a handrail and some benches. The benches face out toward the lower falls, offering a view that's best in winter when the leaves have fallen from the nearby trees to provide a clear line of sight. Continue down the far side of the ridge and stay left at a junction to reach a giant old-growth fir that dwarfs the trees around it. This is the first of several such trees, true forest outliers in terms of their monumental size, scattered along the trail.

Another short climb brings you to a set of wooden steps on the right, leading down to an overlook. A fenced platform provides a great straight-on view of the lower falls, where the river is channeled through a narrow gap in the basalt and then spills out over a rocky face, tumbling into a pool below.

Continue another few hundred yards up the main trail to reach a boardwalk and bridge over the river. This bridge crosses just above the lower falls and provides a good view of the multiple stages of the upper falls, a series of plunge pools dropping through a narrow chasm. A curtain of mist billowing around the corner hints at the top level of the falls, which unfortunately are very difficult to observe from anywhere on the trail.

The bridge makes a good endpoint, for a total of 2.5 miles round-trip when you reach the parking lot. For a longer hike, continue on the far side of the river for about 0.5 mile to reach a junction with gravel Iron Horse Trail. Although this section of the trail is pleasant and well maintained, it rises far enough above the river gorge to be exposed to the sound of the traffic on I-90. It's so close, in fact, that occasional glimpses of asphalt and cars appear through the trees.

Adventurous hikers can continue eastward along the Iron Horse for several miles into the heart of Olallie State Park. This extended hike would make an excellent one-way journey with a shuttle; a trailhead is located at Exit 38, to the right off I-90.

GPS TRAILHEAD COORDINATES

N47° 27.157' W121° 42.316'

From I-90, take Exit 34 and head south on 468th Avenue SE. In 0.7 mile, turn left onto SE 159th Street. The parking lot for Twin Falls Natural Area is at the end of this road in 0.6 mile.

For the alternate Olallie State Park trailhead, take Exit 38 and head south. In 0.1 mile, take the first right into the signed Twin Falls and Iron Horse Trail parking area.

KITSAP PENINSULA AND THE ISLANDS

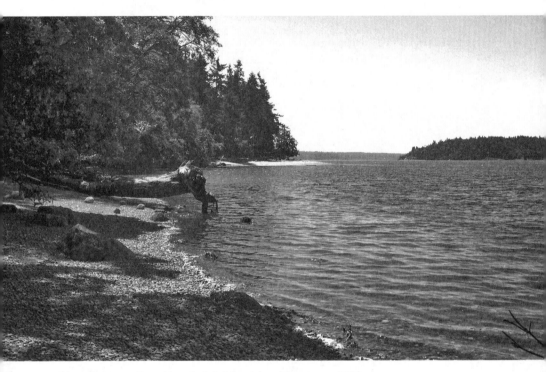

Close Property Beach on Bainbridge Island (see page 176)

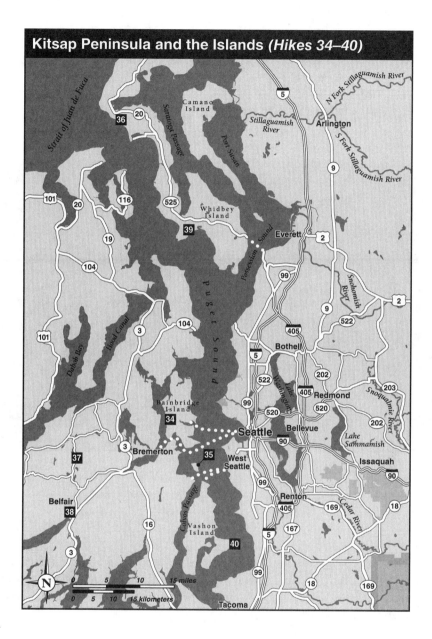

Kitsap Peninsula and the Islands *(Hikes 34–40)*

34 Bainbridge Island:
GAZZAM LAKE
NATURE PRESERVE

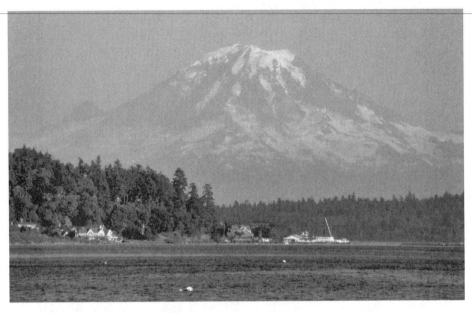

Mount Rainier from Pleasant Beach

In Brief

This diverse hike links three areas: Pleasant Beach, Gazzam Lake Nature Preserve, and Close Property Beach, creating several hiking opportunities. Together they provide a great introduction to the natural environment of Bainbridge, exploring two shorelines and the lowland forest at the island's center.

Description

Bainbridge is only a short ferry ride away, beckoning to downtown Seattle from across the sound. Hordes of tourists make the trip during the warmer months, venturing to the island to enjoy the charms and attractions of the town of Winslow. On a summer's evening, the passage can be nothing short of spectacular, with amazing views of glittering skyscrapers and Mount Rainier during the golden hour before sunset.

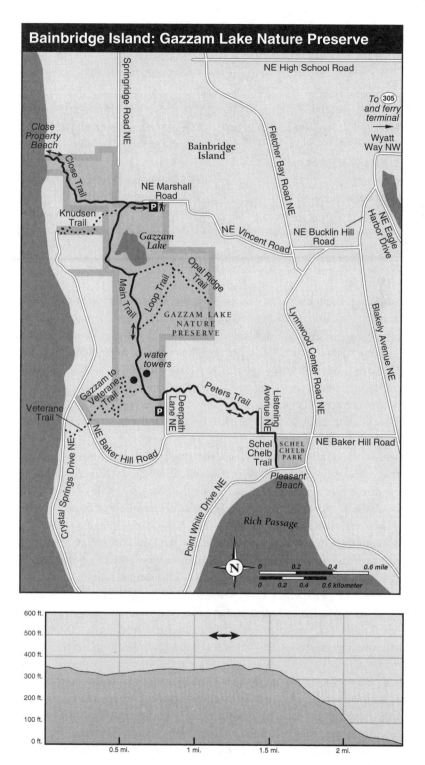

Bainbridge Island: Gazzam Lake Nature Preserve

NE High School Road

Springridge Road NE

To (305) *and ferry terminal*

Wyatt Way NW

Close Property Beach

Bainbridge Island

Fletcher Bay Road NE

Close Trail

NE Marshall Road

P

Knudsen Trail

NE Vincent Road

NE Bucklin Hill Road

NE Eagle Harbor Drive

Gazzam Lake

Opal Ridge Trail

Main Trail

Loop Trail

GAZZAM LAKE NATURE PRESERVE

Lynnwood Center Road NE

Blakely Avenue NE

water towers

Gazzam to Veterane Trail

Peters Trail

Listening Avenue NE

Veterane Trail

P

Deerpath Lane NE

NE Baker Hill Road

Crystal Springs Drive NE

NE Baker Hill Road

Schel Chelb Trail

SCHEL CHELB PARK

Pleasant Beach

Point White Drive NE

Rich Passage

N

| 0 | 0.2 | 0.4 | 0.6 mile |

| 0 | 0.2 | 0.4 | 0.6 kilometer |

600 ft.

500 ft.

400 ft.

300 ft.

200 ft.

100 ft.

0 ft.

0.5 mi.   1 mi.   1.5 mi.   2 mi.

DISTANCE & CONFIGURATION: 5.0-mile out-and-back to Pleasant Beach; 2.0-mile out-and-back to Close Property Beach	HIKING TIME: 1–3 hours
	ACCESS: Hikable year-round, daily, sunrise–sunset; no fee for parking or trail access. Check ferry schedules.
DIFFICULTY: Easy–moderate	WHEELCHAIR TRAVERSABLE: No
SCENERY: Scenic wetland lake and two beaches with views over Puget Sound	MAP(S): USGS *Bremerton East*
	FACILITIES: No facilities at either trailhead
EXPOSURE: Shaded on trails, exposed on beaches	
	DOGS: Allowed on-leash except on Peters Trail to Pleasant Beach
TRAFFIC: Moderate; limited parking space	
	CONTACT: 206-842-2302; biparks.org /biparks_site/parks/gazzam-lake.htm
TRAIL SURFACE: Dirt trail and rocky beaches	LOCATION: Bainbridge Island

Yet most Bainbridge visitors never venture far beyond the ferry terminal at Eagle Harbor and don't see the less-developed part of the island. That is a shame because there's a lot out there worth seeing, as this hike proves. Although getting to the trailhead requires bringing a car across the water, it is still worth the extra cost and effort.

Figuring out the main trailhead can be a little tricky because several gravel roads and driveways converge in the general area. Look for a large sign reading GAZZAM LAKE PARK WILDLIFE PRESERVE on the left; the actual parking area is about 20 yards before that. Walk through a metal gate on the left-hand continuation of the approach road to begin your hike.

After only 0.1 mile, you will reach a well-signed junction. From here, you can head to either the Close Property Beach or Gazzam Lake Nature Preserve. Although the main hike to the lake is on the left, the straight-ahead option down to the beach is a recommended side trip and can even make a suitable stand-alone destination for hikers with only minimal time at their disposal.

To explore the Close Property, a now-public parcel of once-private beachfront land, stay on the wide and obvious main track past a collection of social trails that lead to houses on the right. The trail is marked with occasional reddish-brown posts as it winds through a pleasant, relatively open forest of second-growth maples and Douglas firs. The first views of the water appear through the trees to the left as the trail noticeably steepens.

At a confusing fork, be sure to avoid a singletrack trail heading down toward the water on the left. Although this looks like the correct path, it actually leads into private property. The correct way is shown with a hiker sign, to the right, curving unexpectedly uphill.

The descent resumes around the next bend as the trail drops into a large gully. There are some very large firs and cedars in this area, standing among the massive stumps of some of their fallen brothers. The sinuous route finds its way down to a viewpoint that looks across the waters to Illahee and the Kitsap Peninsula. A brick-and-stone foundation is visible just off the trail to the right, although the structure is off-limits to the public.

The final approach to the beach is through some big roots sticking out over the sand. Bainbridge Parks owns approximately 550 feet of waterfront property here, with barnacle-covered rocks, seasonal seeps, and tree branches jutting out toward the water.

Explore the scenic beach on your own. If you venture beyond the park land (note that the boundary is unmarked and difficult to identify), be sure to stay below the high-water line so as not to trespass on local residents' private property. When you are finished, return up the hill the way you came.

To explore the main section of Gazzam Lake Nature Preserve, follow the other trail from the signed junction mentioned earlier. This wide, easy-to-follow trail heads south through the woods.

Within 0.25 mile, a small clearing appears on the right with a large glacial erratic boulder at its center. This unusual location sometimes sports a number of stick figurines, giving the whole area a creepy feel, like a scene from *The Blair Witch Project*.

After another 0.25 mile, a short spur on the left provides the first access to the lake itself. However, the views of the water are quite limited, and the surface is largely obscured by grasses, lilies, and reeds. Fishing and boating of any kind are also prohibited, meaning that despite the limited sight lines, viewing the lake is about the only waterfront activity available.

Amazingly, Gazzam Lake has frozen over so completely in the past that local residents were able to ice skate freely across its surface. Home movies from the late 1940s attest to this unlikely occurrence, which is hard to imagine now, even on the darkest winter day. Although snow and subfreezing temperatures are still recorded, it would take an extended spell of temperatures well below zero to freeze a lake of this size to a sufficient depth for skating, a weather pattern essentially unheard of in this temperate area.

After another 0.25 mile, a second spur to the lakeshore appears on the left, followed by a significant junction, where the main trail splits. This junction provides the opportunity to complete a loop on the way back, but for now stay to the right. Reach a second junction 0.5 mile farther along, where this alternate trail rejoins the main trail from the left.

Gazzam Lake Nature Preserve is essentially flat, making the travel easy, with only a few gradual ups and downs. Watch and listen for woodpeckers in the trees; they are frequently seen in this area.

A half mile past the second loop junction, a pair of graffiti-covered concrete water towers flanks the trail, followed by a gate and then the southern trailhead with room for a few cars. This location makes an obvious turnaround point, although it is worth following the alternate side loop mentioned above for a little variety on the return.

More-adventurous hikers can explore farther and reach the water at Pleasant Beach by following Peters Trail, which leaves the small parking area to the left. Unlike the other trails in the area, it was not previously a road and is thus a true singletrack. It is also open only to hikers; no horses or bicycles allowed.

Peters Trail immediately crosses a long driveway and then begins in earnest under the trees, where its dirt surface undulates through the vegetation. It eventually starts to head downhill, passes by a small wetland area, and then gets squeezed between encroaching pieces of private property before finally ending on a road, adjacent to some new development.

From the trail's end, head downhill on the access road, which is Listening Avenue NE. Turn left at the next intersection onto busy NE Baker Hill Road and then look for a hiker-icon sign on the far side, where another trail leads into the trees. Note that if you reach a sign for the awkwardly named Schel-Chelb Creek and Pleasant Beach Watershed Surface and Stormwater Management Area, you have gone too far; the trail is about 20 yards back.

The last section of trail leads you through thick brush and snakegrass on a mixed surface of dirt and crushed shells. It eventually ends on Point White Drive NE, with Pleasant Beach just on the other side, bookended by some fine waterfront homes. From the beach, you have wide views directly south to Point Glover and Wautauga Beach, on the far side of Rich Passage. Watch for Washington State Ferries heading through the channel on their way between Seattle and Bremerton, and head up the beach to the right for an impressive view of Mount Rainier to the southeast, if the weather is clear.

Nearby Activities

Established in 1979 and currently occupying one of the oldest buildings on the waterfront in Winslow, the Pegasus Coffee House is a Bainbridge favorite. Although Pegasus has other outlets in downtown Seattle, the Bainbridge location at 131 Parfitt Way SW (a block south of Winslow Way W, several blocks west of the ferry terminal) is where it all began. Along with their signature, home-roasted blend, they even offer live music on the weekends. They also run the Harbor Public House, just up the street, a noted restaurant with a lively history. For more information, call 206-842-6725 or check its website at pegasuscoffeehouse.com.

GPS TRAILHEAD COORDINATES
N47° 37.497' W122° 33.963'

Take the Seattle Ferry to Bainbridge Island. Visit the official ferry website for directions and schedules (wsdot.wa.gov/ferries). Drive off the ferry onto Olympic Drive and turn left onto Winslow Way. Soon turn right onto Madison Avenue and left onto Wyatt Way, which eventually bends to the left. Stay right on Bucklin Hill Road where Eagle Harbor Drive branches left and then turn right to remain on Bucklin Hill Road at the next junction. Go straight to stay on Bucklin Hill Road when the main road bends to the left and becomes Lynwood Center Road. At a T-intersection with Fletcher Bay Road, quickly go left then right onto Vincent Road. Then turn left onto Marshall Road and proceed to the trailhead parking area on the left.

For the alternate trailhead, veer left from Bucklin Hill Road onto Lynnwood Center Road. Then turn right onto Baker Hill Road and right again onto Deerpath Lane, then proceed to a small parking area for four to five cars.

35 Blake Island Marine State Park

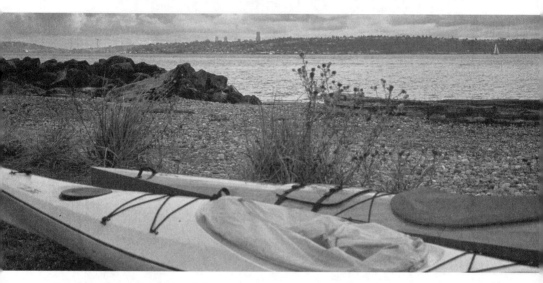

Sea kayaks on Blake Island shore

In Brief

Located in clear view of the Space Needle and just 8 miles from downtown Seattle, Blake Island is nonetheless a remote destination that's only accessible to those who can cross its moat of Puget Sound waters. Anyone making the journey, however, will be richly rewarded with the opportunity to explore the island's history, wildlife, and natural setting. Blake Island Marine State Park is so close to the city, yet so far away.

Description

Although there are multiple places to moor a private boat along Blake Island's shoreline and you can pull up almost anywhere if arriving by sea kayak, the best landing spot is the marina at Tillicum Village. Located on a prominent point on the island's northeast corner, the village commands a view of most of the Seattle skyline to the east, Bainbridge Island to the north, and Vashon Island to the south. On a clear day, look for many of the Cascade Mountain range's peaks above the city, including Mount Rainier. From this sea-level vantage point, the massive ice-clad volcano shows its entire vertical relief, rising 14,411 feet into the sky.

Tillicum Village has been the focal point for visitors to the island since its official opening in July 1962, aimed to coincide with the Seattle World's Fair. The large crowds at

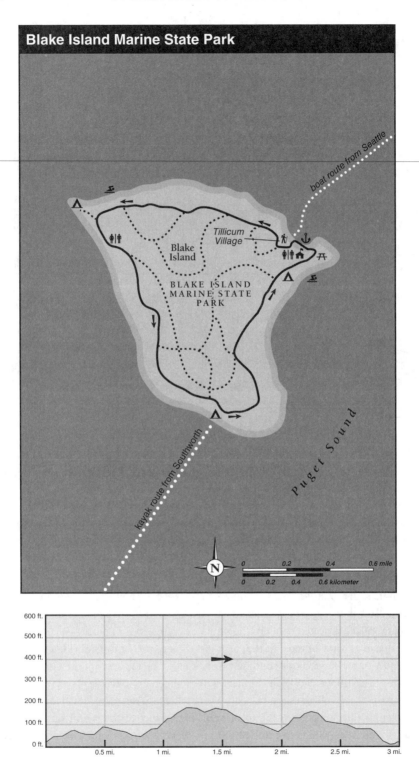

DISTANCE & CONFIGURATION: 3.0-mile loop around the perimeter (many side-trip options)

DIFFICULTY: Easy

SCENERY: Plant life, wildlife, beaches, local history, Tillicum Village and lodge, kayaking; views across Puget Sound

EXPOSURE: Mostly shaded

TRAFFIC: Moderate (low in off-season)

TRAIL SURFACE: Dirt

HIKING TIME: 2–3 hours

ACCESS: Hikable year-round (a few private boat tours scheduled in winter months), daily, 8 a.m.–sunset; no fee for parking or trail access; moorage fees at Tillicum Village marina

WHEELCHAIR TRAVERSABLE: No

MAP(S): Posted at Tillicum Village; USGS *Seattle South*

FACILITIES: Toilets, water, picnic areas, seasonal gift shop, and café at Tillicum Village

DOGS: Allowed on-leash

CONTACT: 360-731-8330; parks.state.wa.us/476/Blake-Island

LOCATION: Blake Island

the fair site never materialized on the island, however, starting a series of rocky financial years for the village's managers and investors. Further problems plagued the development through its first decade, including the seasonal nature of the business, struggles with the Seattle Chamber of Commerce, and the power that private tour companies had over access via their boats.

Nonetheless, despite massive debt and cash-flow problems, founder Bill Hewitt refused to file for bankruptcy, believing he owed it to the family and friends who had backed him financially to make the project successful. His persistence paid off in the end: Tillicum Village eventually turned a profit and still operates under the guidance of the Hewitt family today.

The heart of Tillicum Village is a massive wooden longhouse, modeled on the traditional style of the Northwest Coast American Indian tribes. Inside the structure, salmon is cooked on cedar stakes over an alder-wood fire and served to guests in the dining area while they watch *Dance on the Wind*, an interpretive stage show. Totem poles and murals decorate the interior and exterior of the building, and American Indian artists can sometimes be observed at work inside. The entire development does not reflect the culture of any one tribe in particular, but instead incorporates influences from groups ranging geographically from the Chinooks of northern Oregon to the Kwakwaka'wakws of British Columbia and the Tlingits of southeastern Alaska.

The attractions of the village were sufficient for President Bill Clinton to select the site to host the historic Asia Pacific Economic Cooperation meeting in November 1993, where world leaders from around the Pacific Rim met to discuss their future economic development while enjoying the traditional hospitality of their hosts.

The story of Blake Island predates Tillicum Village by centuries, though. The island was once the ancestral camping ground of the Suquamish tribe, and local legend holds that the great Chief Seattle was born there. Captain George Vancouver was the first European explorer to visit the area, in 1792, a trip that resulted in many prominent geographic

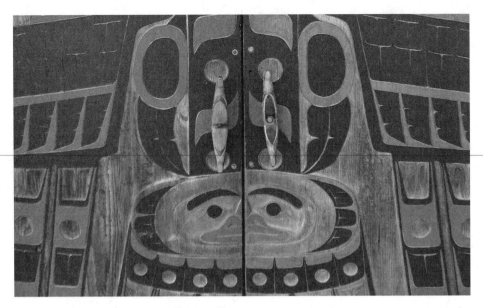

Ornate longhouse doors at Tillicum Village

landmarks throughout the Pacific Northwest being named after members of his crew. However, Blake Island was not named until 1841, in honor of George Smith Blake, who was head of the U.S. Coast Guard survey at the time.

William Trimble purchased the island around 1900 and turned it into a private estate. For many decades afterward, the land passed in and out of the hands of various owners with mixed property claims, until it was acquired by the state in 1959 and reborn as Blake Island Marine State Park. By chance, the competing legal interests kept the southern end of the island from ever being logged, leaving an impressive stand of old-growth forest for current visitors to enjoy.

To explore the island for yourself, find the trailhead on the northwest side of the village, just past the visitor center, and begin a counterclockwise loop. A network of trails laces the center of the island, but the perimeter trail makes a great hike that quite literally reaches every corner of the park, including its three campsites: one adjacent to Tillicum Village, one on the westernmost point, and the last on the southernmost point, facing Vashon Island.

The trail is a reclaimed dirt road, making it wide and easy to follow. Wooden benches offer staggered vantage points for viewing the water. And early on, some interpretive signs identify various plant species along the way.

The lowland growth here shares some similarities with forests at higher elevations in the Cascades, including a large number of Douglas firs, hemlocks, and cedars. Other species here, however, are unique to the coastal environment, including the majestic red-barked madrones, which are particularly prevalent along the shoreline; look for an exceptional grove of these trees adjacent to the southern campground.

Because this is an island, you need only to follow the shoreline to complete the loop and end up back where you started, regardless of the various junctions you might encounter along the way. For most of its length, the trail stays above the waterline and occasionally turns in toward the island's interior. On the western side, it climbs to near the island's highest point, at approximately 225 feet.

Watch out for wildlife along the way, including deer, elk, and raccoons. Eagles, ospreys, and owls are just a few of the bird species that can be spotted in the trees overhead. Marine life, abundant in the surrounding waters, includes seal pups that sometimes rest on the beaches.

There are many options to extend or shorten your hike by using the various trails through the island's interior. You may also choose to relax at a picnic table at one of the campsites, or enjoy the volleyball pits, playgrounds, or other recreational facilities available at Tillicum.

Nearby Activities

Private-tour operators offer boat trips from downtown Seattle to Tillicum Village throughout the year. Package deals typically include a buffet featuring traditional American Indian–style baked salmon, the *Dance on the Wind* stage show, and some free time to explore on your own. For more information, visit argosycruises.com/tillicum-village.

GPS TRAILHEAD COORDINATES

N47° 32.499' W122° 29.010'

See the Tillicum Village website (argosycruises.com/tillicum-village) for information on camping, moorage for private boats, and schedules for public tour boats. However, a great way to reach Blake Island is by sea kayak; the best launch points are the Vashon Island ferry dock and the Southworth ferry dock (see Washington State Ferries website for schedules and driving directions: wsdot.wa.gov/ferries). The shortest open-water crossing is the Southworth route, at about 1 mile. The park at Southworth has a sandy beach launch point at the end of a dead-end street adjacent to the north side of the ferry dock. No matter how you reach the island, the loop trail can be accessed from any of the three camping areas (see map), but the recommended starting point is at Tillicum Village.

To get to Pier 55, the departure point for Argosy Cruises, take I-5 S to Exit 165A. Use the right lane to merge onto Sixth Avenue, and in 0.1 mile turn right onto James Street. In 0.3 mile turn left onto Yesler Way, and go 0.1 mile. Turn right onto Alaskan Way. In 0.2 mile turn left onto Madison Street and make an immediate right to return to Alaskan Way. Pier 55 is on the left.

To reach Pier 55 from I-5 N, take Exit 164B, and turn right onto Edgar Martinez Drive S. In 0.2 mile turn right onto First Avenue S/Dave Niehaus Way, and go 0.4 mile. Make a slight left onto Railroad Way S, which becomes Alaskan Way. In 0.6 mile turn left onto Madison Street and make an immediate right to return to Alaskan Way. Pier 55 is on the left.

36 Ebey's Landing State Park and National Historical Reserve

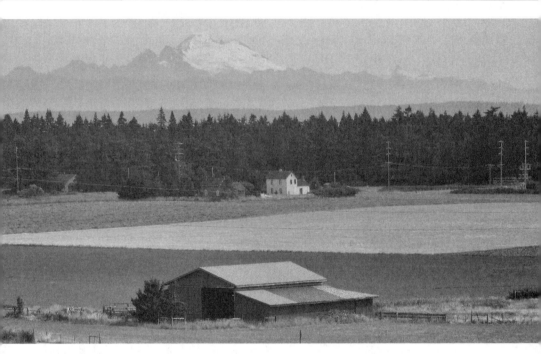

Barn and Mount Baker from Ebey's Prairie Trail

In Brief

Ebey's Landing is one of the most spectacular and historically significant locations any-where on Puget Sound. Reminiscent of the golden hills above San Francisco Bay, the high bluffs provide sweeping views of the water from the Olympic Peninsula to Vancouver Island. Bald eagles perch in the trees overhead, and the long stretch of driftwood-strewn shoreline around Perego's Lagoon is any beachcomber's dream.

Description

Isaac Ebey landed on the western side of Whidbey Island in 1850, drawn by a geographi-cally unusual grassland he found just north of Admiralty Head. (Unfortunately, he was decapitated some years later by members of the Haida tribe as a result of an ongoing

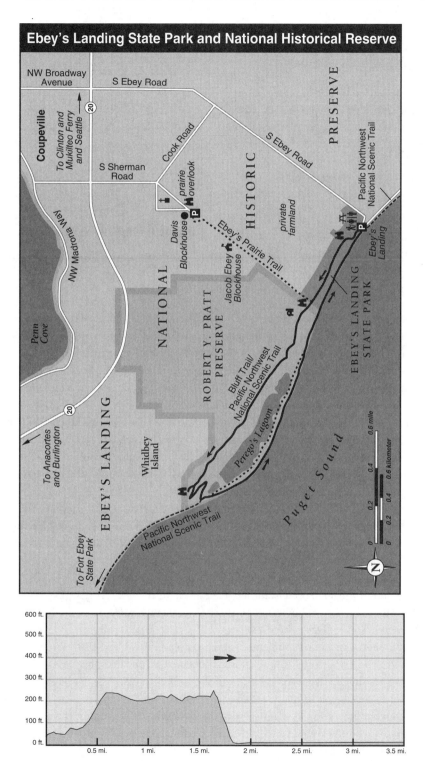

Ebey's Landing State Park and National Historical Reserve

DISTANCE & CONFIGURATION: 3.5-mile loop (plus 1.7-mile optional out-and-back side trip)	**ACCESS:** Hikable year-round, daily, 8 a.m.–sunset; Discover Pass required to park at state park lot, but free parking available along the road outside the lot. Check ferry schedules.
DIFFICULTY: Moderate	
SCENERY: Bird-watching, beach walking, colorful Perego's Lagoon, spectacular ocean views from Bluff Trail, beachcombing, driftwood	**WHEELCHAIR TRAVERSABLE:** No
	MAP(S): USGS *Coupeville*
EXPOSURE: Exposed the entire way	**FACILITIES:** Toilet at trailhead; no drinking water
TRAFFIC: Medium	**DOGS:** Allowed on-leash
TRAIL SURFACE: Half dirt, half sandy beach	**CONTACT:** 360-678-6084; nps.gov/ebla
HIKING TIME: 2–4 hours	**LOCATION:** Coupeville

dispute.) The open prairie did not have to be cleared of trees for development, a particularly valuable commodity among the dense virgin forests of the Pacific Northwest, making it the perfect place for a farm. A century and a half later, the property is mostly unchanged, with the open fields still in use for agriculture and the beaches below retaining much of their original wild and untouched state. Visitors can expect to leave with great memories and photographs (not to mention their heads).

Ebey's Landing was established in 1978 as the first U.S. National Historical Reserve, and even from the access road it's easy to see why the government thought the area was worth preserving. Apart from its considerable historical value as one of the oldest non-native settlements in Washington State, the beauty of the natural surroundings is obvious in the steep headlands that stretch up and down the coast.

Start hiking from the northern end of the parking lot through the dry grass above the sandy beach and then climb some wooden stairs to the right. The entire hike forms an elongated loop, which is easier to travel in the counterclockwise direction by starting up the bluff and then returning along the shoreline.

The stairs lead up to the working farmland of Ebey's Prairie, where the trail skirts the western end of the alfalfa fields and begins to ascend the bluff. A designated area is set aside for model-glider hobbyists, who fly their graceful aircraft over the beach and the fields on updrafts and ocean breezes.

A wooden fence marks the end of the privately owned farmland. From this point, Ebey's Prairie Trail heads inland along the fence to reach Sunnyside Cemetery, a worthwhile side trip that adds 1.7 miles to the total distance. The cemetery houses the graves of Isaac Ebey and many other early pioneers and is guarded by the historical Davis Blockhouse, a square-timbered structure built for defending the area. Beyond the fence, the land is owned and protected by The Nature Conservancy as part of the Robert Y. Pratt Preserve.

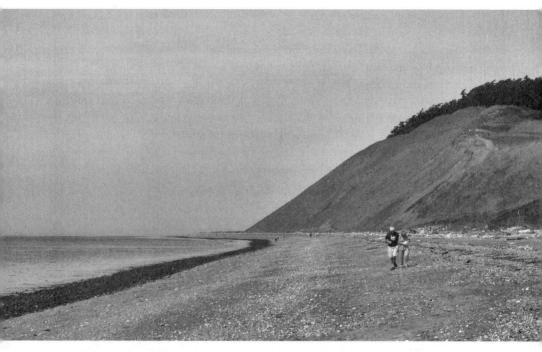

Beach below the bluff

Bluff Trail continues uphill into the preserve through a mix of wildflowers, Oregon grape, and reedy grasses, leveling off about 200 feet above the beach. From the top, the views are unparalleled across Admiralty Inlet to Port Townsend, the high peaks of the Olympic Range, Dungeness Spit, and the noticeably barren Protection Island. Victoria and Vancouver Island lie across the Strait of Juan de Fuca to the north. In between, all manner of oceangoing vessels sail by, including freighters, ferries, pleasure craft, and even the occasional aircraft carrier or submarine.

You can look straight down on kelp fronds growing in the greenish water just off-shore and the vibrant mix of earth tones that surround the shallows of Perego's Lagoon, which becomes visible as the trail pushes north. The lagoon usually looks like a lake, fully separated from Puget Sound by a thin strip of beach, but the outer barrier is occasionally breached by high waters from the sea.

Many species of birds reside on the bluff, including gulls, sparrows, robins, and thrushes. Watch for bald eagles that sit in the stunted and twisted trees on the top of the headlands and survey the water below for fish and other prey. Coyotes make rare appearances on the exposed slope as well, quickly disappearing into the woods.

Bluff Trail dead-ends at a high lookout with a good view to the south, back the way you came. Descend on a sandy trail that switchbacks down to the beach just before the viewpoint. The main advantage of completing the loop in the counterclockwise direction is taking this slope downhill, instead of up.

On the shore, it is possible to continue north along the bottom of the cliffs as far as Fort Ebey State Park, a little more than 2 miles away. This portion of the seashore is generally deserted, an undisturbed beachcomber's paradise that's passable during just about any tide. Arranging a car shuttle at the end allows for a great one-way hike.

However, the standard return along the beach also has plenty to offer. The sun-bleached driftwood is stacked so deep it looks like a mammoth boneyard, sure to keep children occupied for hours. Treasures of all kinds can be found in the sand along the way, especially when the tide pools are exposed between the barnacle- and algae-covered rocks.

Nearby Activities

Ebey's Landing is bracketed by two fascinating former military installations: Fort Ebey State Park to the north and Fort Casey Historical State Park to the south. Underutilized Fort Ebey features an extensive concrete bunker system above an unspoiled beach. The more popular Fort Casey also has a concrete bunker, impressively capped by two massive guns still aimed out over Admiralty Inlet, as well as a historical lighthouse, open playing fields, and the famous Fort Casey Inn, converted from the original World War I officers' quarters. Both parks are right off WA 20. For more information, visit the Fort Casey and Fort Ebey websites at parks.state.wa.us/505/fort-casey and parks.state.wa.us/507/fort-ebey.

GPS TRAILHEAD COORDINATES

N48° 11.545' W122° 42.514'

Visit the official ferry website for schedules (wsdot.wa.gov/ferries). From I-5 N, take Exit 182 for WA 525, toward the Mukilteo Ferry. Continue on WA 525, also signed as Mukilteo Speedway, 8.1 miles to the town of Mukilteo and drive onto the ferry to Clinton on Whidbey Island. Once in Clinton, continue on WA 525, which eventually becomes WA 20, 27.9 miles to Coupeville. On the outskirts of Coupeville, turn left off WA 20 onto S. Ebey Road. In 0.3 mile, continue straight where another road bends left, and follow Ebey Road all the way to the shoreline, another 1.4 miles. The parking area for Ebey's Landing is on the right, where Ebey Road turns left to follow the beach.

Ebey's Landing can also be reached from the northern end of Whidbey Island. Take I-5 to Exit 230, and head west on WA 20. In 11.7 miles turn left to stay on WA 20, and go 16.4 miles. Turn right onto WA 20, and go 9.2 miles. Turn right onto S. Ebey Road. You will reach the trailhead in 1.7 miles.

37 Green Mountain State Forest

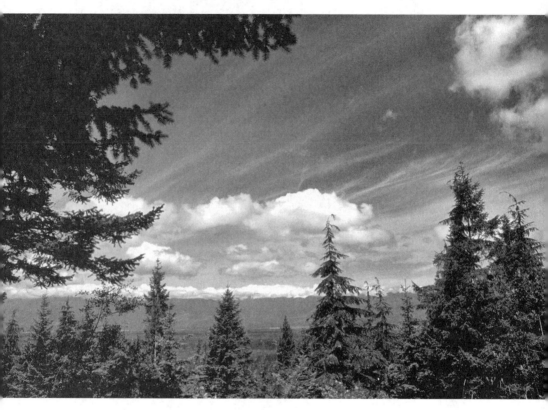

Summer sky from Green Mountain summit

In Brief

The Kitsap Peninsula has numerous hiking options, but there is only one Green Mountain, a prominent high point in the middle of a mostly flat and low-lying landscape. Luckily, the second-highest peak in the region provides plenty of good reasons to visit, other than just its exclusivity, including an extensive network of trails and great summit views.

Description

The Kitsap Peninsula is full of recreation opportunities, with a host of campgrounds, boat launches, and parks. Many Seattle residents keep waterfront cottages on the shores

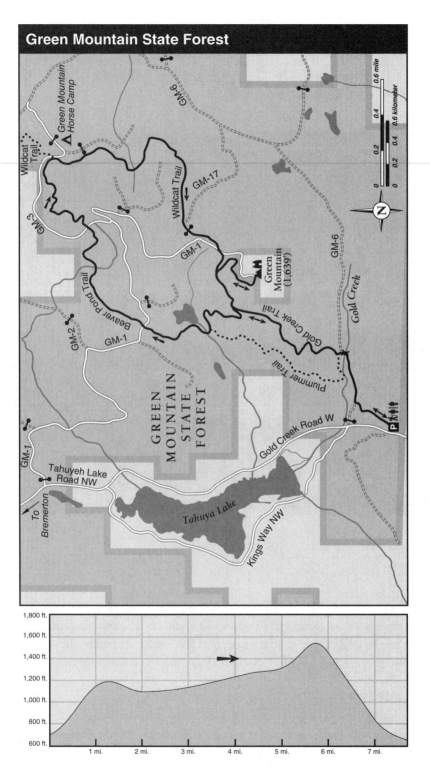

Green Mountain State Forest

DISTANCE & CONFIGURATION: 7.7-mile loop; 4.0-mile out-and-back to summit	**TRAIL SURFACE:** Dirt
	HIKING TIME: 3–7 hours
DIFFICULTY: Moderate–difficult	**ACCESS:** Hikable year-round; Discover Pass required for parking
SCENERY: Summit views west to the Olympic Mountains and east to Seattle over Puget Sound; ponds and marshes; wildflowers	**WHEELCHAIR TRAVERSABLE:** No
	MAP(S): USGS *Wildcat Lake*
	FACILITIES: Toilet at trailhead; no drinking water
EXPOSURE: Mostly shaded (a few exposed sections)	**DOGS:** Allowed on-leash
TRAFFIC: Moderate (note that trail is open to bikes, horses, and motorcycles, though seldom seen)	**CONTACT:** 360-825-1631; dnr.wa.gov /GreenMountainTahuya
	LOCATION: Bremerton

of the Hood Canal or on any of a number of popular lakes and flock across Puget Sound each weekend in the summer for the chance to get away. Despite the undeveloped landscape outside Bremerton, public trails that climb to significant peaks on Kitsap are few and far between.

The obvious exception is Green Mountain State Forest, a managed woodland run by the Washington Department of Natural Resources. At the heart of the 6,000-acre forest are the twin summits of Green and Gold Mountains, the two highest points on the peninsula. Gold might hold a slight edge in altitude, but Green is the one to visit, featuring an extensive network of multiuse trails, a central campground, and wide-ranging views from the summit. If you're looking for a hike on Kitsap, this is the place to go.

The slopes of Green Mountain are still considered a working forest, so selected stands of trees are periodically harvested for timber. Because it is not a protected wilderness area, the trails serve a range of recreational users, including hikers, equestrians, mountain bikers, and even all-terrain vehicle riders and motorcyclists. Luckily, the mountain is sufficiently large and spread out that conflicts between groups are rare, and natural geographic segregation helps to keep human-powered visitors separate from engine-powered ones most of the time.

The Gold Creek Trailhead sits about 0.25 mile from the site of an older one; it was reborn as part of a grand improvement plan initiated in the mid-1990s to combat the vandalism, abuse, and neglect that were then plaguing the state forest. The spacious parking lot is now well maintained, providing room for plenty of vehicles and a latrine. A radio tower on the ridge to the northeast marks the destination of the hike on the mountain's summit.

The dusty trail begins at the northern end of the parking lot through the stumps of a former clear-cut, elevation 650 feet. Foxgloves, daisies, and many other wildflowers fill the field with color in the summer as the path runs through several forks in the low brush. Follow a series of blue and white TRAIL signs to find the best way. Turn right on abandoned gravel road GM-6 (which leads up from the old trailhead), and soon cross chattering Gold Creek on a sturdy footbridge with railings.

Immediately over the bridge, make a sharp left onto Gold Creek Trail and climb a short rise. The trail is marked with a low vertical post in the ground, typical for the area. As part of the recent rehabilitation, many unofficial trails have been blocked off and closed; they're visible as you continue ascending on the dry, sandy tread. Stay right to remain on Gold Creek Trail past a junction with Plummer Trail, turn left at a small clearing, and then choose either path at a strange fork whose two branches converge again another 0.25 mile up the hill.

The surrounding ecosystem—with madrones, rhododendrons, salal, and low, scrubby trees as the norm—is quite different from a typical Cascade lowland environment. Much of the difference can be attributed to the Olympic Mountains only 20 miles to the west, which cast a substantial rain shadow over the region and keep it drier than its latitude would generally indicate.

Near 1,300 feet, cross beneath some old power lines with a west-facing view down to Tahuya Lake and the Olympics beyond. Descend slightly to a major intersection, about 1.5 miles from the trailhead. To the right, Gold Creek Trail continues uphill and joins Vista Trail to the summit, providing a short out-and-back option. This is also the return route for the extended loop to the top, which is described below.

Turn left down the hill on Beaver Pond Trail and then head back around to the right (north). Ferns appear in the understory and small creeks flow down the mountainside, shaded by tall trees that slow evaporation. Continue straight to remain on Beaver Pond Trail past Plummer Trail and then cross a creek and turn right, heading upstream. The first beaver pond (one of two swampy, stagnant pools full of reeds, lilies, and downed logs) appears soon after.

Cross foxglove-lined road GM-1 at an elevation of just more than 1,000 feet. Despite the presence of motorcycles and all-terrain vehicles elsewhere on the mountain, the only sounds you are likely to hear in the forest are natural: birds singing, frogs croaking, insects buzzing. Follow Beaver Pond Trail for another 0.5 mile through a pleasant forest to cross road GM-3 and start climbing again on the far side.

Reach the GM-3 road a second time at a junction with Wildcat Trail from the north. Stay right on the near side of the road to join Wildcat and pass by the Green Mountain Campground in the trees. Noticeably wider and smoother than the single-track Beaver Pond Trail, the Wildcat Trail climbs a mile on the eastern side of the mountain with views out to Seattle and Mount Rainier through some gaps on the left. The radio installation on the top of Gold Mountain appears around a bend, and then the summit of Green Mountain swings into view as well.

Cross road GM-17 near 1,250 feet and then meet GM-1 just above. The trail crosses the road, then runs parallel to it on the left side for 100 yards in a clear-cut before crossing back again. After 0.25 mile through a thick, dark forest of low trees, turn left at a junction with Vista Trail. Pass along the parking lot at the end of GM-1 (it is possible to drive here when the gate near the park entrance is open, usually weekends between 9 a.m. and 6 p.m., June–August) and climb another 200 feet to emerge at the 1,639-foot summit.

Although this is just about 1,000 feet above the trailhead, the total vertical gain via the long loop is closer to twice that distance.

The main, rocky overlook provides views over Gold Mountain to the cranes of Bremerton to the east, with Bainbridge Island, the high-rises of Seattle, and the distant Cascades behind. On a clear day, it is possible to make out the white cone of Mount Baker far off to the north. Past some picnic tables on the western side of the summit, another viewpoint looks out through trees to the Hood Canal and some of the high peaks of the Olympic Range, often veiled by clouds.

Start down on Vista Trail and turn left at the junction with Gold Creek Trail to complete the loop in another 0.25 mile. Return to the trailhead the way you came.

Nearby Activities

Wildcat Lake County Park provides conventional recreation opportunities such as swimming, volleyball, picnicking, and fishing in a scenic lakefront setting. To reach the lake, turn right on Gold Creek Road W from the trailhead and then turn right again on Northwest Holly Road after about 3 miles. The park is another 3 miles on the right, at 9025 Holly Road. For more information, visit the Wildcat Lake County Park website at kitsapgov.com/parks /Parks/Pages/regionalparks/wildcat_lake_cp.htm.

GPS TRAILHEAD COORDINATES

N47° 33.078' W122° 49.642'

From I-5 S, take Exit 165A. Use the right lane to merge onto Sixth Avenue, and in 0.1 mile turn right onto James Street. In 0.1 mile turn right onto Fourth Avenue, and go 0.1 mile. Turn left onto Columbia Street. In 0.3 mile turn left onto Alaskan Way. Immediately turn right into the Seattle Ferry Terminal. Take the ferry across Puget Sound to Bremerton. After exiting the ferry, drive west on WA 304/Burwell Street, and go 1.1 miles. Turn left to remain on WA 304 (now Charleston Boulevard), and go 1.4 miles. Turn right (north) on WA 3, and in 4.2 miles take the Chico Way exit. Turn left onto Chico Way, then in 0.7 mile turn right onto Northlake Way NW. In 0.4 mile, turn right again onto Seabeck Highway NW and continue 2.9 miles to NW Holly Road on the left. Follow Holly Road 4.2 miles, and then turn left onto Tahuya Lake Road (signed Tahuyeh). In 1.2 miles turn left onto Gold Creek Road. In 1.8 miles, after passing Tahuya Lake, look for the Gold Creek Trailhead parking lot on the left.

From I-5 N, take Exit 164B, and turn right onto Edgar Martinez Drive S. In 0.2 mile turn right onto First Avenue S/Dave Niehaus Way, and go 0.4 mile. Make a slight left onto Railroad Way S, which becomes Alaskan Way. In 0.6 mile turn left onto Alaskan Way and into the Seattle Ferry Terminal. From there, follow the directions above.

From Tacoma, take I-5 to Exit 132B. Travel 26.9 miles on WA 16 W, across the Tacoma Narrows bridge, and continue all the way to WA 3 N. Take WA 3 N 6.1 miles to the Chico Way exit; follow the directions above from there.

38 Hood Canal and Theler Wetlands

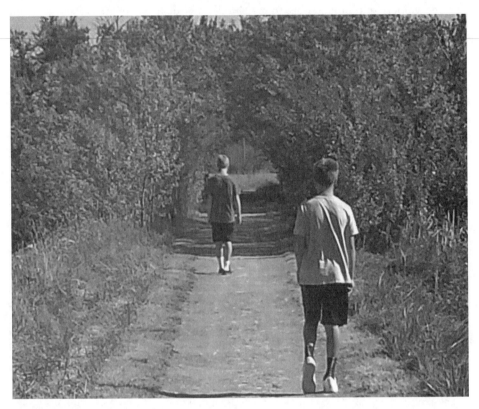

Along the River Estuary Trail

In Brief

Biology, botany, and ecology are just a few of the subjects taught in the living classroom of the Theler Wetlands. With an educational community center and more than 3 miles of trails that explore the saltwater and freshwater marshes at the head of the Hood Canal, even seasoned naturalists are sure to come away from a hike at Theler with new knowledge, understanding, and appreciation of the natural world.

Description

When Samuel Theler deeded his 72-acre wetland property to the local community, it's doubtful he really knew the value of what he was giving away; at that time in the late

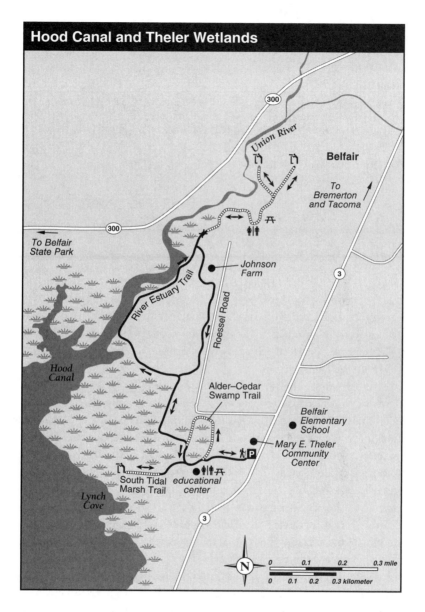

Hood Canal and Theler Wetlands

1960s, there was little popular demand for wetlands preservation. The modern environmental movement was only in its earliest stages, far from the considerable political force it would later become. These days, the Hood Canal Wetlands Project, which includes the Theler Wetlands, has grown to 135 acres and has become a local favorite.

However, in the decades since Theler's generous donation, the Belfair community has frequently squabbled over just how the property should be used and whether or not a related financial trust has been appropriately managed. At the heart of the debate

DISTANCE & CONFIGURATION: 2.8-mile loop on River Estuary Trail; nearly 4 miles to explore all trails	**HIKING TIME:** 1–3 hours
DIFFICULTY: Easy	**ACCESS:** Hikable year-round, daily, sunrise–sunset; no fee for parking or trail access
SCENERY: Education center with interpretive garden, abundant wildlife, birdwatching, and views of scenic marshlands and Hood Canal	**WHEELCHAIR TRAVERSABLE:** Yes, on all trails
	MAP(S): USGS *Belfair*
EXPOSURE: Exposed on Marsh and River trails, some shade on others	**FACILITIES:** Toilet at trailhead; no drinking water
	DOGS: Not allowed
TRAFFIC: High	**CONTACT:** 360-275-4898; thelertrails.org
TRAIL SURFACE: Mostly gravel (barrier-free) with boardwalk over marshlands and swamps	**LOCATION:** 22871 NE WA 3, Belfair, WA 98528

is the regrettably vague directive given by Theler himself about the fate of his land, words that are now interpreted and analyzed with some of the same passion and scrutiny that the Supreme Court might apply to determine the Founding Fathers' original intent in writing the Constitution.

For better or worse, the task of administering the gift fell to the North Mason School District, which chose to devote the land to educational purposes. Whether Sam Theler intended it or not, this forward-thinking decision provides many benefits, both for Belfair residents and for anyone else who visits the wetlands and discovers the natural treasures within.

Park in front of the Mary E. Theler Community Center, named for Sam's wife. Start hiking on the gravel road that runs downhill and enters the preserve through a big gate, barrier-free and wheelchair-accessible like the entire network of trails on the site. Descend through two rock walls to reach a boardwalk through the forest, with many plants common to the area identified along the way, such as skunk cabbage, Pacific bleeding heart, bear grass, twinberry, and serviceberry.

These plants after only a taste of what follows—a comprehensive interpretive garden with enough species that even a serious botanist might be hard pressed to name them all. At the heart of the garden stand several structures: the Mary E. Theler Exhibit Building, the Hood Canal Watershed Center, and the North Mason School District Classroom, all designed to educate and inform the public about the local environment; particular emphasis is placed on programs for children. There is even an outdoor "lecture hall" and a huge gray-whale skeleton hanging overhead.

Three trails head out from the educational center, each worth exploring. South Tidal Marsh Trail runs on an elevated boardwalk over the rim of the canal to the edge of Lynch Cove. Despite dead-ending at a viewing platform after only 0.25 mile, the marsh trail offers plenty to see along the way. Visiting this location during high and low tides

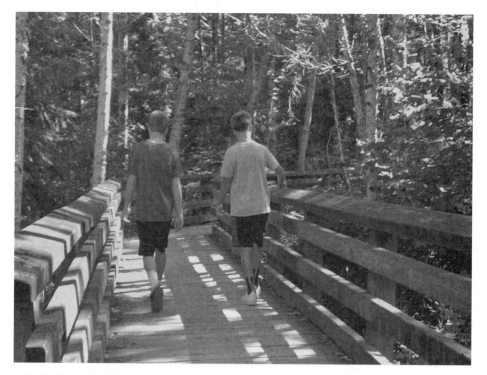

On the boardwalk

can provide vastly different experiences; a huge mudflat hidden beneath the water is exposed only when the tide is out.

This is a great place to watch for ospreys and bald eagles, just a few of the multitude of bird species that visit the area or call it home. A rudimentary list might also include loons, grebes, plovers, sandpipers, gulls, terns, doves, owls, chickadees, hummingbirds, wrens, thrushes, sparrows, and warblers, not to mention the more-common herons, ducks, and geese. The dizzying number of bird species potentially present is a direct testimony to the diversity of life supported in the estuary environment at the heart of the wetlands, where the freshwater of the Union River intermingles with the salt water of the Hood Canal.

Alder–Cedar Swamp Trail offers an alternate look into wetland diversity by showcasing a forested bog, characterized by an abundance of red alders and western red cedars. Along the 0.3-mile boardwalk, interpretive signs provide nuggets of interesting information, such as the true definition of a swamp: a wetland with a tree canopy. Sword ferns are common in the damp understory, also favored by frogs and other small amphibians.

River Estuary Trail is the longest option and offers the best hike, heading 1.4 miles upstream along the Union River and then back across the bottomlands to create a 2.8-mile loop. The trail starts out toward the river on a raised berm with wetlands on both sides that are a perfect habitat for a variety of ducks. A sea of cattails, grasses, and reeds grows out of the shallow water, along with some nasty-looking thistles and blackberry bushes at the edge. Benches line the trail, providing plenty of opportunity to rest and observe the surroundings.

The trail continues to the edge of the broad and shallow river, then follows the bank to the northeast on gravel and boardwalk through the wetlands. During the fall run, salmon can be observed swimming upstream to spawn, and several other species of fish populate the river year-round. A good set of polarized lenses can help make them easier to spot through the surface glare. But the fish do not make themselves too obvious, lest they end up as food for raptors that watch carefully overhead.

Proceed up the river to where the trail forks. Each branch soon leads to a dead end with a viewing platform, and both are worth exploring. From here, retrace your steps to a junction and then turn left toward the Johnson Farm, which borders the Theler property. Follow the wide path as it roughly parallels NE Roessel Road until it brings you back to where you began.

Nearby Activities

Belfair State Park provides many recreational opportunities along the Hood Canal shoreline, including a freshwater lagoon for swimming. The park is 3 miles west of the town of Belfair on N. Shore Road/WA 300, which runs right along the canal. A public boat launch is 2 miles farther along. For more information, visit the Belfair State Park website at parks .state.wa.us/475/Belfair.

GPS TRAILHEAD COORDINATES

N47° 26.293' W122° 50.163'

From I-5 S, take Exit 165A. Use the right lane to merge onto Sixth Avenue, and in 0.1 mile turn right onto James Street. In 0.1 mile turn right onto Fourth Avenue, and go 0.1 mile. Turn left onto Columbia Street. In 0.3 mile turn left onto Alaskan Way. Immediately turn right into the Seattle Ferry Terminal. Take the ferry across Puget Sound to Bremerton. After exiting the ferry, drive west on WA 304/Burwell Street, and go 1.1 miles. Turn left to remain on WA 304 (now Charleston Boulevard), and go 1.4 miles. Turn left (south) on WA 3, and after merging onto WA 3, continue 9.1 miles through Gorst to the town of Belfair. The trailhead is located in the parking lot of the Mary E. Theler Community Center, 1 mile past the main intersection in Belfair, on the right (west) side of WA 3 across from Belfair Elementary School.

From I-5 N, take Exit 164B, and turn right onto Edgar Martinez Drive S. In 0.2 mile turn right onto First Avenue S/Dave Niehaus Way, and go 0.4 mile. Make a slight left onto Railroad Way S, which becomes Alaskan Way. In 0.6 mile turn left onto Alaskan Way and into the Seattle Ferry Terminal. From there, follow the directions above.

From Tacoma, take I-5 to Exit 132B. Travel 26.9 miles on WA 16 W, across the Tacoma Narrows bridge, and continue all the way to WA 3 S. Take WA 3 S for 8.9 miles to Mary E. Theler Community Center.

39 Useless Bay Park and Double Bluff Beach

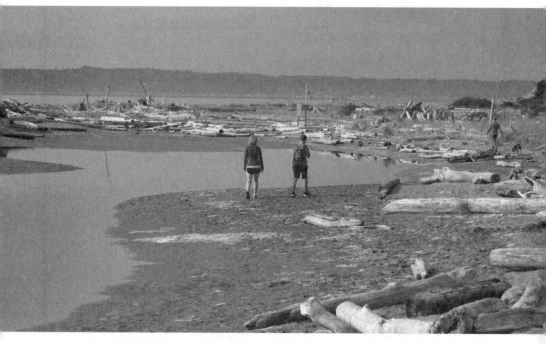

Shoreline at Useless Bay

In Brief

Useless Bay is a true oddity, the only hike in this book without any semblance of a trail. Instead, the bay provides a few miles of wild saltwater shoreline on Puget Sound for free wandering and discovery. An out-and-back trip on the beach to Double Bluff makes a good 4-mile round-trip hike, but many visitors will find the plentiful and welcome distractions along the way to be worthwhile destinations in and of themselves.

Description

Useless Bay joins Point No Point, Deception Pass, and Cape Disappointment in a long list of colorful geographic place names given to locations on the rugged coast of the Pacific Northwest; the terms were typically assigned by early seafaring explorers who had trouble navigating the region's notoriously hazardous currents and stormy seas. For

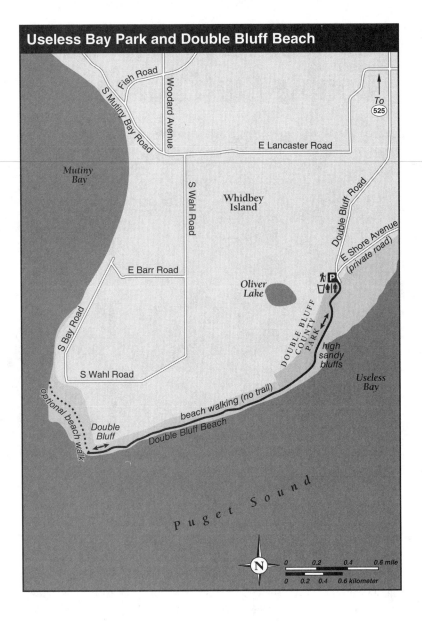

Useless Bay Park and Double Bluff Beach

land-based visitors to these spectacular settings, however, there is little connection to the sailors' troubles—and Useless Bay is no exception. The tidal mudflats that likely make the bay useless for anchoring purposes make it anything but useless for beach-bound adventurers, who can find all manner of marine riches along the shore.

Although the beach at Useless Bay can be hiked at any time, it is best to plan your trip for an ebb tide, when the beach is effectively twice its normal size and the flourishing life below the high-water line is exposed. Check local tide charts for more information.

DISTANCE & CONFIGURATION: 4.0-mile out-and-back (can be extended beyond Double Bluff)	**ACCESS:** Hikable year-round, daily, sunrise–sunset; no fee for parking or trail access. Check ferry schedules.
DIFFICULTY: Easy	**WHEELCHAIR TRAVERSABLE:** No
SCENERY: Abundant marine life at lower tides, beach walking, beachcombing, driftwood, seashells; views across Puget Sound all the way to Seattle	**MAP(S):** USGS *Hansville*
	FACILITIES: Toilets and water at trailhead
EXPOSURE: Exposed the entire way	**DOGS:** Allowed off-leash after the first 500 feet (must be leashed up to that point)
TRAFFIC: Low after leaving the crowds near the parking area	
	CONTACT: 360-679-7335; tinyurl.com /doublebluff
TRAIL SURFACE: Sandy beach	
HIKING TIME: 3–4 hours	**LOCATION:** Freeland

The Useless Bay Tidelands are technically part of the Washington State Park system, but the land is not shown as a park on most maps and the area remains undeveloped, except for a few facilities adjacent to the parking lot. Private beachfront houses run along the shore to the east toward Deer Lagoon and Sunlight Beach, with small pleasure craft moored out on the water. If you arrive at low tide, these boats might be resting on the mud, which stretches almost 0.25 mile away from the shore without any significant drop-off.

The extensive shallows are formed by the prominent point at Double Bluff, which intercepts northbound tidal currents in Puget Sound and forces the flow into Useless Bay to deposit sand and dirt while sheltering the bay from southbound currents that might otherwise carry the sediment away. These same two forces also result in the high quantities of flotsam and jetsam that collect on the shore, noticeably more than on the typically west-facing beaches up and down the coast of Whidbey Island.

From the parking lot, head west along the sand toward the high bluffs. Although dogs must be leashed for the first 0.25 mile, beyond a prominent windsock four-footed explorers are as free to wander as their two-legged companions, who swim, wade, dig for clams, poke around in the logs and grasses above the high-water line, and participate in a host of other recreational activities on the water's edge.

The sandy cliffs rise almost 300 feet above the beach at the nearest headlands, forming a natural psychological barrier for most visitors. Once you are around the point and the parking lot has disappeared from view, the shoreline receives very little traffic. Surprisingly, the Seattle skyline is visible straight out to the south, poking above the intervening landmass of the Magnolia neighborhood about 25 miles away. Nonetheless, the city seems very distant and far removed from this piece of remote and wild coast.

A staggering variety of marine life can be found on the beach. Bird-watchers will enjoy spotting such diverse species as bald eagles, belted kingfishers, grebes, terns, goldeneyes, and great blue herons. Harbor seals occasionally swim by or even come up on the land.

But it is the smaller life forms that tend to be the most interesting, particularly in the intertidal zone. At first glance, it might seem there is not much to see, yet patient inspection reveals entire worlds of activity, suggesting the emergence of primordial life from the ocean millions of years ago. All manner of cockles, mussels, and barnacles cling to the rocks, fighting for space with anemones and other mollusks. Green seaweed and algae provide shelter for scampering crabs, and multiple tide pools hide minnows, snails, and starfish. Buried clams spray water in mini-fountains from beneath the sand, giving away their hidden positions, while insects swarm overhead.

Fascinating shells, castoffs from bottom-dwelling organisms in deeper water, are everywhere as well. Most are bleached as white as the ubiquitous driftwood and come in standard clam-like shapes and sizes, but less common fans, spirals, and cones appear in exotic colors such as red, brown, and even purple. Plenty of evidence of human marine activity also ends up at Useless Bay—some welcome and some not—but it is always interesting to speculate how these items might have come to be tossed up here by the waves.

The hike to Double Bluff at the western end of the bay is only 2 miles one way, but covering the distance can be deceptively difficult and time consuming. Walking through the sand and rocks is much slower than walking on a firmer and smoother surface, there is virtually no shade or protection from the sun, and almost everything along the way invites lengthy contemplation. It will be particularly hard to get children all the way to the end because they will find so much of interest en route. However, if the 4-mile round-trip journey to Double Bluff is not enough, it is possible to continue around the point and hike northward along the next beach, below some nice waterfront houses.

GPS TRAILHEAD COORDINATES
N47° 58.935' W122° 30.856'

Visit the official ferry website for directions and schedules (wsdot.wa.gov/ferries). From I-5 N, take Exit 182 for WA 525, toward the Mukilteo Ferry. Continue on WA 525, also signed as Mukilteo Speedway, 8.1 miles to the town of Mukilteo and drive onto the ferry to Clinton on Whidbey Island. Once in Clinton, continue 8.6 miles on WA 525 to Double Bluff Road on the left just before the town of Freeland. Drive 1.9 miles to the end of Double Bluff Road, where Shore Avenue bends left, and find the Double Bluff day-use parking area. Additional parking is also available along Double Bluff Road, if necessary.

40 Vashon Island:
POINT ROBINSON AND
MAURY ISLAND MARINE PARK

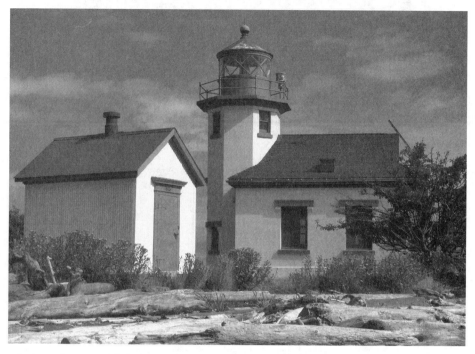

Point Robinson Lighthouse

In Brief

This attractive out-and-back hike along a pristine beach provides a real taste of island life to visitors. Starting at the historical Point Robinson Lighthouse, the trail runs along the shore about 1.5 miles to Maury Island Marine Park, with a host of interesting discoveries to be made along the way.

Description

Many Seattle residents think of Vashon and Bainbridge together, linked in people's minds as neighboring islands across Puget Sound to the west. Yet they are actually quite different, each with its own unique character and style. Much of Bainbridge is simply an upscale suburb of Seattle, with a ferry that lands right downtown, bringing crowds of

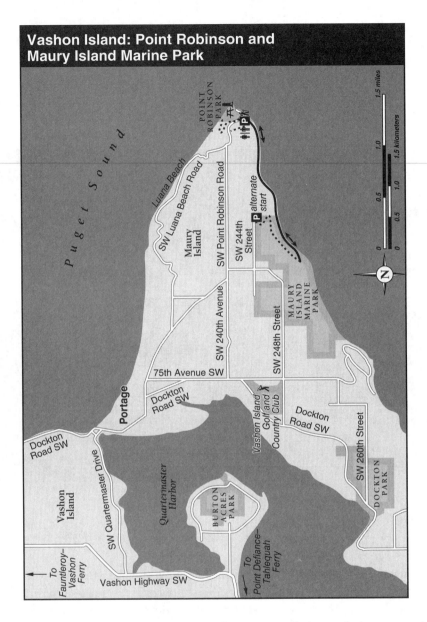

Vashon Island: Point Robinson and Maury Island Marine Park

daily commuters who retreat back across the water to their stately homes at night. Vashon, on the other hand, retains a rural character and receives far fewer visitors. Most of its outbound ferry traffic gets dropped at Fauntleroy, located, inconveniently for commuters, at the southern end of West Seattle.

This means that the typical mainlander is far more familiar with Bainbridge and far likelier to have traveled there. Vashon, on the other hand, is the sort of place that many people from Seattle have always meant to visit but have never actually seen. This hike should be the draw that finally motivates them to go.

DISTANCE & CONFIGURATION:
3.0-mile out-and-back from lighthouse;
1.5-mile point-to-point from Maury Island
Marine Park

DIFFICULTY: Easy–moderate

SCENERY: Historical lighthouse, marine
life, bird-watching, solitude, views across
Puget Sound

EXPOSURE: Exposed on beach and
shaded on trails

TRAFFIC: Light

TRAIL SURFACE: Dirt trail, gravel trail,
and sandy beach

HIKING TIME: 2–3 hours

ACCESS: Hikable year-round; no fee for
parking or trail access. Check ferry schedules. Consult a tide chart before hiking, as
beach may be impassable at high tide.

WHEELCHAIR TRAVERSABLE: No

MAP(S): USGS *Vashon*

FACILITIES: Toilet at trailhead; no
drinking water

DOGS: Allowed off-leash on beach but
must be on leash on the Maury Island
Marine Park trails

CONTACT: 206-463-1323; vashonparks
.org/point-robinson or 206-477-4527;
tinyurl.com/mauryislandmp

LOCATION: 3705 SW Point Robinson
Road, Vashon, WA 98070

Note that the southeastern part of Vashon consists of a peninsula only narrowly connected to the rest of the island. This peninsula is not truly separate, but it is nonetheless called Maury Island, which can add to geographic confusion in the area.

The recommended route starts at Point Robinson Park, where there are two parking lots, an upper and a lower. Both are OK to use, but the lower lot can fill up quickly and has a gate that is closed dusk to dawn, which makes the upper lot a more flexible option for many visitors.

Either way, begin the actual hike on the beach below the lower parking lot. Be sure to admire the historical Point Robinson Lighthouse, originally built in 1885 to help guide boat traffic in the southern end of Puget Sound. The light station has been operated by the Vashon Park District since 1997, offering the Keepers' Quarters for vacation rentals. For more information on staying in these classic buildings, contact the park district directly at 206-465-3180 or visit vashonparks.org. There are also occasional guided tours of the lighthouse during the summer season.

In addition to sporting a lighthouse, Point Robinson hosts many bird species found nowhere else on Vashon that make their way here from other parts of Puget Sound. Practiced bird-watchers frequent the area just for that reason, so keep your eyes peeled as you explore along the beach.

As you head south along the shore, countless watercrafts pass by on your left. Although marine navigation is now typically done by GPS, it's easy to see why a lighthouse was built at Point Robinson, which juts far out into Puget Sound and forms the easternmost point of Vashon Island. Despite the offshore channel being only about 2 miles wide, it is over 200 feet deep, allowing the occasional container ship to pass by on its way to the Port of Tacoma, seemingly way too close to shore for safety. Despite the

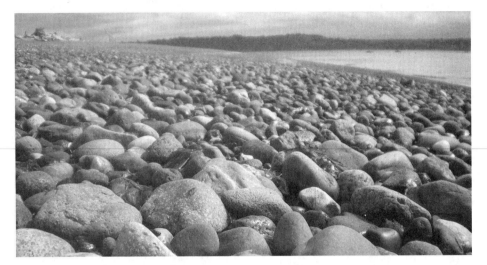

Pebbles on the beach

passage of these huge craft and the continuous cycle of air traffic in and out of Sea-Tac Airport across the water, this section of beach nonetheless feels quite remote.

Heavy piles of sun-bleached driftwood on the sand attest to the volume of items that wash up here, making the beach a collection of marine treasures for those willing to look. Be sure to stay on public land, bounded by the high-tide line. You will find beach travel slower than hiking on a regular trail, thanks to the tricky footing and the endless side attractions that draw your attention, from starfish and tide pools to ducks and great blue herons.

Steep bluffs rise on the right, reaching as high as 50 feet above the beach. This part of Vashon sits in the island's own rain shadow, leaving sandy soil that is good for madrones. Look for their signature red, peeling bark and long limbs reaching out overhead toward the water. Round, baseball-sized rocks lie underfoot, mixed in with driftwood, clamshells, and whatever else has recently washed ashore.

Pass by some interesting waterfront homes on the right, being sure to stay far enough away that you do not trespass on private property. Some feature elaborate decks above the beach that look out toward Mount Rainier and are decorated with tropical flourishes like tiki torches and hammocks. A particularly large and prominent house sits close to water and is visible almost from the very beginning of the hike, notable for its bright green roof. This house can serve as a useful judge of the total distance to be covered, sitting just about halfway between Point Robinson and the turnaround.

A wooden pier once stood at Maury Island Marine Park, although it was removed in August 2008 to prevent carcinogens leaching from the creosote pilings into the surrounding water. The project was controversial, as local divers felt the pier provided a needed habitat for marine life and posed little if any significant threat to the environment. Nonetheless, the pier is now gone, meaning it is necessary to find the gravel road and parking lot on the right to identify the recommended endpoint for the hike.

From here most hikers will be content to return along the beach the way they came, but it is possible to extend the hike by either continuing along the beach or heading up the hill on the gravel road to explore the upper section of the marine park. However, be aware that the main trail rises steeply some 500 feet to the top and offers little in the way of additional views.

Another option is to return to the lighthouse and then continue northward on the other side along Luana Beach. As long as you stay below the high-tide line, you are free to hike and explore wherever you want.

Finally, the upper parking lot at Point Robinson serves as a trailhead for two short side trails, both worth exploring. The North Loop circles through a number of grassy campsites, complete with picnic tables and the occasional view to the northeast, while the South Loop runs on a surface mostly of dirt and culminates at a bluff-top overlook where Des Moines is visible across the sound through a grove of cliff-hugging madrones. On both loops, be sure to watch out for stinging nettles and poison oak, each common on Vashon.

Nearby Activities

Located on the west side of Vashon Highway SW where it crosses SW Cemetery Road at the island's center, the Vashon Island Coffee Roasterie is a public meeting place, general store, and historical landmark all in one. They also serve some top-flight coffee, freshly brewed with select fair-trade beans from around the world. For more information, call 206-463-9800 or visit tvicr.com.

GPS TRAILHEAD COORDINATES
N47° 23.226' W122° 22.560'

Visit the official ferry website for directions and schedules (wsdot.wa.gov/ferries). From I-5, take Exit 163A, and merge onto the West Seattle Bridge. In 2.6 miles, continue onto Fauntleroy Way SW, and go 3.3 miles. Turn right into the Fauntleroy Ferry Terminal. Take the ferry to Vashon Island. Drive off the ferry onto Vashon Highway SW, and continue 7.8 miles to SW Quartermaster Drive; turn left. Travel 1.4 miles, then turn right onto Dockton Road SW. After another 0.6 mile, go straight onto SW Point Robinson Road. Drive 1.4 miles and turn left to stay on Point Robinson Road. Continue 1.2 miles to a T-intersection, and drive 0.4 mile to the park. The gate closes at sunset, so park in the upper or lower lot based on your schedule and space availability.

For the alternate trailhead at Maury Island Marine Park, from SW Point Robinson Road, go 1.4 miles, and turn left to stay on SW Robinson Point Road. Immediately turn right onto 59th Avenue SW. In 0.2 mile, turn left onto SW 244th Street and continue 0.3 mile to the well-signed trailhead on the right.

From Tacoma, take I-5 to Exit 132A. Keep left and merge onto WA 16 W, and go 3.0 miles. Take Exit 3. Continue onto Bant Boulevard, and then turn right onto WA 163/N. Pearl Street. In 3.0 miles, make a slight right onto the Point Defiance–Tahlequah ferry. In Tahlequah turn left onto Vashon Highway SW. In 1.8 miles veer right to stay on Vashon Highway, and go another 3.9 miles. Turn right onto SW Quartermaster Drive, and follow the directions above from there.

NORTH OF SEATTLE

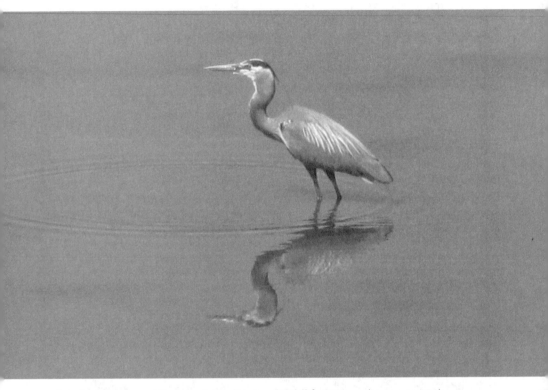

Great blue heron at Spencer Island Natural Wildlife Reserve (see page 258)

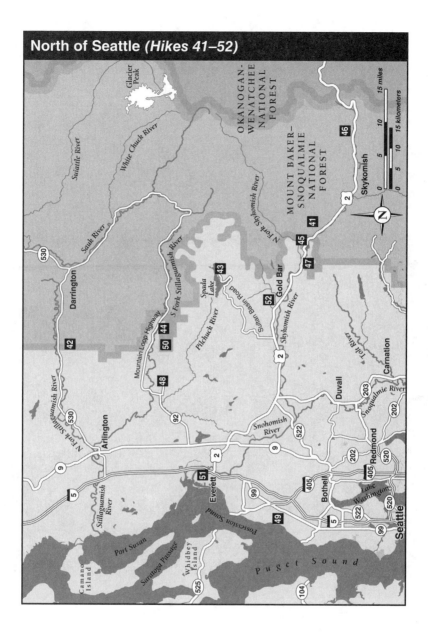

211

41 Barclay Lake, Stone Lake, and Eagle Lake

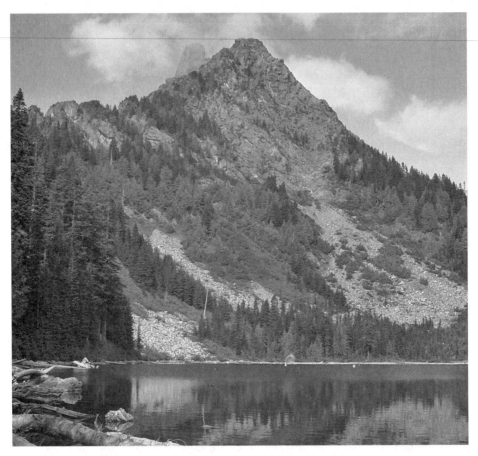

Merchant Peak above Eagle Lake

In Brief

This is the best of hikes, this is the worst of hikes. Well, not really. But it is a tale of two trails. The first offers a relaxing walk through beautiful forest to reach Barclay Lake, and the second continues on a rough and steep climb to remote Eagle Lake, less than 2 miles farther but much harder to reach. In between, unheralded but scenic Stone Lake rests in a high mountain saddle.

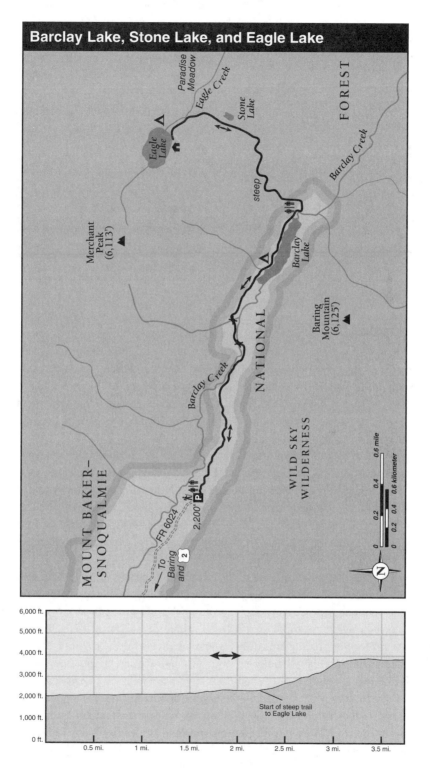

Barclay Lake, Stone Lake, and Eagle Lake

Start of steep trail
to Eagle Lake

DISTANCE & CONFIGURATION:
4.5-mile out-and-back to Barclay Lake;
7.5-mile out-and-back to Eagle Lake

DIFFICULTY: Easy Barclay Lake to
difficult Eagle Lake

SCENERY: Plant life, subalpine meadows, wildflowers (in Paradise Meadow),
old cabin; mountain views

EXPOSURE: Mostly shaded, some exposure in Paradise Meadow

TRAFFIC: Heavy to Barclay Lake,
low to Eagle Lake

TRAIL SURFACE: Dirt with some
rocky sections past Barclay Lake

HIKING TIME: 3–8 hours

ACCESS: Hikable spring–fall (Eagle Lake,
summer–fall); NW Forest Pass required
for parking

WHEELCHAIR TRAVERSABLE: No

MAP(S): Green Trails *Monte Cristo 143*;
USGS *Baring*

FACILITIES: Toilet at trailhead; no
drinking water

DOGS: Allowed on-leash

CONTACT: 360-677-2414; www.fs.usda
.gov/recarea/mbs/recarea/?recid=17874

LOCATION: Baring

Description

The Barclay Lake Trailhead sits in the middle of several impressive high peaks, most
notably the rocky spires of Baring Mountain and Mount Index and the crags of Gunn and
Merchant peaks, which give some indication of the character of the surrounding terrain.
However, the trail to Barclay Lake is much less demanding than the environment would
make it seem and is accessible to almost anyone. Reaching Eagle Lake, on the other hand,
requires physical exertion and route-finding skills.

Maintained by the Skykomish Ranger District of the Mount Baker–Snoqualmie
National Forest, the trail is open solely to hikers and begins from the eastern end of the
parking lot next to the information board. Right away the path plunges into the dark
woods. Despite being largely second growth, the trees here look like they're from a pri-
meval forest straight out of *Grimm's Fairy Tales*. Mosses, ferns, and fungi cover the trees
and the ground, making it is easy to imagine trolls, elves, and other mythical creatures
hiding in the shadows along the way.

A bushwhacking route leads off to the right within the first 0.5 mile. This difficult-to-
follow path is not for the inexperienced and is used by climbers attempting the western side
of Baring Mountain, where a steep scramble up a gully offers the easiest access to the top.

The trail roughly follows Barclay Creek, which runs through the valley on its way
to the south fork of the Skykomish River just northwest of the town of Baring. In dry
spells the stream may have little or no flow, although the size of the creek bed suggests
that during spring runoff it can become a raging torrent. The trail crosses the creek on
a footbridge built in 2003, funded by the nonprofit Spring Family Trust for Trails. This
organization seeks to preserve the Washington wilderness that Ira Spring loved and
revealed to the world through his photographs and tireless lobbying before his death
from cancer at age 84.

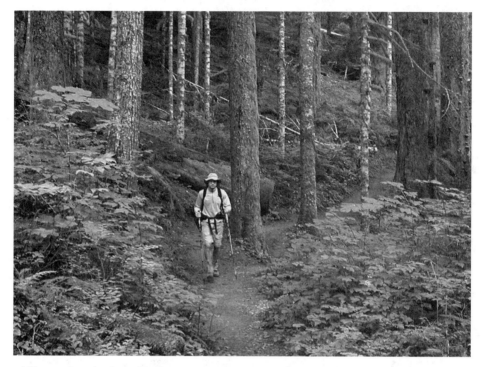

Hiker on Barclay Lake Trail

The trail gently undulates through the woods, gaining elevation so gradually it can be difficult to tell that the overall trend is uphill. After a little more than a mile, it reaches the northern shore of Barclay Lake, where several excellent campsites are tucked among the trees. The lake lies directly below the massive northern face of Baring Mountain, whose cliff faces look like the walls and towers of a giant fortress. At 6,125 feet, the summit is more than 3,700 feet straight up, all exposed rock. There is a noticeable echo off the far wall for anyone willing to disturb the peace to test it out. Unfortunately, the lake has generally muddy shores, making it less than a great place to swim.

For many hikers, this friendly destination makes an excellent turnaround point. If you are seeking additional challenge and solitude, continue around the shore to find the route to Eagle Lake up the ridge to the north. The Eagle Lake Trail is not shown on most topographic maps and can be tricky to locate and follow. Look for an unmarked trail heading straight up the hill to the left, just past the path to the toilet. If you reach the inflow creek to the lake at the last campsite, you have gone too far.

The boot-beaten track starts immediately uphill, and is marked intermittently by some ribbons, although these can be unreliable. Expect to do some route finding as you climb through fallen logs, dirt, and needles. If you lose your way, your best bet is to continue uphill and angle to the right. As long as you stay on the western side of the creek, eventually you should recover the trail.

Enter a boulder field 0.5 mile up, near 3,200 feet. These boulders continue in sections most of the way to Stone Lake, some 700 feet higher. The trail is easier to follow here than below, thanks to a series of cairns, although the general trend is the same as before: straight uphill. Near 3,400 feet, the trail crosses the creek and continues ascending on its eastern side. Look behind you for a great view of Baring Mountain across the Barclay Lake basin.

The trail finally relents at the southern end of Stone Lake—really just a pond; its name is probably derived from a rockslide that reaches into the clear water on the eastern shore. The route reaches a relatively high point here and then descends on the far side into Paradise Meadow and the Eagle Creek Valley.

Paradise Meadow sits in a vast subalpine bowl, surrounded by Townsend Mountain (5,936') to the north, Merchant Peak (6,113') to the west, and Eagle Rock (5,615') at the far eastern end of the valley. Indian paintbrush and wild blueberry bushes stretch along Eagle Creek, among grasses, flowers, and stunted pines. The trail crosses the creek several times through some muddy sections as it winds northwest.

At 3,888 feet, Eagle Lake is slightly higher than Stone Lake and almost twice as big as Barclay. A good tent campsite is located where the trail first reaches the lake on its eastern side, and an old cabin is also available for public use about 200 yards around the shoreline to the southwest. The cabin has collected a host of equipment and junk over the years, but the front porch is a great place to rest and gaze out over the lake. Fish jump out of the clear water, chasing nymphs and bugs on the surface; bleached deadwood lines the shore. The rocky face of Merchant Peak rises directly above the western end, although the true summit is not visible from here. Return the way you came.

Nearby Activities

The Washington State Department of Fish and Wildlife operates a salmon hatchery on the Wallace River in Gold Bar. The public is allowed to tour the working facility and see various types of smolts in their tanks before they're released into the wild. The hatchery is at 14418 383rd Ave. SE; 360-793-1382. Look for a big brown sign for the State Salmon Hatchery on US 2, across from the West Gold Bar rail station at milepost 27.

GPS TRAILHEAD COORDINATES
N47° 47.554' W121° 27.561'

On I-5 at the northern end of Everett, take Exit 194 for US 2 E. Travel 35.2 miles east on US 2 through the towns of Monroe, Sultan, Startup, and Gold Bar to reach the turnoff to Index, and continue on US 2 another 5.5 miles to the tiny town of Baring. Take a left onto 635th Place NE, immediately crossing railroad tracks. This road becomes Forest Route 6024 and dead-ends 4.3 miles from US 2 at the Barclay Lake Trailhead and parking area.

42 Boulder River Trail

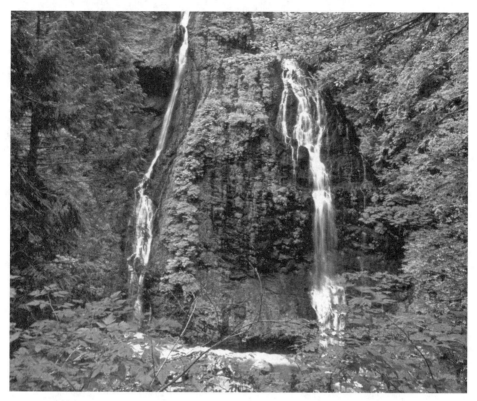

Waterfalls along Boulder River Trail

In Brief

Boulder River Trail brings together a great combination of unlikely elements. Old-growth forests and breathtaking waterfalls can be found in many wilderness areas in the Cascades, but the minimal elevation gain and year-round access available here are two pleasant surprises that make Boulder River stand alone.

Description

The Boulder River Wilderness juts out from the Mount Baker–Snoqualmie National Forest west of the town of Darrington, separating the north and south forks of the Stillaguamish River. In between, Whitehorse Mountain and Three Fingers reach close to 7,000 feet, the centerpiece of a rugged collection of peaks that is crossed by only a single road, the Mountain Loop Highway through Barlow Pass to the east.

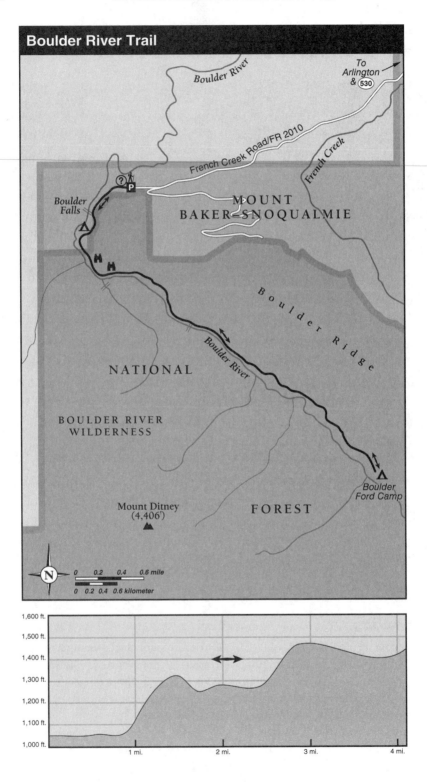

Boulder River Trail

DISTANCE & CONFIGURATION:
8.4-mile out-and-back to Boulder Ford Camp; 2.0-mile out-and-back to waterfalls

DIFFICULTY: Easy–moderate

SCENERY: A low-elevation year-round river-trail hike in a wilderness area with old-growth forest, stunning waterfalls, and two trailside backcountry camps

EXPOSURE: Shaded

TRAFFIC: Low–medium

TRAIL SURFACE: Dirt (progressively degrades with distance from trailhead; very muddy in spots, especially after rains)

HIKING TIME: 4–6 hours to Boulder Ford Camp; 1–2 hours to waterfalls

ACCESS: Hikable year-round; NW Forest Pass required for parking

WHEELCHAIR TRAVERSABLE: No

MAP(S): Green Trails *Granite Falls 109*; USGS *Meadow Mountain*

FACILITIES: Toilet about 1 mile up French Creek Road; no drinking water

DOGS: Allowed on-leash

CONTACT: 360-436-1155; www.fs.usda .gov/recarea/mbs/recarea/?recid=17732

LOCATION: Arlington

Yet Boulder River Trail penetrates the area via a gentle valley without meeting any significant barriers for almost 5 miles, providing an exceptional opportunity to explore some of the mountain wilderness without the usual toll of sweat and muscle. Better still, the hike is much milder than its location would suggest: In winter, the low elevation keeps the trail mostly snow-free; in summer, the forest canopy provides plenty of shade even on the hottest days, and the river is always nearby for a quick dip.

Although this is a federally designated wilderness, permits are not required for entry. However, there is a self-registration kiosk at the western end of the trailhead parking lot to assist in tracking usage and help the U.S. Forest Service manage the area.

The trail starts on an old gravel road cut into the side of the slope by local pioneers. A small rocky cliff band runs alongside on the left, the exposed backbone of Boulder Ridge, which forms the northern side of the Boulder River Valley and reaches its high point at 4,378-foot French Peak. The road actually hangs out over the valley at one point, supported by some heavy timbered beams, although it is difficult to notice unless you look carefully. The river can be heard down the valley to the right, and occasionally seen through gaps in the forest of red alders and moss-covered cedars and maples. Some giant stumps hint at the huge trees that once grew here but were harvested long ago.

The trail bends around to the south and reaches a side trail to an old cabin site in the ferns to the right, about 0.5 mile from the trailhead. Not much remains of the cabin, except parts of the foundation, but the clearing where it once stood now serves as a good place to camp. Boulder Falls can usually be heard thundering in the river below, but unfortunately, it is not visible from here. An indistinct use trail descends to the water's edge down a steep sandy cliff and provides the best opportunity to view the cascade, but this route is not recommended.

The true wilderness boundary lies just past the campsite, where the trail soon fades to a rocky singletrack and gradually approaches the river. After another 0.25 mile, a spectacular waterfall tumbles down the sheer rocky face of the gorge on the opposite side, split into two distinct forks before meeting the green, churning waters of the Boulder River in a pool at the bottom. The total drop easily exceeds 75 feet as the water plunges down through a hanging garden of moss and plants clinging to the face of the cliff and fed by the constant spray. Note, however, that these falls may not be running during the dry season.

This noteworthy landmark and possible turnaround point goes unnamed on regional topographic maps, which instead tend to prominently label the hidden Boulder Falls; this can lead to some confusion. The situation is further complicated by a second, smaller waterfall on another side creek about 0.25 mile farther up the valley.

Continue upstream, climbing through roots and rocks until the river is far below. Occasional glimpses of some of the surrounding high peaks appear through the forest, which is now beginning to show some of the signs of true old growth. The tree species are typical for the lowland Cascades, including silver fir, western hemlock, and Douglas fir. Watch for a particularly large western red cedar on the right-hand side that has been neatly hollowed out, a natural playhouse in the woods that is irresistible to children. Below the giant trees, the forest floor displays an impressive collection of virtually every type of fern native to the Pacific Northwest, fed by the heavy precipitation and dampness of the river valley. Expect the footing to be muddy and wet, as creeks and streams drain down from Boulder Ridge and frequently flood short sections of the trail.

The hike meanders up and down along the northern bank of Boulder River for several miles altogether, sometimes far above the water level and other times much closer to it. A number of good swimming holes appear below, although they are not always easily or safely accessible.

Boulder Ford Camp is the effective turnaround point, where the trail reaches a campsite right next to the river at an elevation of 1,450 feet. Note that this is less than 500 feet higher than the trailhead, although the frequent ups and downs along the way make the total vertical gain closer to twice that distance.

It is theoretically possible to continue beyond the camp and head for Tupso Pass to the south, but that requires fording the river, finding the overgrown and deteriorating trail on the far side, and then essentially bushwhacking steeply uphill 1.5 miles or more, which few if any hikers would realistically enjoy—or should even consider. The camp does provide a good place to relax, with plenty of rocks and logs to sit on while watching the river flow. When you are ready, retrace your steps to the beginning.

GPS TRAILHEAD COORDINATES

N48° 15.024' W121° 49.041'

From I-5 north of Everett, take Exit 208 for WA 530, and head east. Drive 3.7 miles, and turn left onto WA 530, then immediately turn right onto WA 530/Burke Avenue. In 19.8 miles, just after milepost 41, turn right onto French Creek Road. Continue on this road 3.7 miles to the parking lot and trailhead for Boulder River Trail.

43 Greider Lakes

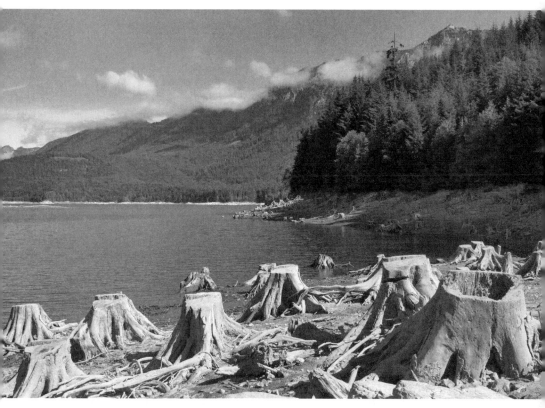

Exposed stumps at Spada Lake

In Brief

The two Greider Lakes nestle among a crown of rugged mountains, rocky cliffs, and sharp peaks. The high alpine scenery and isolated feel of the setting provide a wilderness experience more typical of the remote North Cascades than of the ranges only 30 miles east of Everett.

Description

In 1965 Culmback Dam was completed and the Spada Lake Reservoir was born. Serving the needs of most of Everett and Snohomish County, the reservoir collects runoff from the Upper Sultan River Basin before sending it through a pipeline to the Lake Champlain Reservoir for filtration and treatment.

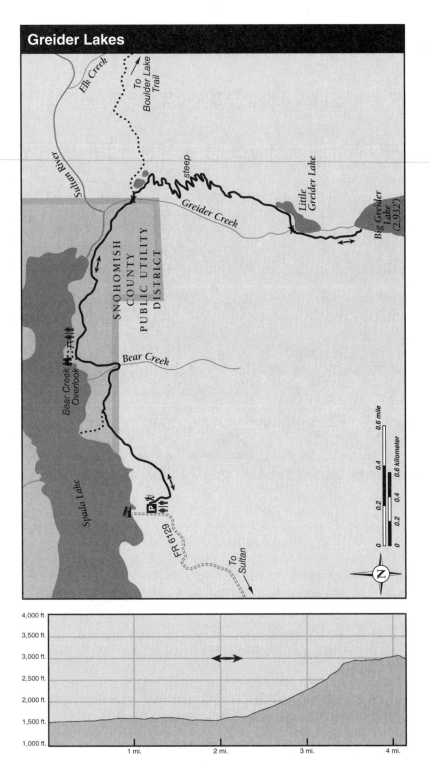

Greider Lakes

DISTANCE & CONFIGURATION: 8.6-mile out-and-back	**HIKING TIME:** 4–8 hours
DIFFICULTY: Difficult	**ACCESS:** Hikable late spring–early fall, daily, sunrise–sunset; all vehicles must register (free) at the Olney Pass entrance into the Spada Watershed
SCENERY: Two mountain lakes with camp spots, ponds, river access, large reservoir (restricted uses)	**WHEELCHAIR TRAVERSABLE:** No
EXPOSURE: Shaded most of the way with some exposure at the lakes and on the lower trail	**MAP(S):** USGS *Mount Stickney*
	FACILITIES: Toilet at trailhead
TRAFFIC: Low	**DOGS:** Allowed on-leash
TRAIL SURFACE: Flat old dirt road and steep dirt trails	**CONTACT:** 425-783-1712; snopud.com/?p=1955
	LOCATION: Sultan

Like many other man-made bodies of water, Spada Lake invites public recreation. However, access and use are highly regulated in order to protect the water quality downstream. Swimming and wading in the lake are forbidden, as is any other activity where one's body might contact the water. Pets face similar prohibitions, and only electric boats are allowed on the lake's surface. Gasoline-powered vessels and even inflatables are not allowed.

With these tight restrictions, not too many visitors can find the means or motivation to enjoy the lake's offerings. The long drive up the gravel Sultan Basin Road doesn't help much either, which often leaves the area largely underused.

And just in case the access wasn't hard enough already, the road along the lakeshore to the trailhead is closed permanently to motor vehicles beyond the South Shore Parking Area, adding 2 miles to the hike each way. Although flat and easy, this extra distance filters out another group of potential users and provides an additional layer of isolation at the end. Thanks to the long approach and the absence of the drone of powerboats on the reservoir, hikers on the Greider Lakes Trail will feel as if civilization is far away.

From the South Shore Parking Lot, the trail heads east through a pleasant second-growth forest. This promising start is something of an illusion, however, because the trail emerges again from the trees very quickly onto the decommissioned road.

The road continues east along the lakeshore, although the lake itself is only intermittently visible through the trees. Expect to cross multiple creek beds along the way through short arroyos, providing quick up-and-downs on the otherwise flat surface. In season, watch for a profusion of pink and purple flowers, including fireweed, foxglove, and hardhack.

The abandoned Nighthawk lake access point appears down a short spur to the left after 0.6 mile. Continue up the road for another 0.6 mile, crossing substantial Bear Creek along the way, to arrive at the Bear Creek Overlook, complete with toilet, picnic tables, and an excellent viewpoint over the reservoir. This is a good place for a rest in either direction.

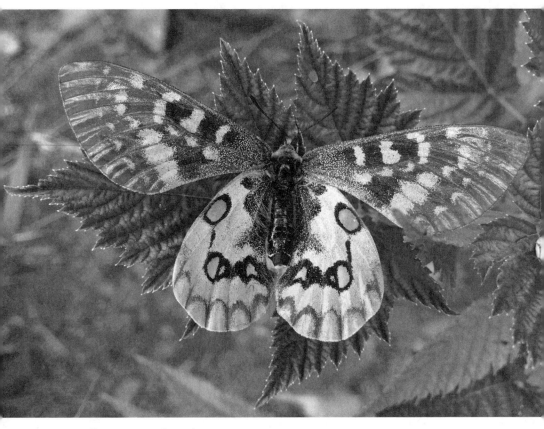

Butterfly at Big Greider Lake

In another 0.4 mile, an unnamed creek presents a second substantial river crossing. At a time of high water, it may be necessary to use an informal bypass route that heads uphill into the woods on the right and rejoins the road on the far side.

Beyond this creek, Spada Lake fades into a series of braided channels, which is the reservoir inflow from the main fork of the Sultan River. The old road then crosses Greider Creek on a bridge and reaches a clearing, signed on the right by the Washington Department of Natural Resources (DNR) as the Greider Lakes Trailhead. The old road continues to a trailhead for the Boulder Lake Trail, but that trail is overgrown and in disrepair, so its future is uncertain.

The elevation at the Greider Lakes Trailhead is about 1,500 feet, essentially the same as at the South Shore Parking Area. The flatness that led to this point doesn't last much longer, however. After passing by some ponds and a wetland area, the trail soon begins a steep, switchbacking climb up the mountainside. Watch for roots, rocks, and other obstacles underfoot, especially where they may be concealed by heavy brush overgrowing the path.

The brush can offer a harvest of wild berries in the summer and fall, a pleasant wayside treat, but that also makes this good bear country, so use all appropriate cautions. As you climb, the understory eventually begins to thin and the route becomes easier to follow as you enter some old-growth forest. The uphill pace does not relent, however, and some exposed drop-offs down the side of the mountain can be hazardous to the unwary. Although parts of the trail are well developed, with water bars, boardwalks, and even wooden steps, others are still quite rough.

After about 1.5 miles uphill, reach a relative saddle near 2,800 feet. Little Greider Lake is only a short distance farther along on the now mercifully flat trail. There are several good campsites along the lake's northwestern shore, most equipped with fire rings, grills, and tent platforms. Open solely to backpackers, these campsites are a stark contrast to the shores of Spada Lake Reservoir, where only day use is allowed. The best access to the water of Little Greider is from the sites farthest along.

From Little Greider Lake, the massive rock wall below Greider Mountain is visible to the south, appearing deceptively close. It's hard to imagine that a larger body of water sits in a separate bowl between Little Greider and these cliffs, but another 0.5 mile of moderate climbing brings you to Big Greider Lake, more than twice the size of its sister. To get there, cross the Little Greider Lake outflow on a bridge over a logjam with views straight down Greider Creek and then proceed up the frequently overgrown trail.

Big Greider, at 2,932 feet, also features many fine campgrounds, although access to the shore is limited. The lake sits in a craggy, high-alpine cirque, bounded on three sides by talus, rocks, and impressive cliffs. It was once possible to follow a side trail that climbed the slope to the west to reach a good viewpoint above Big Greider Lake, but that trail has been lost with time and lack of use.

Return the way you came, taking care to resist the temptation of cooling off in Spada Lake Reservoir, no matter how hot and sweaty you might become.

GPS TRAILHEAD COORDINATES
N47° 58.422' W121° 36.803'

On I-5 at the northern end of Everett, take Exit 194 for US 2 E. Travel 22.9 miles east on US 2 through the town of Sultan. Just after the town, turn left onto Sultan Basin Road, and follow it 13.3 miles. Make a slight right and go straight onto Forest Route 6120, and in 2.3 miles, continue on FR 6129 for 2.5 miles to the trailhead at the South Shore Boat Launch on Spada Lake. Be sure to stop at Olney Pass and register your vehicle (free) when you enter the Spada Watershed.

44 Heather Lake

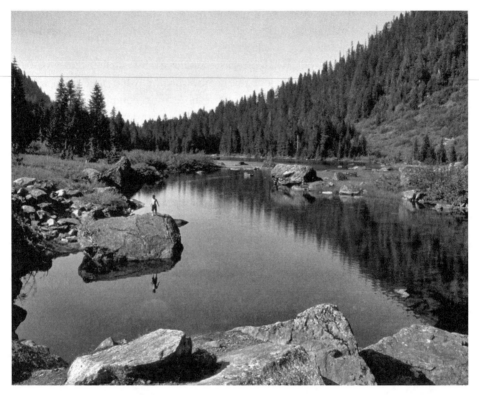

Swimming hole at Heather Lake

In Brief

The trail to Heather Lake offers an interesting and rewarding hike, with just enough challenge to make the swim at the end all the more inviting—at least during high summer. If you prefer solitude, the lake also makes for a worthwhile destination during some of the colder months, thanks to its low elevation and dramatic setting beneath 1,500-foot cliffs.

Description

Heather Lake is the westernmost of a chain of lakes spread out on the northeastern side of Mount Pilchuck, including Bear Lake, Hempel Lake, and Lake Twentytwo, all formed by natural bowls that collect runoff above the South Fork of the Stillaguamish River. Nestled in an impressive cirque, the lake lies less than 1 mile from the top of Pilchuck but almost

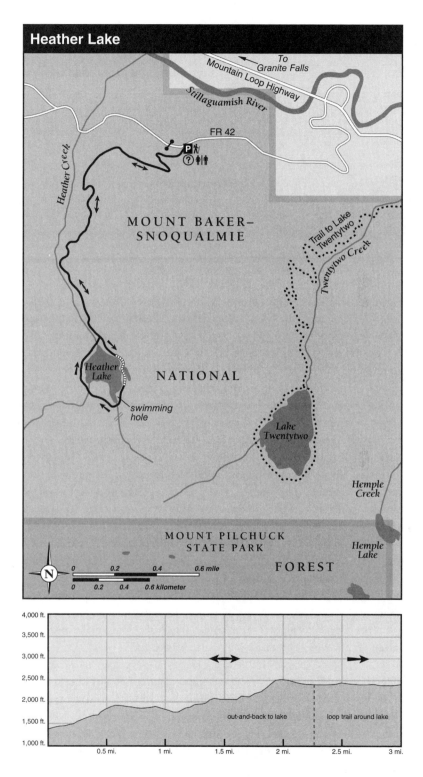

DISTANCE & CONFIGURATION: 5.25-mile balloon	**ACCESS:** Hikable spring–fall; NW Forest Pass required for parking
DIFFICULTY: Moderate	**WHEELCHAIR TRAVERSABLE:** No
SCENERY: Old-growth trees and massive stumps, lake bowl	**MAP(S):** Green Trails *Granite Falls 109*; USGS *Verlot*
EXPOSURE: Shaded in forest, exposed around lake	**FACILITIES:** Toilet at trailhead; no drinking water
TRAFFIC: Heavy (hike midweek, if possible)	**DOGS:** Allowed on-leash
TRAIL SURFACE: Dirt, short scenic boardwalk at lake	**CONTACT:** 360-436-1155; www.fs.usda .gov/recarea/mbs/recreation /recarea/?recid=17754
HIKING TIME: 3–5 hours	**LOCATION:** Granite Falls

3,000 feet beneath it. The summit, however, cannot be seen from the lake, thanks to the high ridges that rise sharply from the southern shore. These ridges funnel the water down into the basin and shade the snowpack, often preserving it late into summer.

From the trailhead on the Mount Pilchuck access road, Lake Heather Trail 701 climbs steadily for 2 miles and 1,200 feet to reach its destination. Find the beginning of the trail next to the information board, across the gravel road from the main parking pullout. On a summer weekend expect to see cars parked along both sides of the road, as hikers aim to reach the lake at the hottest part of the day. Some of the crowds can be avoided by getting an unusually early or late start, but it might prove too cold to swim when you reach the lake.

The trail begins its ascent through a damp second-growth forest, where the moss-laden trees appear velvety and bearded. Scattered along the way is a series of enormous cedar stumps, evidence of what the forest used to be in its old-growth heyday. Many still show the notches where the loggers anchored their springboards as they cut down the trees by hand in the early 20th century. The height of the current trees, a few actually growing out of the stumps themselves, gives some idea of the massive size these ancient wonders would have attained.

Like many trails in this part of the Mount Baker–Snoqualmie National Forest, the path is well traveled and well taken care of, with water bars and lining logs where needed. The current route replaces an older trail whose traces are occasionally visible along the way, but there is never any question about which way to go.

The forest floor is littered with deadfall, showing every stage of decay and rebirth imaginable; this includes some old-growth cedars still enduring on either side of the trail near the halfway point to the lake. These impressive trees stand straight as Greek columns, rising far above the surrounding canopy.

The trail narrows to singletrack and crosses a creek near the 2,000-foot level. Expect some mud in this section even in the driest part of the year. This is not Heather Creek, the lake's outflow that roughly parallels the trail to the west but which the trail never reaches, despite the frequently audible sound of running water.

With just 0.25 mile remaining, reach the trail's high point at 2,500 feet and then start a short descent through a marshy area into the Heather Lake basin. The high trees obscure most of Mount Pilchuck, but glimpses of its rocky ridges are periodically visible through the upper branches. Finally reach the lake at 2,395 feet.

A loop trail continues another 0.75 mile, completing a circuit around the shoreline. All sides of the lake are worth visiting, and you may need to explore on your own to find the best spot. A series of sandy beaches on the northern side of the lake is particularly popular for swimming, but the far end also offers some excellent opportunities where boulders from an old rockslide reach the deep water, allowing for jumping and diving. Segmented snake grass growing out of the water is fun for children, who will enjoy wading among the stems and looking for fish and frogs.

Heather Lake is not particularly deep, but the water never really warms too much, especially in the years when the snow lingers well into July. Even a shallow dive will show the marked difference between the surface water and the icy layers beneath. Although it might be refreshing after a sweaty hike, it could turn hypothermic under the wrong conditions, so be careful, especially with children. A pack towel is a great accessory to bring along for when you are finished.

For the adventurous, a scramble up the rockslide to the south leads to the steep face of the cirque itself. Poke around to find various small waterfalls running down the cliff and into the rocks, and look back down for a commanding aerial view of the lake.

Nearby Activities

There are multiple amenities and services available in Granite Falls, where the Mountain Loop Highway meets WA 92. As you enjoy a posthike meal or drink, look for Mount Pilchuck, clearly visible, towering over the eastern end of town.

GPS TRAILHEAD COORDINATES

N48° 4.962' W121° 46.497'

On I-5 at the northern end of Everett, take Exit 194 for US 2 E. Head east 1.9 miles on US 2, and exit left onto WA 204, which climbs to the town of Lake Stevens. In 2.7 miles, at the intersection with WA 9, turn left (north). Proceed 1.7 miles to a right turn onto WA 92 toward Granite Falls. In 8.5 miles, in Granite Falls, turn left onto N. Alder Avenue, which becomes Mountain Loop Highway. In 11.9 miles, after passing Verlot and immediately after crossing the Stillaguamish River, go right on Mt. Pilchuck Road/Forest Route 42. Travel on this paved and gravel road 1.4 miles to a parking area on the right across the road from the Heather Lake Trailhead.

45 Heybrook Ridge and Lookout Tower

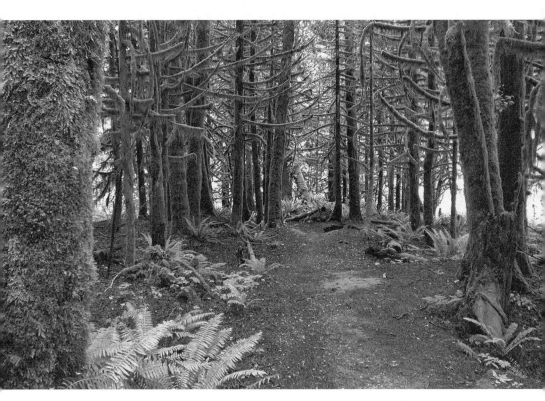

Mossy trees along the trail

In Brief

This short and sweet hike can easily be completed in a single morning or afternoon, including plenty of time spent both lingering on the trail along the way and enjoying the sweeping views of the lower Skykomish River Valley and its stunning surrounding peaks from the fire lookout at the top.

Description

It's not hard to see why Heybrook Ridge was chosen for a fire lookout. Like all such sites, the ridge has a nearly perfect location for observing a wide swath of the surrounding

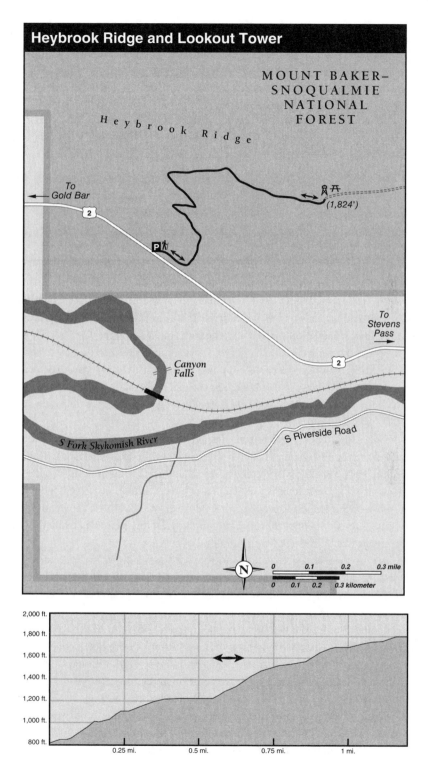

Heybrook Ridge and Lookout Tower

Heybrook Ridge

MOUNT BAKER–
SNOQUALMIE
NATIONAL
FOREST

To
Gold Bar

(1,824')

2

To
Stevens
Pass

2

Canyon
Falls

S Fork Skykomish River

S Riverside Road

N

| 0 | 0.1 | 0.2 | 0.3 mile |

| 0 | 0.1 | 0.2 | 0.3 kilometer |

2,000 ft.
1,800 ft.
1,600 ft.
1,400 ft.
1,200 ft.
1,000 ft.
800 ft.

0.25 mi.   0.5 mi.   0.75 mi.   1 mi.

DISTANCE & CONFIGURATION: 2.8-mile out-and-back	snow-covered at the top in winter); NW Forest Pass required for parking
DIFFICULTY: Moderate	**WHEELCHAIR TRAVERSABLE:** No
SCENERY: Eight-story fire-lookout tower with observation deck below the cabin; stunning views of Mount Index and other nearby mountains	**MAP(S):** Green Trails *Index 142*; USGS *Index*
EXPOSURE: Mostly shaded	**FACILITIES:** None at trailhead
	DOGS: Allowed on-leash
TRAFFIC: Moderate	**CONTACT:** 360-677-2414; www.fs.usda .gov/recarea/mbs/recreation/hiking /recarea/?recid=17886
TRAIL SURFACE: Dirt	
HIKING TIME: 2 hours	
ACCESS: Hikable year-round (may be	**LOCATION:** Index

countryside—the impressive lower Skykomish River Valley. But unlike most lookouts, which typically extract a heavy toll in sweat and labor for access, Heybrook, at 1,824 feet, is one of the lowest-elevation towers anywhere in the Washington Cascades. Instead of making the grueling climbs most U.S. Forest Service staffers have to endure to reach their posts, often while hauling water and supplies, to reach Heybrook you need walk little more than a mile of trail from busy US 2. For the generally unencumbered day hiker, the 1,000-foot climb right outside of Index is a wonderful gift, a true big-mountain view that is almost too easy to attain.

Heybrook Ridge Trail could not be simpler to follow, as it is completely devoid of junctions, side trips, and alternate routes all the way to the top. Start out from the trailhead, heading east, parallel to the highway, and then turn left up the hill. Despite being a long way inland, the forest here is only 800 feet above sea level and is typical of the lowlands on the western slope of the Cascades. Moss grows like thick velvet, draped over every exposed inch of the host trees. Passing underneath the branches while the sunlight filters through is like hiking in a living cathedral of green.

The footing soon becomes rough and rocky as the trail gets steeper and generally trends north. Giant erratic boulders and a few exposed slabs of polished rock hint at the area's ancient glacial history, while some stumps between the tall trees recount the more recent effects of man upon the landscape.

After about 0.5 mile, follow a broad bend around to the right. Amazingly, at just more than 1,200 feet, this is already the halfway point in terms of both horizontal distance and vertical gain. Once through the turn, the trail continues to climb through stately Douglas firs until it reaches the crest of a broad ridge. Although the forest prevents any views, the ground drops gently away on the left toward the North Fork of the Skykomish River.

Follow the southern side of the ridge for another 0.25 mile to abruptly emerge at the top of a brush-laden chute. The summit is only a few steps farther, just up the hill to the left where the high fire lookout rises above the trees.

The commanding wooden tower has been through various permutations and renovations since its original construction in 1925. Most recently refurbished in the 1990s, Heybrook Lookout now stands about 70 feet high. The tower is usually open for public access to the outdoor observation level, just below the cabin; a staircase zigzags up the eight stories to reach it.

The deck provides a grand view. Directly across the valley to the south, Mount Index's three jagged peaks (north, middle, and main) dominate the skyline. The steep rock walls below the long summit ridge rise more than 2,500 feet straight up from the forest below. Lake Serene rests at the bottom of the huge wall, although it is several hundred feet higher than the Heybrook Lookout and therefore not visible from this vantage. The whitewater of Bridal Veil Falls, the lake's outflow, can be discerned, tumbling down through the trees. Mount Persis stands behind Mount Index to the right, and has a similar rocky summit ridge.

A section of US 2 is visible to the east, below the distinctive twin spires of Mount Baring, two sharp points thrust into the sky. At 6,125 feet, Baring is about 200 feet higher than Index and 5,000 feet above the South Fork of the Skykomish, which runs along the highway. On the northern side of Baring, Gunn Peak and Merchant Peak stand across the Barclay Creek Valley.

The view to the north is largely obscured by trees and nearby ridges, although there are many prominent peaks in that direction. To the west, it is possible to see beyond the end of the valley and onto the flatlands around Monroe and on toward Puget Sound.

Below the lookout, a pair of picnic tables near the trees to the east offers a good place to sit down and have something to eat, although the only view they provide is of the tower itself. The gravel surface underneath connects to a network of U.S. Forest Service roads continuing eastward along the ridge, which some hikers may find worth exploring, although there is no better vista to be found than the one here.

Nearby Activities

On your way home, try the Mountain View Diner at the eastern end of Gold Bar for a filling posthike meal. The diner serves up a variety of hearty plates and attracts an interesting mix of customers, both locals and tourists. Look for the Mountain View along the southern side of US 2, or call 360-793-3345 for more information.

GPS TRAILHEAD COORDINATES
N47° 48.501' W121° 32.101'

On I-5 at the northern end of Everett, take Exit 194 for US 2 E. Travel 35.2 miles east on US 2 through the towns of Monroe, Sultan, Startup, and Gold Bar to reach the turnoff to Index. Continue on US 2 another 2 miles to the parking lot and trailhead on the left (north) side of US 2, across from the Mount Baker–Snoqualmie National Forest sign.

46 Iron Goat Trail

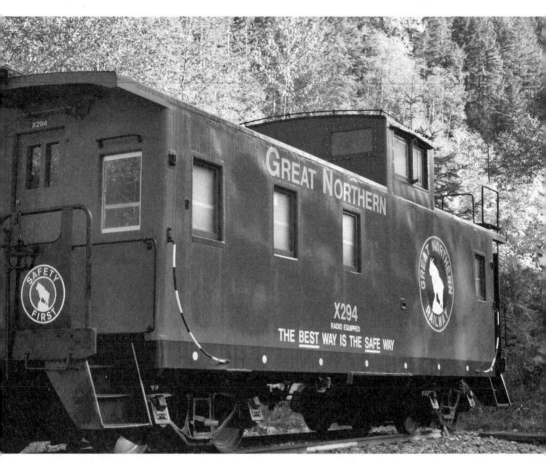

Great Northern railcar at the interpretive center

In Brief

History and nature converge on Iron Goat Trail unlike anywhere else, a tribute to both the beauty of the environment in its pristine condition and to man's amazing ability to transform it. Hiking the Iron Goat is like exploring a living museum in the wilderness, showcasing some great engineering achievements and the men who changed the world by building them. Throw in wildflowers, high mountain views, and a virtually flat, single-track trail, and the Iron Goat is an absolute must for any Washington State hiker.

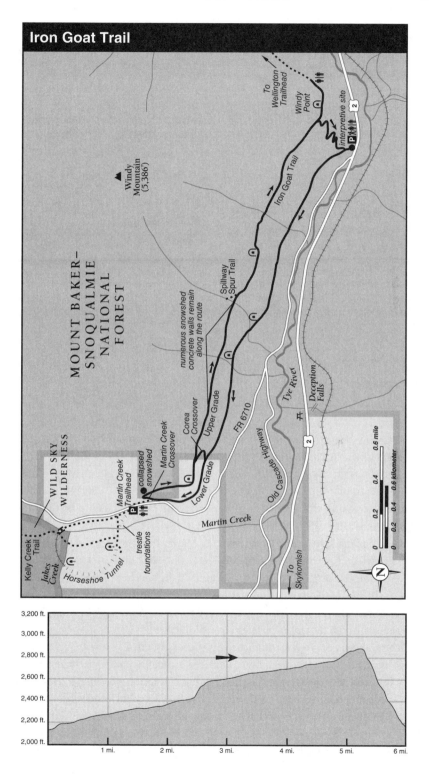

Iron Goat Trail

DISTANCE & CONFIGURATION: 6.0-mile loop with side options	**WHEELCHAIR TRAVERSABLE:** Yes, on the lower grade between Scenic and Martin Creek parking lots
DIFFICULTY: Moderate	**MAP(S):** Green Trails *Stevens Pass 176*; USGS *Scenic*
SCENERY: Historical railroad (including tunnels, snowshed walls, and artifacts), interpretive signs, wildflowers, well-maintained hiking trail; numerous viewpoints	**FACILITIES:** Toilet at trailhead; no drinking water
EXPOSURE: Mostly shaded	**DOGS:** Allowed on-leash
TRAFFIC: Medium	**CONTACT:** 360-677-2414; www.fs.usda .gov/recarea/mbs/recarea/?recid=17892 or irongoat.org
TRAIL SURFACE: Mostly dirt; with short sections of boardwalk and gravel	**LOCATION:** Skykomish
HIKING TIME: 3–6 hours	**COMMENTS:** Iron Goat Trail is still a work in progress, requiring volunteer labor and donations for maintenance and expansion. For more information or to become involved in the project, visit the official Iron Goat Trail website at irongoat.org.
ACCESS: Hikable late spring–fall; NW Forest Pass required for parking at Wellington and Martin Creek trailheads, but not main trailhead at interpretive center	

Description

Many people believe Stevens Pass was named for Isaac Stevens, the first governor of the Washington Territory from 1853 to 1857. But it is actually a tribute to railroad engineer John F. Stevens, who managed the construction of more than 1,000 miles of James J. Hill's Great Northern Railway at the end of the 19th century. Hill, sometimes called The Empire Builder of the Northwest, hoped to lay track from Saint Paul, Minnesota, all the way to Seattle to link the rich natural resources around Puget Sound to the markets of the east. But to realize this dream, a difficult Cascade crossing had to be built, and Stevens had the answer.

Stevens had made his name by discovering Marias Pass through the Rocky Mountains with the help of an American Indian guide in late 1889. At only 5,300 feet, Marias was the lowest-elevation crossing of the Rockies, located on the southern edge of what is now Glacier National Park. Managing to find the pass in frigid winter weather, Stevens saved the Great Northern millions of dollars and the need to travel hundreds of extra miles on a circuitous route through the notoriously rugged Bitterroot Range.

Hill counted on Stevens to duplicate his success in the Cascades, but it was actually Stevens's assistant, C. F. B. Haskell, who located a suitable pass in 1890 and named it in honor of his boss. In a rush to get the trains running as fast as possible, a tricky route was chosen across the mountain gap using eight separate switchbacks; this later proved to be extremely hazardous. Heavy snowfall and frequent avalanches often closed the tracks in winter, prompting Stevens to oversee construction of what is now known as the First Cascade Tunnel, a 2.6-mile passage under the Wenatchee Mountains and a remarkable engineering achievement. A series of snowsheds was built over long sections of the track and additional tunnels were later added for further protection, each constructed under difficult and dangerous conditions.

All of this history is close enough to touch on Iron Goat Trail, which follows the old right-of-way used by the Great Northern and gets its name both from the Great Northern logo, a mountain goat on a precipice, and from the idea of trains as iron horses.

There are three trailheads on the Iron Goat, one at Martin Creek, another about 6 miles east at Wellington, and the recommended one halfway in between at the interpretive site; each is at a pivotal point on the former railway. Martin Creek once housed an exceptional, U-shaped tunnel, known as the Horseshoe Tunnel, where trains crossed between the lower and upper grades just west of the current trailhead. At the other end, Wellington sits next to the western entrance to the First Cascade Tunnel on the site of one of the worst rail accidents in US history. On March 1, 1910, a massive avalanche swept two trains down the mountain and took half the town of Wellington with it, killing 96 people. Afterward, the settlement was renamed Tye to try to erase the connection between the name Wellington and the disaster, but the name Wellington is now in use once again. Finally, the interpretive site sits near where the historical settlement of Scenic once stood, an important rail town also known for its curative hot springs.

The trail starts west from the interpretive site on the lower-grade trail. Remain on the lower grade past a junction, which is the return route from Windy Point coming down the mountain. Watch for a beautifully restored black-and-white post marking mile 1,720, as measured from the eastern terminus of the line in St. Paul. These highly visible posts can be found at each mile interval and are useful for gauging distance.

A long concrete wall on the uphill side of the trail is all that remains of a significant snowshed, the first of many along the way. Today, it is hard to imagine the serious avalanche danger that would have prompted construction of these sheds, as a forest of Douglas firs and western hemlocks now covers the mountainside. However, the steep slopes were once stripped bare, cleared by logging and forest fires that were frequently started by sparks from passing locomotives, leaving the denuded land unable to adequately hold the wet and heavy snowpack. Despite the regrowth of the forest, a massive landslide during 2008 convincingly demonstrated that even today the slope is not as stable as it might seem.

Amazingly, the footing feels almost perfectly flat, although trains once struggled to climb this stretch. The trail runs at an average 2.2% grade, meaning it gains 2.2 vertical feet for every 100 horizontal feet—steep for rail travel but imperceptible to hikers.

The first of the Twin Tunnels, a pair of gaping holes blasted through the side of the mountain, eventually appears on the right, past milepost 1,719. Stand next to the mouth to get a true sense of the size of the opening and imagine the trains chugging through. Just past the tunnels, an elegant footbridge crosses a steep slope above the forest.

Reach a junction after another mile, signed MARTIN CREEK CROSSOVER (to Upper Grade), just short of the Martin Creek trailhead. Turn up the slope to the right through a lush forest of maples, alders, and ferns, and then turn right again onto the upper grade, about 120 feet farther up the side of the mountain. The upper grade is narrower

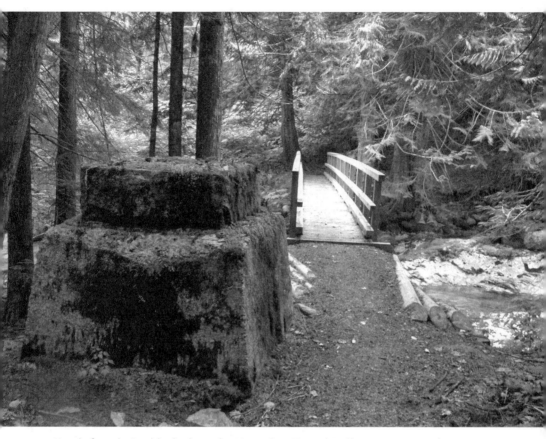

Trestle foundation block along the Horseshoe Tunnel Trail

than the lower grade and starts next to the rotting timbers of a collapsed snowshed. Note that it would have required a train to travel a little more than 1 mile through the Horseshoe Tunnel to gain the same altitude.

For the next 3 miles, the Iron Goat continues to offer a host of historical, archaeological, and natural delights too numerous to name and best left to each individual to discover. Rotting timbers, towering concrete snowshed walls, metal debris, old work camps, stone supports, and more gaping tunnels are all among the treasures to be found along the way, scattered between the trees and wildflowers. Perhaps inspired by the engineering feats of the original laborers, the restoration work on the trail itself shows a great level of inventiveness and creativity, often taking advantage of buried railroad supports, concrete pilings, and other relics.

Frequent viewpoints look south over the Tye River Valley to the right and the Alpine Lakes Wilderness beyond. Watch and listen for the trains of the Burlington Northern Santa Fe line that still run in the valley below; they're what's left of the Great Northern after several mergers with other railroads. The trains are headed for the Second Cascade Tunnel, whose inauguration in 1929 caused the abandonment of the entire upper line that has now been reclaimed as the Iron Goat Trail. The second tunnel runs underneath Big Chief Mountain and the Stevens Pass ski area for 7.8 miles, the longest tunnel in the Western Hemisphere at the time of its building and still the longest anywhere in the United States— yet another engineering marvel of the railway through Stevens Pass.

Although the signed downhill route back to the interpretive site is up at the beginning of the Windy Point Tunnel, it is worth continuing past the turn to an excellent overlook near the opposite end. The 0.25-mile tunnel was dug in 1913 to ease the passage around this dangerous, exposed curve on the edge of 5,386-foot Windy Mountain. The viewpoint looks straight down on US 2, the old townsite at Scenic, and the western mouth of the Second Cascade Tunnel. And if nature should happen to call, an open-air latrine down the slope to the right provides a spectacular view from "the throne."

Ambitious hikers can continue eastward from here as far as Wellington on an out-and-back route, but most will be content to complete the loop by returning straight down the slope from Windy Point at the signed junction.

Nearby Activities

The Wellington trailhead provides three additional points of interest, all easy to reach and within 0.25 mile of the parking area: the western entrance to the First Cascade Tunnel; the avalanche disaster site; and the all-concrete snowshed, whose columns provide one of the most unusual hiking experiences anywhere in Washington for those passing underneath. The alternate Wellington trailhead is located on Forest Route 050, 2.8 miles down the Old Stevens Pass Highway, which begins on the left (north) side of US 2 between mileposts 64 and 65.

The Martin Creek trailhead provides access to the Horseshoe Tunnel Trail, which explores the massive rail switchback from the upper grade to the lower grade that was in use before the completion of the Second Cascade Tunnel in 1929. Watch for moss-covered, concrete foundation blocks in the forest, all that remains of the two high trestles that once carried trains here. As with the rest of the Iron Goat, expect to find various other rail artifacts and points of interest along the way. The Martin Creek trailhead can be reached by driving about 3 miles west on FS 6710 from the interpretive site or by hiking west along the lower grade from the Martin Creek Crossover and then crossing the road.

GPS TRAILHEAD COORDINATES
N47° 42.670' W121° 9.770'

On I-5 at the northern end of Everett, take Exit 194 for US 2 E. Travel 57.9 miles east on US 2 through the towns of Monroe, Sultan, Startup, Gold Bar, and Baring toward Stevens Pass. Just past milepost 58, turn left into the Iron Goat Interpretive Site parking lot.

47 Lake Serene and Bridal Veil Falls

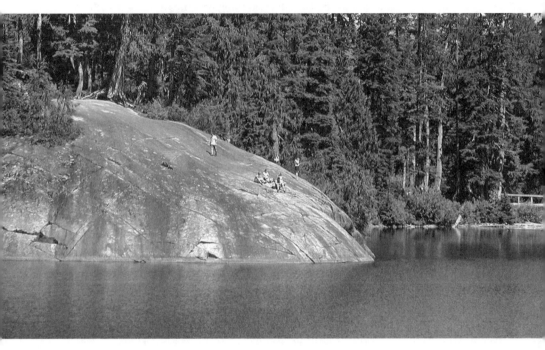

Lunch Rock at Lake Serene

In Brief

Lake Serene might be the perfect swimming hole. With a fantastic location below the northern wall of Mount Index, crystal-clear water, and a collection of sun-soaked boulders along the shore for diving, it's hard to imagine any better place to spend a summer's day. The tough hike in only adds to the experience, keeping away the worst of the crowds and making the swim seem that much more inviting.

Description

The Washington Cascades are blessed with countless lakes, tarns, and ponds, but there are precious few that can rival Lake Serene. The location is unforgettable, in a bowl at the bottom of the sheer 3,000-foot northern face of Mount Index. Although the peak's

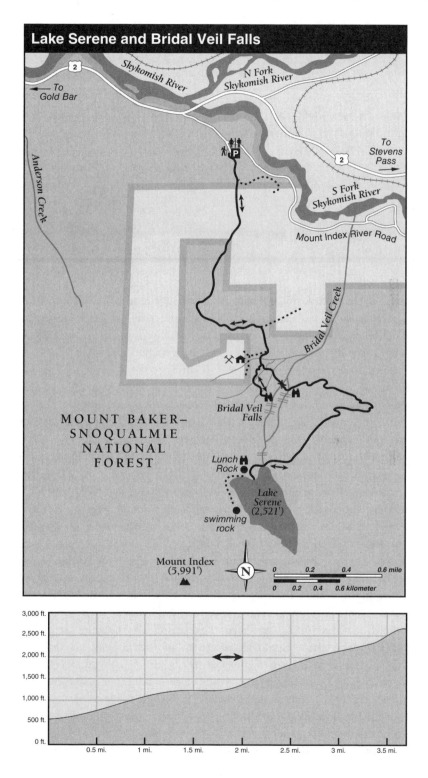

DISTANCE & CONFIGURATION: 7.4-mile out-and-back to lake; 3.4-mile out-and-back to the falls	**HIKING TIME:** 4–6 hours
	ACCESS: Hikable late spring–fall; NW Forest Pass required for parking
DIFFICULTY: Difficult	**WHEELCHAIR TRAVERSABLE:** No
SCENERY: Bridal Veil Falls, Lake Serene under the high walls of Mount Index, old-growth forest; views across the Sky-komish Valley	**MAP(S):** Green Trails *Index 142*; USGS *Index*
	FACILITIES: Toilet at trailhead, no drinking water
EXPOSURE: Mostly shaded	**DOGS:** Allowed on-leash
TRAFFIC: High	**CONTACT:** 360-677-2414; www.fs.usda .gov/recarea/mbs/recarea/?recid=17900
TRAIL SURFACE: Dirt, with slippery rocks and roots in places	**LOCATION:** Index

signature crags can be easily identified from almost anywhere in the Skykomish Valley, it's the view straight up from the lake that truly shows the mountain's massive vertical relief. If that's not enough, the lake is directly fed by melting snow and ice, leaving the water clean, pure, and cold—and unbelievably refreshing on a hot, sunny day.

If Lake Serene were just off the road, it surely would be overrun every summer weekend and a good portion of the rest of the time as well. Thankfully, access to this alpine treasure needs to be earned, and not everyone is prepared to pay the price. All potential visitors must first complete a strenuous 3.7-mile hike with a 2,000-foot elevation gain. Yet for anyone seeking a shorter journey, thundering Bridal Veil Falls makes a great alternate destination for less than half the effort, an amazing added bonus among an embarrassment of riches.

The trail begins at an altitude of just less than 600 feet on an old road with a very rocky surface. The road forks within the first 0.25 mile, connecting to a larger network of reclaimed vehicle-access points all along the southern side of the Skykomish Valley. Stay right, following a sign with a hiker symbol.

The forest here is in shade most of the time, shielded from the sun by the high walls of Mount Index to the south and the thick canopy of alders and big-leaf maples overhead. Expect the trail to be wet and muddy all year and for the trail to cross several small creeks and streams as it climbs through the trees on a shallow incline.

At about 1.5 miles from the trailhead, the road branches a second time. Once more stay right, following a hiker sign, and then reach another intersection soon after. The right branch enters a small maze of gravel roads exploring an old copper-mining claim. A ruined prospector's cabin is shown on some maps, but it is not easy to find. The main route starts a gradual descent toward Bridal Veil Creek on the left.

The signed trail to Middle Bridal Veil Falls comes up a few hundred yards farther along. Although the side trip adds more than 0.5 mile and 300 feet of vertical gain to the total hiking distance, it should be considered an absolute must for everyone.

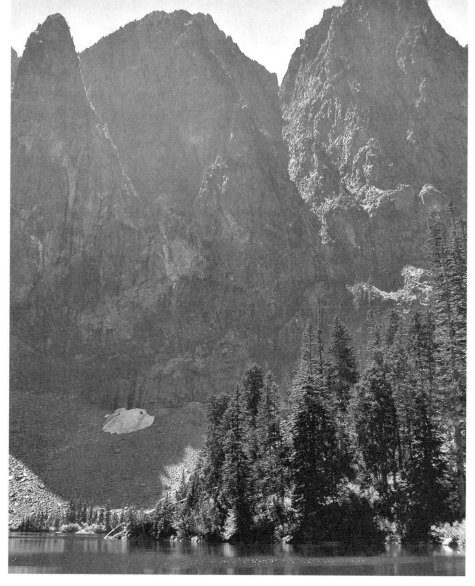

Mount Index from Lake Serene

The rugged singletrack to the falls climbs steeply through rocks and roots, staging a direct assault on the mountainside. A set of wooden stairs leads to the spectacular cascade, where Bridal Veil Creek plunges down a giant slab of exposed rock, tossing curtains of mist out over the Skykomish Valley. Unless the water is very high, it is possible to walk out onto the rocks below the falls or cross to the far side to get a better view. Use caution and stay well back from the edge, however, as the rocks are wet and slippery.

The falls make a great place to rest, with plenty of space to sit down and enjoy the thundering water and the great view across the valley from the 1,500-foot vantage. Look for the cliffs on the opposite side; known collectively as the Index Town Wall, they are popular with rock climbers.

For some hikers, Bridal Veil Falls makes a worthwhile destination all on its own, and this is their turnaround point. Yet beautiful Lake Serene still awaits, another scenic jewel some 1,000 feet above.

Descend from the falls to return to the main trail, and then follow the sign to Lake Serene, 2 miles away. Cross Bridal Veil Creek on a sturdy footbridge with a view of the impressive lower falls through the trees to the right, a slide falls similar in form to the middle falls farther up. The trail runs below yet another waterfall in the next 0.25 mile, close enough that anyone passing underneath is sure to feel the spray.

Beyond this point, the trail gives up any pretense of moderation and starts on a demanding and relentless climb. The mountainside is so steep as to allow only seven major switchbacks before the top, resulting in many sections with wooden stairs and other aids to ease the ascent. The sheer slope also makes logging very difficult, with old-growth western hemlock still standing here that would have been cut long ago in the flats closer to the bottom of the valley.

At 2,400 feet, emerge from the trees to meet a view of Mount Index straight ahead and the Skykomish River far below to the right. Another mucky 0.25 mile of climbing leads to the crest of the trail and then, at last, the shoreline of the lake.

Cross the outflow stream to the right on a wooden bridge and proceed to the Lunch Rock, a broad slab of unmistakable granite overlooking the eastern shore where most hikers congregate. It is also possible to scramble farther around the edge of the lake to some substantial boulders at the bottom of the talus field below the rock walls of Mount Index. The tricky crossing is worth it for the improved solitude and excellent diving platforms on the far side.

The massive face of Index tends to keep much of Lake Serene in shadow later in the day, but when the morning sun shines down unobstructed, the setting is glorious. The emerald waters of the lake can almost look like the Caribbean, in contrast to the forbidding walls of Cascade rock just behind. Amazingly, there are some climbing routes up Mount Index that start from the lake, but they are extremely difficult and hazardous and are rarely attempted. For most hikers, reaching the lake will be reward enough.

GPS TRAILHEAD COORDINATES

N47° 48.544' W121° 34.427'

On I-5 at the northern end of Everett, take Exit 194 for US 2 E. Travel 34.8 miles east on US 2 through the towns of Monroe, Sultan, Startup, and Gold Bar. Just past milepost 35 (immediately before the bridge over the South Fork Skykomish River), turn right onto Mt. Index Road. In 0.3 mile, turn right into the parking lot for Lake Serene Trail.

48 Lime Kiln Trail

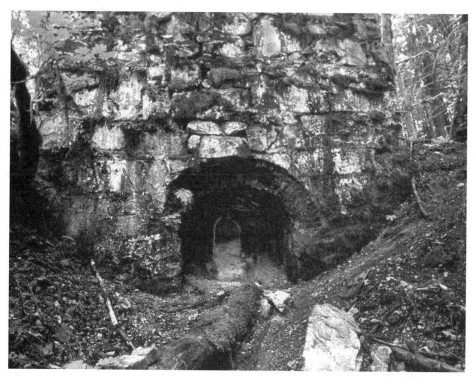

Front view of the limekiln

In Brief

Despite its laid-back demeanor, the quiet town of Granite Falls was once a thriving economic hub. The local railway disappeared long ago with the logging and mining firms it used to serve, but many archaeological remnants of the industrial-era operation still remain, waiting to be discovered by those who know where to look. This hike runs along the southern side of the Stillaguamish River, exploring the region's colorful past and culminating at the unique ruins of an old limekiln standing in the beautifully regenerated forest.

Description

Access to the south fork of the Stillaguamish between Granite Falls and Verlot has generally been restricted to the river's northern bank. The rich history of the southern side was largely hidden, refusing to give up its secrets to the casual visitor.

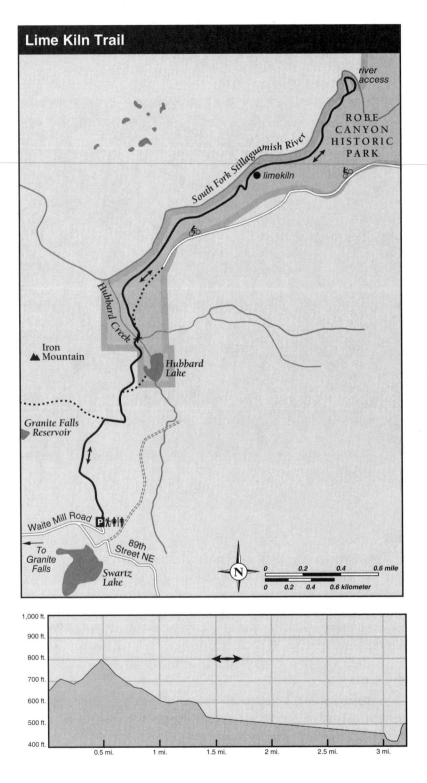

Lime Kiln Trail

DISTANCE & CONFIGURATION: 6.4-mile out-and-back to river; 4.8-mile out-and-back to limekiln	**ACCESS:** Hikable year-round, daily, 7 a.m.–sunset; no fee for parking or trail access
DIFFICULTY: Easy–moderate	**WHEELCHAIR TRAVERSABLE:** No
SCENERY: Historical limekiln and old artifacts along a little-used rail-trail; views down to South Fork Stillaguamish River; access to riverbank	**MAP(S):** Green Trails *Granite Falls 109*; USGS *Granite Falls*
EXPOSURE: Mostly shaded; exposed along a portion of dirt road	**FACILITIES:** Toilet at trailhead; no drinking water
TRAFFIC: Low–medium	**DOGS:** Allowed on-leash
TRAIL SURFACE: Mostly dirt with a couple of sections of gravel	**CONTACT:** 425-388-6600; snohomish countywa.gov/Facilities/Facility/Details /Lime-Kiln-Trailhead-95
HIKING TIME: 4–5 hours	**LOCATION:** Granite Falls

All that changed in the fall of 2004 with the inauguration of Lime Kiln Trail, center-piece of the Robe Canyon Historic Park. The trail circles around the eastern side of Iron Mountain on an easement through private land to join the former route of the Everett and Monte Cristo Railway. From there, the route penetrates deep into the canyon on the river's high southern bank before ending at the location of a former bridge, now long since disappeared. Although this is the end of the trail, the park continues linearly along the river canyon for several more miles to the original Robe townsite. Hopefully, future development will extend Lime Kiln Trail to the east where it can be linked with Old Robe Trail and other trails originating from around Verlot.

Until then, Lime Kiln Trail still makes a great hiking destination on its own, combining the beautiful natural environment with a window into the region's fascinating history. The trail's builders also took extra care in construction and development, crafting a well-designed journey into the wilderness.

Look for the trailhead at the northern end of the parking lot and start hiking through a dark forest of ferns and low maples. About 0.25 mile in, a sign marks the beginning of some private property. It is particularly important to stay on the trail through this section, although a tangled and virtually impenetrable mess of salmonberry bushes on either side effectively prevents passage anywhere but along the footpath.

Stay right at a junction, signed for Robe Canyon Park and Lime Kiln, and emerge onto a wide gravel road. Follow the old logging road downhill to the right at the next intersection and then bear left to reach a fork. Both of these turns are clearly marked. Stay left for another 0.25 mile to reach the signed entrance to Robe Canyon Historic Park, the end of the passage through the private property. The trail reenters the trees and shrinks back to singletrack on a rough surface of gray and reddish rocks, now about a mile from the trailhead.

Cross a wide wooden bridge over Hubbard Creek. The creek flows out of Hubbard Lake, just through the trees to the right, although not visible from here. On the far side

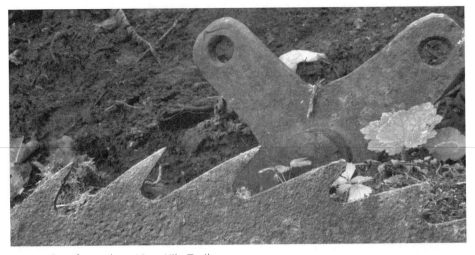

Rusted artifacts along Lime Kiln Trail

of the bridge, the trail surface returns to gravel road for another 0.25 mile, where a singletrack heads left into the trees, signed for Lime Kiln Trail. This turn is the start of the hikers-only section, although mountain bikers and equestrians can continue along the road until it ends.

Descend along Hubbard Creek toward the Stillaguamish River and find the start of the old Everett and Monte Cristo Railway, built in the early 1890s and abandoned in 1934. Turn right to join the old railroad grade, hardly distinguishable from the previous trail except for its flatness.

The river runs at the bottom of the canyon, about 100 feet below to the left. Large cedars and big-leaf maples grow from the steep slope, spreading their branches at eye level along the trail, an unusual vantage point for inspecting the forest canopy. Ferns gather in sheltered glades where side creeks flow down on their way to meet the Stillaguamish.

At first, evidence of any former human activity is hard to find, with only the occasional piece of rusted debris or cable poking up through the dirt. Soon after entering the Cutoff Junction historical site, however, all manner of cast-off items can be found scattered beneath the trees. Look for pieces of ceramic plates, bowls, and glass jars, along with bricks, leather boots, and even old iron-stove components. Particularly striking is a large number of rusted circular-saw blades, whose jagged teeth stand in high contrast with the softer textures and smooth edges of the natural forest. These fascinating relics are testaments to the strange transformation that takes place when worthless junk is left anywhere for a sufficiently long period of time—it turns into something of great interest and value.

The history lesson culminates at the old limekiln, which stands about 20 feet high. Limekilns date back at least to the ancient Egyptians, who used lime mortar for their stone buildings; this kiln, however, is a textbook example of the design for such structures used during the Industrial Revolution. The tower is built on a slope to facilitate the addition of limestone to the top, with wood and other burning materials fed into a fire through an opening on the side. Powdered lime would be removed from the main access arch at the bottom, which now faces the trail. The final product would be used for a host of applications, including construction, agriculture, and cleaning.

The kiln's gray rock walls are now covered in green mosses, lichens, and ferns, giving it the appearance of something out of the ruined civilizations of the Mayas, Incas, or Aztecs. It's easy to forget that it has only been standing for about a century.

The trail continues past the limekiln another 0.7 mile through some former logging sites to reach a fork, the beginning of a short loop. Continue right for a few hundred yards to a viewpoint over the river, where the Everett and Monte Cristo Railroad once crossed to the far side of the canyon on a bridge. Almost all evidence of the span has disappeared, inviting speculation as to where the two ends might have been anchored in the rocks and on what angle the structure crossed the water.

This is the end of the trail and the turnaround point for the hike, at least pending further development of the Robe Canyon Historic Park. The hoped-for future linking of Lime Kiln Trail with Old Robe Trail would require construction of another bridge over the river.

On the way back, be sure to explore the short loop from the last junction that leads down through salal and low brush to the riverbank. With a little effort, it is possible to scramble down to the rocks on the riverbed, a great place to enjoy some rest and relaxation.

Nearby Activities

It is possible to explore a section of Old Robe Trail on the opposite side of the river. The trail passes through Old Robe townsite and then follows the abandoned Monte Cristo Railroad track for about 1.5 miles before becoming impassable. To reach the Old Robe Trailhead, take the Mountain Loop Highway out of Granite Falls, travel about 7 miles, and look for a brick monument and shoulder parking area on the right side of the road. Find more information at tinyurl.com/robecanyonhp.

GPS TRAILHEAD COORDINATES

N48° 4.641' W121° 55.964'

On I-5 at the northern end of Everett, take Exit 194 for US 2 E. Head east 1.9 miles on US 2, and exit left onto WA 204, which climbs to the town of Lake Stevens. In 2.7 miles, at the intersection with WA 9, turn left (north). Proceed 1.7 miles to a right turn onto WA 92 toward Granite Falls. In 8.5 miles, in Granite Falls, turn right onto S. Alder Avenue, and continue 0.3 mile to a T-intersection. Turn left onto Menzel Lake Road, signed for Lake Roesiger. In 0.9 mile, turn left onto Waite Mill Road. In 0.7 mile, after the school bus turnaround, stay left on a gravel road that climbs uphill. Look for the entrance to the parking area on the left signed for Robe Canyon Historic Park and Lime Kiln Trail.

49 Meadowdale Beach County Park

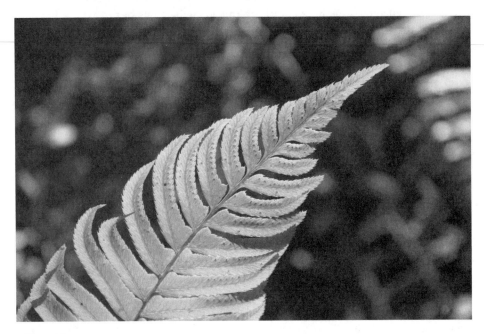

Sword fern

In Brief

Meadowdale is a valuable rarity among the many good Puget Sound beachfront parks, thanks to restricted road access to the shore. This makes it a great choice for hikers, who will enjoy the descent on an easy trail along Lunds Gulch Creek, which runs through a beautiful forest on the way to the beach.

Description

Not surprisingly for a waterfront parcel of land in the heavily developed Edmonds region, Meadowdale Beach Park passed through many private hands before being acquired by the Snohomish County Parks and Recreation Department in 1968. Of the private owners, the most significant was surely the Meadowdale Country Club, which built and maintained a clubhouse, swimming pool, and other facilities on-site, although most of the evidence of the club is long gone. The memory of John Lund, an early homesteader in the

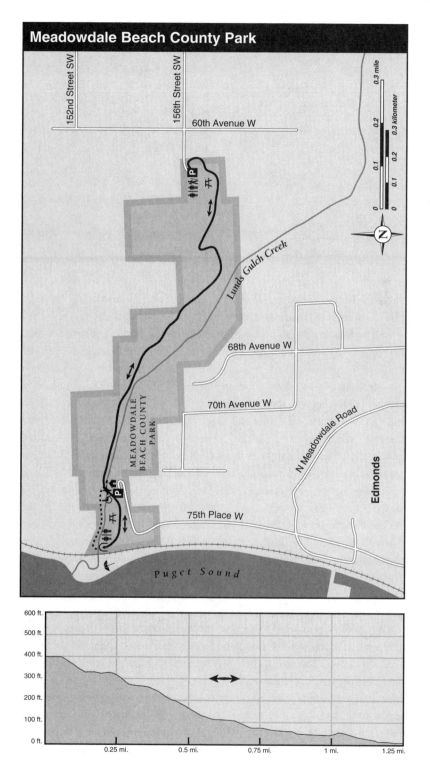

DISTANCE & CONFIGURATION: 2.5-mile out-and-back	before sunset); no fee for parking or trail access
DIFFICULTY: Easy–moderate	**WHEELCHAIR TRAVERSABLE:** Not on main trail, but the lower park near beach has a separate disabled access. See park website for info.
SCENERY: Lunds Gulch Creek, Meadowdale Beach, playfields, and a variety of trees with identification plaques	
EXPOSURE: Shaded along the trail, exposed at the beach	**MAP(S):** USGS *Edmonds East*
TRAFFIC: High	**FACILITIES:** Toilet at trailhead; no drinking water
TRAIL SURFACE: Mixture of dirt and gravel	**DOGS:** Allowed on-leash
HIKING TIME: 1–2 hours	**CONTACT:** 425-388-6600; tinyurl.com /meadowdalebeach
ACCESS: Hikable year-round, daily, 7 .am.–sunset (beach closes 30 minutes	**LOCATION:** 6025 156th St. SW, Edmonds, WA 98026

late 1800s, is more obvious today—the hike runs through Lunds Gulch, carved out over the ages by the waters of Lunds Gulch Creek.

The trail, which starts on the opposite side of the parking lot from a good-sized madrone tree, curves around a broad bend through the field to the east. Start down the wide surface, circling through the grass, and then enter the forest. The gradual descent and smooth trail make this hike a good option for families with small children, who will find the route interesting but not too difficult.

Some wooden stairs and a split rail fence mark the beginning of a steeper descent into the narrow valley of Lunds Gulch. The fern-covered walls rise 200 feet to the rim, and Lunds Gulch Creek soon appears in a gully to the left as the trail runs beneath a mix of maples, Douglas firs, cottonwoods, and alders. Despite its very limited length, the creek carries a number of species of fish, including some salmon that make the run upstream from the ocean to spawn. The mix of freshwater and saltwater at the creek's mouth acts as a tiny estuary, where the young smolts go through the substantial physical changes that allow them to make the transition from life in the freshwater of their birth to that of the saltwater of their adult lives, the unique adaptation of anadromous fish.

Moss-covered big-leaf maples now seem to be the dominant tree species in the forest, but a series of enormous western hemlock stumps near the half-mile mark gives some idea of what the original ecosystem here might have been like. Look for the old springboard notches in the wood, used to support the working platforms the loggers used to fell the ancient giants. A few low-to-the-ground interpretive signs help identify some of the major plant species and point out their distinguishing characteristics, such as the heart-shaped leaves of the black cottonwood.

As you near the beach, high alders lean out over the trail from either side, creating an effect similar to a towering arbor trellis. The setting is magical when the sunlight filters through the living archway to the ground below. The trail emerges from the trees and then crosses the creek on a bridge next to a park ranger station on the left. A road connects the ranger's facility to surface streets on the southern side of the gulch, but access is currently restricted, keeping the crowds away. Only disabled individuals who would otherwise be unable to descend the longer trail from the top are permitted to use this approach. Pass through a grassy clearing with a picnic shelter and a volleyball pit and then head into a short concrete tunnel under railroad tracks to finally reach the beach.

Note that the tunnel is frequently flooded by the creek and may be completely impassable at times. Even at best, there may be no way to get through without getting your feet wet, so always proceed with caution. Do not attempt to bypass the tunnel by crossing the railroad tracks above; it is both dangerous and illegal.

Lunds Gulch Creek empties into Possession Sound through the sand, depositing the sediment and runoff it has collected along its course. At low tide, a tiny barrier island serves as a breakwater just offshore and numerous small tide pools are exposed, ripe for examination. Pieces of sun-bleached driftwood are scattered around the gravelly beach, cast up by the whims of the tide.

Much like the more popular beaches at Golden Gardens and Carkeek parks to the south, Meadowdale is a great place to watch the sun set over the Olympic Mountains. Just to the northwest, Possession Point marks the extreme southeastern end of Whidbey Island, and the northern tip of the Kitsap Peninsula sits straight out to the west.

Spend any length of time along the water, and there is a good chance that a freight train will come thundering up the tracks. The sight and sound of the locomotives hauling a mile-or-more-long chain of cars certainly does not enhance the wilderness aspect of the hike, but the spectacle is thrilling nonetheless.

The beach serves as a frequent haul-out site for harbor seals that come up on shore from the water to help regulate their body temperatures, interact with other individuals, and rest or sleep. Young pups that have not yet learned to fear people are particularly vulnerable while on land and should not be disturbed, especially if they are nursing. Seals may potentially be found here at almost any time of year.

After exploring the beach, retrace your steps up Lunds Gulch Creek to the trailhead. You will need to climb back up the 400 feet lost on the descent to complete the round-trip journey of approximately 2.5 miles.

GPS TRAILHEAD COORDINATES
N47° 51.432' W122° 18.998'

From I-5, take Exit 183 for 164th Street SW, and head west. In 1.3 miles 164th Street SW curves north and crosses over WA 99. In 0.8 mile from the curve, turn right onto 52nd Avenue W, and go 0.5 mile. Turn left onto 156th Street SW and proceed 0.6 mile straight into the Meadowdale Beach County Park parking lot.

50 Mount Pilchuck State Park

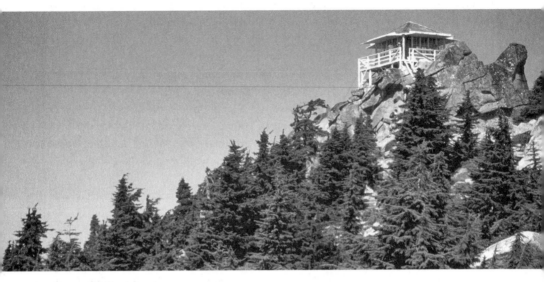

Mount Pilchuck Lookout

In Brief

Though the only man-made structure here is the summit lookout, Mount Pilchuck could not be any better designed even if it had been specifically planned and constructed by hand. When it comes to getting the most bang for your buck, no other peak offers such great rewards for so little effort. This landmark hike should not be missed.

Description

Most 5,000-foot peaks near Seattle rise so steeply and abruptly they require some 4,000 feet of climbing to reach the summit. Thanks to an approach road that winds high above the Stillaguamish River Valley, 5,324-foot Mount Pilchuck can be crested via a relatively short trail with only 2,200 feet of vertical gain. Once you attain the lookout, the view is so grand it seems all of western Washington is spread out below you.

At an altitude of more than 3,100 feet, the parking lot alone offers impressive views, and some people drive up the road just to take a look. To the northeast, Three Fingers Mountain rises high above the Stillaguamish (which locals call the Stilly), and several vantage points look straight up through the trees at Pilchuck's rocky pinnacle. The lot has plenty of space, so even on the busiest days there is a good chance there will be room. Expect those busy days to come quite frequently, especially in the summer, as the trail is suitable for hikers of all kinds, including many children and pets.

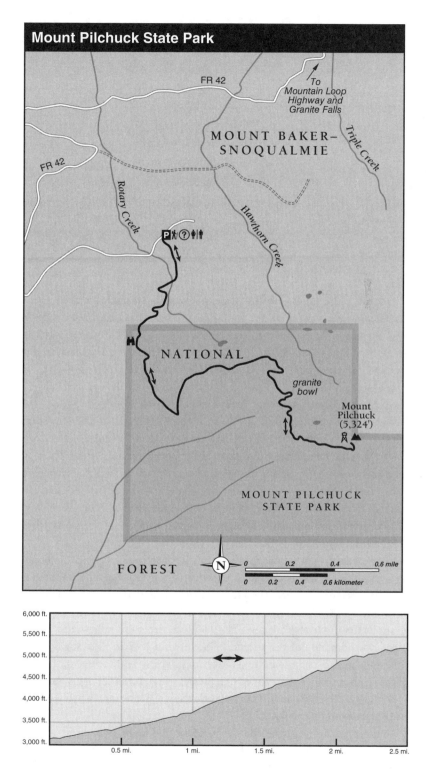

Mount Pilchuck State Park

FR 42

To
Mountain Loop
Highway and
Granite Falls

Triple Creek

MOUNT BAKER–
SNOQUALMIE

FR 42

Rotary Creek

Hawthorn Creek

NATIONAL

granite
bowl

Mount
Pilchuck
(5,324')

MOUNT PILCHUCK
STATE PARK

FOREST

N

0   0.2   0.4   0.6 mile

0   0.2   0.4   0.6 kilometer

6,000 ft.
5,500 ft.
5,000 ft.
4,500 ft.
4,000 ft.
3,500 ft.
3,000 ft.

0.5 mi.   1 mi.   1.5 mi.   2 mi.   2.5 mi.

DISTANCE & CONFIGURATION: 5.0-mile out-and-back	**ACCESS:** Hikable summer–fall (road remains snowed-in during spring); NW Forest Pass required for parking
DIFFICULTY: Moderate	
SCENERY: Scenic trail, historical lookout cabin open to public; summit views	**WHEELCHAIR TRAVERSABLE:** No
	MAP(S): Green Trails *Granite Falls 109*; USGS *Verlot*
EXPOSURE: Shaded on about half the route; lookout cabin provides shelter at the summit	
	FACILITIES: Toilet at trailhead; no drinking water
TRAFFIC: Heavy (hike midweek, if possible)	**DOGS:** Allowed on-leash
TRAIL SURFACE: Dirt and rock, large boulders	**CONTACT:** 360-793-0420; parks.state .wa.us/548/Mount-Pilchuck
HIKING TIME: 3–5 hours	**LOCATION:** Granite Falls

Unfortunately, the sheer number of people passing through the area causes some problems beyond heavy traffic on the trail. This trailhead has had some break-ins, so be sure not to leave any valuables in the car.

Marked as Mount Pilchuck Trail 700, the route originates at the western end of the parking lot next to the information board and is posted at 3 miles in length, one way, although it is actually closer to 2.5 miles. For the first 100 yards, the trail is as wide and rocky as a gravel road, but it soon narrows as it climbs to the south.

The area is jointly administered by Washington State Parks and Recreation and the U.S. Forest Service. Watch for a sign marking the entrance to Mount Pilchuck State Park nestled next to some reeds and huge skunk cabbage plants after 0.25 mile. The trail is well maintained and worn, with regular water bars for drainage and a raised surface lined by logs on either side. Steps have been built in several areas where needed, and the uphill grade is moderate and relatively easygoing for about the first mile. Occasional viewpoints open out to the west through a mixed forest of young conifers interspersed with some far older trees and sun-bleached snags.

Near 3,600 feet, the path picks its way through a large boulder field, the beginning of a rocky surface that continues most of the way to the top. Fortunately, steady views appear as well. Each one is better than the last, especially in the last mile, which is by far the steepest and most demanding.

The trail exits the forest for good at 4,000 feet, emerging into a vast granite bowl beneath the northern side of the summit. The lookout is visible far above, silhouetted against the sky on the highest crag. The setting here is spectacular and geologically unusual for the area, like a piece of the High Sierras lifted from California and dropped at the edge of the western Cascades. Pikas whistle their alarm from the white rocks, while several small tarns shimmer below.

The route skirts the western side of the exposed granite, passing by the ruins of a tramline that once served the summit. Weathered timbers, giant bolts, and rusted pulleys are all visible along the way, evidence of the hardships of building high in the mountains before the advent of the helicopter.

Wrap around to the southern side of the mountain before reaching the final ridge. Traverse the ridge, scramble through the last few boulders, and then clamber up the ladder to the lookout. The climb can be a little tricky, but there is no real exposure and everyone should be able to complete it.

The handsome lookout has a long history, intimately tied to the development of the area. The first access trail up Mount Pilchuck was constructed along Black Creek and Pinnacle Lake in 1909, ascending the peak's eastern flank. A more direct 7-mile route was established within a year from near the town of Robe, crossing the Stillaguamish River on a hand-driven cable car. Much of that route is not too far from the trail still in use today.

In 1921 the first lookout was completed on the summit. Subsequent redesigns and renovations occurred in 1941, 1971, and 1989, bringing it to its current form as a year-round hiker's shelter. Heavy snow shutters can be lowered over the windows in winter to shield the building and its occupants from storms and the brunt of the wind. The Everett chapter of The Mountaineers is responsible for the most recent remodeling of the structure as well as its current upkeep, a great service to the public.

Inside the cozy shelter, benches line the walls beneath the 360-degree windows, a perfect place for lunch. Informational panels recount the history of the lookout with text and photographs, and panoramic displays indicate the countless landmarks on all sides.

The view offers a virtual who's who of the high peaks of the central Washington Cascades, including Baker, Shuksan, Three Fingers, Whitehorse, El Dorado, Glacier, Sloan, Big Four, Dickerman, Pugh, and Rainier. To the west, the town of Granite Falls lies directly below, with Everett, Lake Stevens, Camano Island, and Puget Sound out to the Olympic Peninsula beyond. Enjoy your rest on top of the world before starting the descent.

Nearby Activities

There are multiple amenities and services available in Granite Falls, where the Mountain Loop Highway meets WA 92. As you enjoy a posthike meal or drink, look for Mount Pilchuck, clearly visible towering over the eastern end of town.

GPS TRAILHEAD COORDINATES
N48° 4.244' W121° 48.847'

On I-5 at the northern end of Everett, take Exit 194 for US 2 E. Head east 1.9 miles on US 2, and exit left onto WA 204, which climbs to the town of Lake Stevens. In 2.7 miles, at the intersection with WA 9, turn left (north). Proceed 1.7 miles to a right turn onto WA 92 toward Granite Falls. In 8.5 miles, in Granite Falls, turn left onto N. Alder Avenue, which becomes Mountain Loop Highway. In 11.9 miles, after passing Verlot and immediately after crossing the Stillaguamish River, go right on Mt. Pilchuck Road/Forest Route 42. Travel on this paved and gravel road 6.9 miles to the parking area.

51 Spencer Island Natural Wildlife Reserve

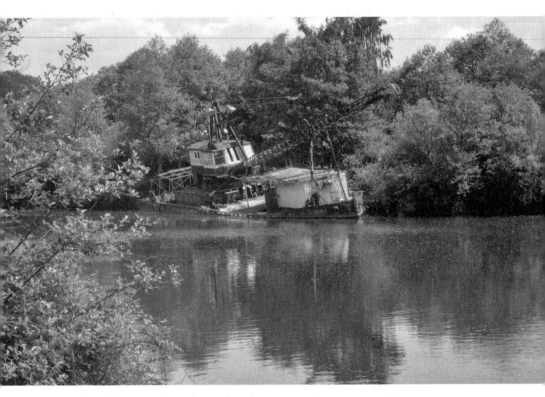

Abandoned boat on Steamboat Slough

In Brief

Spencer Island sits at the center of the biologically flourishing Snohomish River Estuary, home to countless animals and plants, including more than 350 known species of birds. A series of trails explores the rich life of the wetlands, great for naturalists, birdwatchers, and hikers.

Description

Just north of downtown Everett, freshwater from the mouth of the Snohomish River mingles with the salt water of Possession Sound, creating a highly dynamic environment and

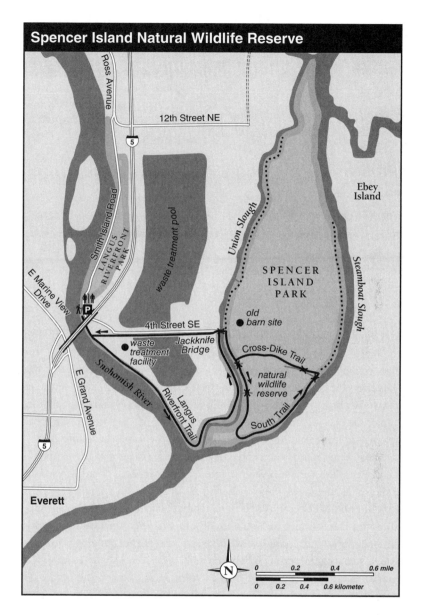

Spencer Island Natural Wildlife Reserve

Ross Avenue

12th Street NE

5

Ebey
Island

Smith Island Road

LANGUS
RIVERFRONT
PARK

waste treatment pool

Union Slough

Steamboat Slough

E Marine View
Drive

SPENCER
ISLAND
PARK

P

old
barn site

4th Street SE

waste
treatment
facility

Jackknife
Bridge

Cross-Dike Trail

E Grand Avenue

Snohomish River

Langus
Riverfront Trail

natural
wildlife
reserve

South Trail

5

Everett

N

| 0 | 0.2 | 0.4 | 0.6 mile |

| 0 | 0.2 | 0.4 | 0.6 kilometer |

forming critical habitat for hundreds of species. However, these same dynamic forces are frequently not so kind to the land itself. Rising and sinking saltwater tides coupled with seasonal flooding cause the ground to endlessly shift and erode, only to be built up somewhere else. Sitting at the center of the estuary, Spencer Island often gets the brunt of the relentless waters, and in many ways, it continues to exist thanks only to an extensive series of dikes and levees designed to keep the river and the ocean at bay.

DISTANCE & CONFIGURATION: 4.0-mile figure eight plus optional northern-island trails	**ACCESS:** Hikable year-round, 7 a.m.–sunset; no fee for parking or trail access
DIFFICULTY: Easy and flat	**WHEELCHAIR TRAVERSABLE:** Yes, on the paved Langus Riverfront Trail and a short accessible trail from the bridge onto the island that leads to a viewpoint.
SCENERY: Wildlife watching and bird-watching, wetlands, interpretive board-walk trails, river and mountain views	**MAP(S):** USGS *Everett*
EXPOSURE: Mostly exposed	**FACILITIES:** Toilet at nearby Langus Riverfront Park; no drinking water
TRAFFIC: Medium	**DOGS:** Not allowed
TRAIL SURFACE: Mixture of dirt, gravel, pavement, and boardwalk	**CONTACT:** 360-568-2482; tinyurl.com/spencerisland
HIKING TIME: 2–4 hours	**LOCATION:** Everett

The system is certainly not fail-safe, though, and the largely wood-chip dikes are in constant need of repair. The fragility of the system was graphically displayed in 2003, when catastrophic damage from several large breaches and a fire smoldering within one of the dikes caused the closure of several key trails and significantly altered the landscape. Although two key bridges were finally rebuilt in 2008, recovery and construction work—both to repair the considerable damage and also for ongoing maintenance to prevent further problems—continue and should be expected for the foreseeable future.

Just as the island sits at the center of the swirling waters of the estuary, so, too, does it lie in the middle of a mix of government jurisdictions, creating a strange juxtaposition of conflicting uses. The southern half is administered as a Natural Wildlife Reserve by Snohomish County Parks and Recreation, while the northern half, run by the Washington Department of Fish and Wildlife, is open for hunting in season. Yet even with this apparently paradoxical division, the island remains a great place to explore the fascinating Snohomish Estuary.

From the parking lot, there are two different ways to reach the island. The most direct route is on Fourth Street SE heading straight to the Jackknife Bridge, a little more than 0.5 mile to the east. However, a more interesting route to the bridge leads along the river to the south on Langus Riverfront Trail and then back up the shoreline of the Union Slough, about 1.5 miles altogether.

Langus Riverfront Trail promises little in the way of a natural experience at the start, as it is fully paved and almost directly under I-5. The first 0.5 mile is only marginally better, with significant industrial development on the far shore and along the path bordering the Everett wastewater facility on the left. The exposed treatment pools can occasionally be glimpsed through the trees, and unfortunately, the odor tends to waft over the trail unless merciful winds blow it back the other way.

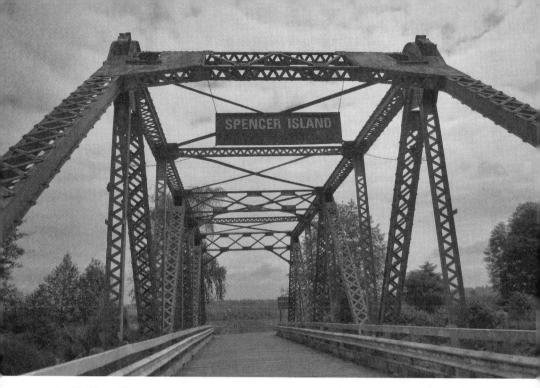

Jackknife Bridge

However, things start to improve a little farther along, where tangled blackberry bushes and some benches appear on either side. By the time you reach Union Slough, after 0.8 mile, the setting becomes much more pleasant. Follow the slough northward through grasses, reeds, and trees, looking out over the southern end of Spencer Island just across the water to the right.

Jackknife Bridge spans Union Slough where the trail joins Fourth Street SE to the parking lot. Cross the bridge to reach the island at a well-signed junction on the far side. The ruins of a barn once sat straight ahead among a sea of cattails, but almost nothing remains of the structure, which was once the heart of the now-closed cattle-ranching operation that spawned the original set of dikes to hold back the water. A boardwalk near the old barn site leads to an interpretive sign.

It was once possible to complete a 3.5-mile grand loop all the way around the island, but the damage to the dikes in 2003 unfortunately eliminated that popular route. However, it is still possible to complete a smaller loop around the island's bottom half, linking South Trail and Cross-Dike Trail. These trails are in the natural reserve and away from bicyclists, dogs, boats, and hunters, so they are sure to provide the most attractive option for the majority of hikers.

Start south on the dirt trail, a right turn as you step off the bridge. Another short interpretive boardwalk leads to an overlook on the left, with excellent views over the reeds; helpful information about the marsh ecosystem is provided by easy-to-spot displays. On a clear day, a chain of prominent peaks is visible in the Cascades, including Whitehorse

Mountain, Three Fingers, and Mount Pilchuck, with Mount Baker rising far to the north. If the wind is calm, look for reflections of the snow-clad peaks in the still waters below.

Just past the boardwalk, Cross-Dike Trail leads off to the left on a raised berm through the center of the island. For now, continue along Union Slough on South Trail. Soon you will reach a bridge (likely seen earlier from Langus Riverfront Trail on the opposite bank) that may host bird-watching photographers. The bridge provides a flat and stable tripod platform, necessary for the giant zoom lenses they use.

Bear to the left at the bottom end of the island, now following Steamboat Slough on the levee surface. The trail can be uneven and tricky at times with holes hidden under the grass and vegetation. Some dilapidated houseboats and barges float on the opposite bank, and other watercraft occasionally go by. A collection of snags stands along the trail here, formed when the trees were inundated by water coming over the levees and subsequently died. The trees' loss is the bird-watchers' gain; all manner of avian species like to perch in the bare treetops, especially hawks, eagles, and other raptors that use the high vantages to look for food. Partway up the trunks, man-made bat boxes provide shelter for winged hunters of an altogether different kind.

A bridge connects South Trail to the end of Cross-Dike Trail. Hike over the bridge and then turn left onto the dike itself to explore the heart of the island on the raised embankment, crossing another bridge along the way. With no vegetation other than the low reeds, panoramic views of the area are available on all sides, providing some of the best opportunities for wildlife observation anywhere at Spencer. Ducks and a host of other waterfowl are impossible to miss any time of year. Also, deer, beavers, and even seals and otters can occasionally be spotted.

After completing Cross-Dike Trail, a short walk north returns you to the Jackknife Bridge. From here, it is possible to head straight back to the parking area by following Fourth Street SE and completing the loop, or you may retrace your steps around the longer Langus Riverfront Trail, to the left. You also can head along the near side of Union Slough for a short distance to explore the northern portion of Spencer Island.

GPS TRAILHEAD COORDINATES
N47° 59.634' W122° 10.757'

From I-5 N, take Exit 195 for Marine View Drive, and turn left onto E. Marine View Drive. Continue on Marine View Drive 1.4 miles, then turn left up the curved entrance ramp to WA 529 over the Snohomish River Bridge toward Marysville. In 1.0 mile, take the first right, then immediately turn right again, following signs to Langus Riverfront Park. In 0.3 mile turn left at the stop sign onto Ross Avenue, and continue 0.8 mile past the marinas to another intersection. Veer right onto Smith Island Road. In another 1.0 mile, at the southern end of Langus Riverfront Park, is a parking lot and trailhead under I-5.

52 Wallace Falls State Park

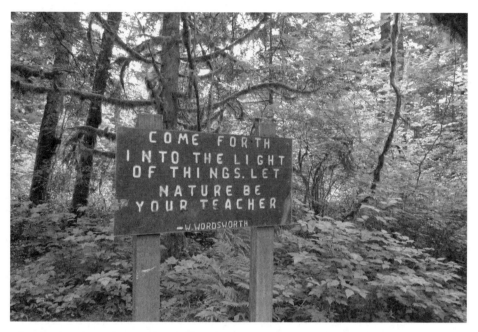

Inspirational words near the trailhead

In Brief

This deservedly popular hike leads to an impressive series of waterfalls in the Skykomish River Valley, several of which drop more than 50 feet and whose centerpiece is the 265-foot Middle Falls. The falls aren't the only attraction, however, as old-growth forest, a wide network of trails, and local history all converge at this year-round park.

Description

From the trailhead, the two most striking features of the landscape are the power lines that stretch along the northern end of the parking lot and the sunset-clock display, the latter reminding day-use visitors to leave before the gates are locked for the night. Needless to say, neither of these items fits into most people's vision of an outdoors experience. The situation doesn't improve much over the hike's first 0.25 mile, where the trail runs eastward beneath the crackling and humming wires on a gravel access road. However, all of that is soon left behind when the trail heads into the trees, revealing the true nature of Wallace Falls State Park.

Wallace Falls State Park

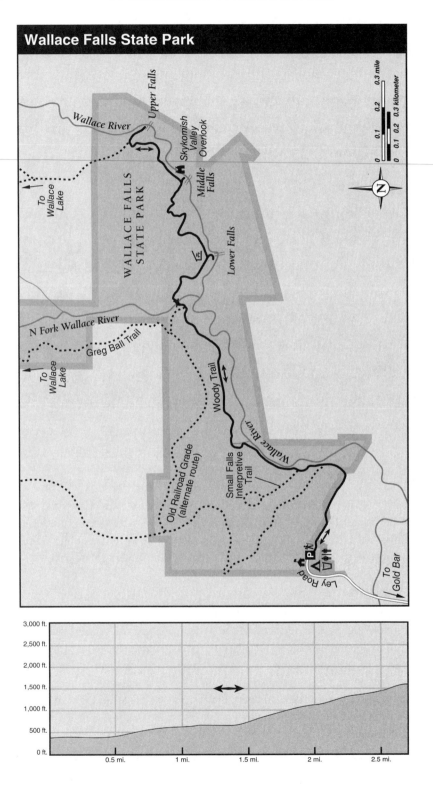

DISTANCE & CONFIGURATION: 4.0-mile out-and-back to Middle Falls; 5.4-mile out-and-back to Upper Falls	**HIKING TIME:** 2–4 hours
	ACCESS: Hikable year-round, daily, 8 a.m.–sunset; Discover Pass required for parking
DIFFICULTY: Moderate–difficult	
SCENERY: Four waterfalls with great vantage points, mossy tree-lined trails, interpretive trail, old railroad grade, and campgrounds	**WHEELCHAIR TRAVERSABLE:** No
	MAP(S): Green Trails *Index 142*; USGS *Gold Bar*
EXPOSURE: Shaded	**FACILITIES:** Toilet at trailhead, water at campground
TRAFFIC: Hike midweek or start early (parking lot fills up on weekends)	**DOGS:** Allowed on-leash
	CONTACT: 360-793-0420; parks.state.wa .us/289/Wallace-Falls
TRAIL SURFACE: Dirt (Woody Trail) and gravel (old railroad grade)	**LOCATION:** Gold Bar

Right away, the trail reaches the first fork. The left branch is the Old Railroad Grade, open to foot traffic, mountain bikers, and equestrians. Head through the gate on the right to access the hikers-only Woody Trail. The path is named after State Senator Frank Woody, a longtime advocate of youth programs at parks like this one.

Beyond the fence, Woody Trail narrows to singletrack and begins a steady ascent along the northern bank of the Wallace River. Moss hangs in thick coats over the trees, heavy enough to be reminiscent of the Hoh Rain Forest on the Olympic Peninsula. The growth of the moss is aided by mist rising from the fast-moving river, keeping the forest here particularly damp.

Small Falls Interpretive Trail branches to the left. Laid out by an Eagle Scout in 1995, the short detour explores a cascading tributary of the Wallace River and explains the methods and history of logging in the area on a series of informative signs.

At the 1-mile mark, the Railroad Grade Cut-Off Trail climbs over a small rise and leads to the Old Railroad Grade Trail. On the way back, this trail provides a good option for creating a small loop, although the route is a mile longer than Woody Trail.

The Old Railroad Grade was once used to haul logs and timber from the forest to the town of Gold Bar, where they could be sent down the Skykomish River or loaded onto the Great Northern Railroad. It was the arrival of James J. Hill's transcontinental Great Northern line in the late 1800s that allowed the town to flourish, firmly connecting it to growing urban centers on both sides of the mountains.

The value that the growing nation placed on the first cross-country rail connections is hard to imagine today, but the story of the Great Northern gives some idea. In order to establish a railroad linking Lake Superior to the Pacific, Hill was granted some 44 million acres of land, slightly more territory than currently makes up the entire state of Washington. The rail line, established in a checkerboard pattern of public and

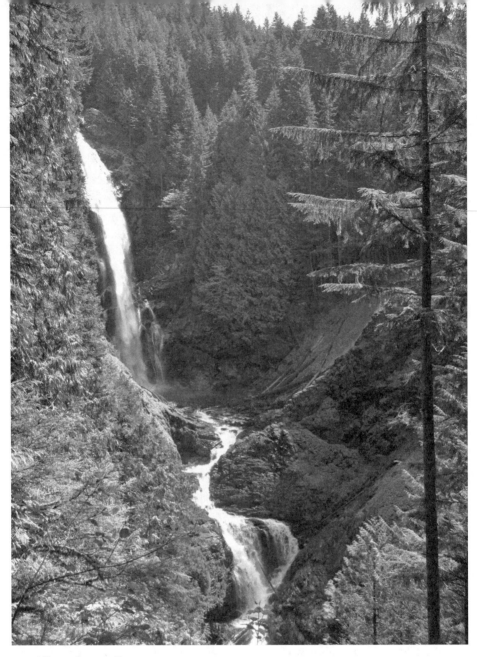

Middle Wallace Falls

private ownership, would travel through a band of land approximately 120 miles wide and more than 2,000 miles long.

James Hill instantly became one of the wealthiest and most powerful men in the United States, controlling with his corporation about 25,000 acres of land for every single mile of track he eventually built—and that was before his crucial railroad had ever made a single transcontinental run. Like so many of the vastly influential men of his time, Hill was a strange mix of monopolist, entrepreneur, and robber baron, depending on how his legacy is viewed. The checkerboard patchwork of land ownership that marks most current timber concessions and continues to shape the landscape of the West is also part of Hill's legacy, dating back to the original system of land grants first set down by the government in 1864.

Continue on Woody Trail and cross the North Fork of the Wallace River at 1.5 miles on a sturdy wooden bridge, and then start a steady climb up the other side through a series of switchbacks. After another 0.3 mile, a picnic shelter provides a good resting point with a view of the Lower Falls, the first of the three main plunges.

Above the picnic shelter the trail becomes more rugged, with exposed roots and rocks. The 2-mile mark is signed with a wooden post in the middle of an uphill section, just short of the fenced overlook for the Middle Falls. At 265 feet, the Middle Falls is one of the highest waterfalls in the state and the most striking anywhere in the park. The river tumbles down through two separate drops, with a series of small pools in between. For some hikers, this makes an excellent turnaround point for a 4-mile out-and-back trip.

Above Middle Falls, the trail becomes steeper and darker, sheltered by the high trees. Even at the height of the summer, it tends to be cool here in the perpetual dusk, among the shadows of the thick growth. Just past the top of the falls, the Skykomish Valley Overlook opens out to the right, providing views of the valley below if the weather is good.

The Upper Falls mark the traditional turnaround point for most hikers, 2.7 miles from and 1,200 feet above the trailhead. The falls themselves are another double-tiered-pool drop like the Middle Falls, although not as high.

With close to 4,800 acres of land, Wallace Falls State Park provides plenty of options for longer and more demanding trips. Above the Upper Falls, the trail climbs another 200 feet to Wallace Lake, 2.5 miles away, with Jay and Shaw Lakes even farther along. Most of this route follows a logging road favored by mountain bikers; it loops back to both the Old Railroad Grade Trail and a network of Department of Natural Resources roads leading all the way to the town of Startup. The hikers-only Greg Ball Trail opened in summer of 2005, roughly following the North Fork of the Wallace River from the end of the railroad grade to Wallace Lake and allowing foot traffic to stay clear of the bikers.

GPS TRAILHEAD COORDINATES
N47° 52.031' W121° 40.706'

On I-5 at the northern end of Everett, take Exit 194 for US 2 E. Travel 27.5 miles east on US 2 through the towns of Monroe, Sultan, and Startup. Once you reach the town of Gold Bar, look for the Wallace Falls State Park sign, and take a left onto First Street. In 0.4 mile turn right onto May Creek Road, and in 0.7 mile stay left at the fork to get on Ley Road. In 0.4 mile stay left again at the end of Ley Road to enter the state park parking lot.

SOUTH OF SEATTLE

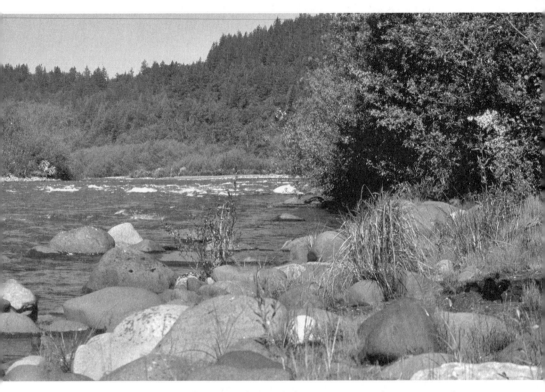

White River at Scatter Creek access above Mud Mountain Dam (see page 295)

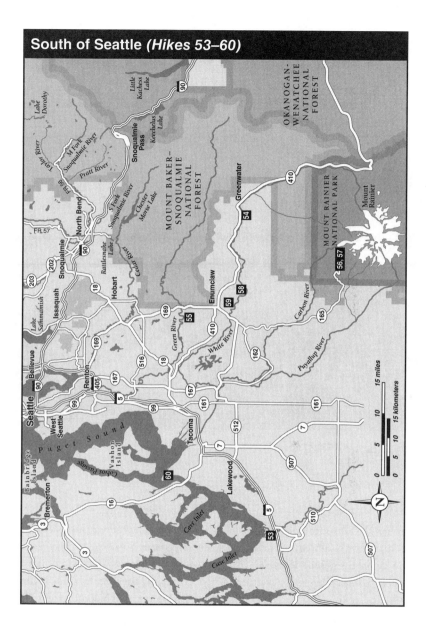

53 Billy Frank Jr. Nisqually National Wildlife Refuge

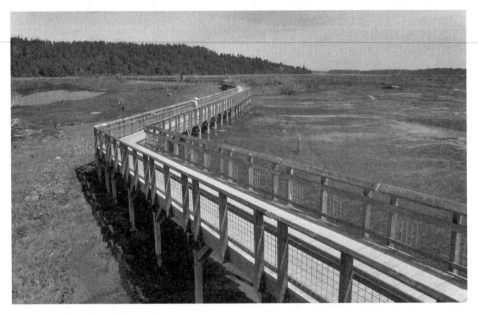

Estuary Boardwalk Trail

In Brief

Far from its glacial source on the southern side of Mount Rainier, the Nisqually River empties into Puget Sound in a broad delta. Once a working farm, the site has become one of the finest bird-watching locations in the Puget Sound region, although many people come purely to enjoy the natural setting. Whether looking specifically at the birds or not, hikers will find an interesting walk that explores a wide range of habitats and wildlife.

Description

Anyone who has frequented the I-5 corridor between Tacoma and Olympia has sped by the sign for the Nisqually National Wildlife Refuge countless times and probably not given it a second thought. A special place, the refuge was established in 1974 to protect migratory birds. More than 200 species, many federally listed as threatened or endangered, have been observed in the refuge's 3,000 acres. Winter brings particularly high numbers of visitors to see migratory birds, but there are plenty during other seasons as well.

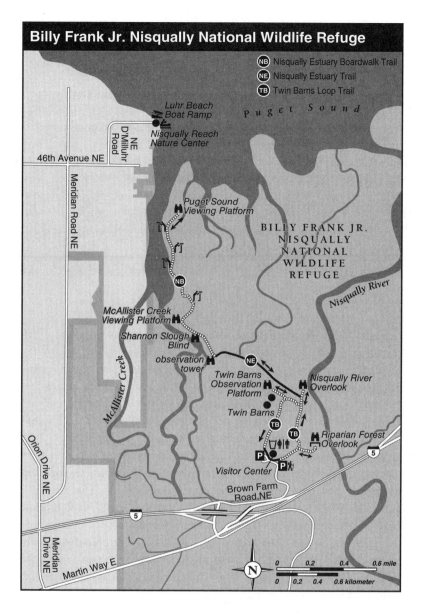

The refuge is open year-round from sunrise to sunset, although there are some trail closures during the hunting season from October to January. Note that dogs, bicycles, fires, camping, and jogging are all prohibited here, but many of the trails are wheelchair accessible, including boardwalk trails at Twin Barns Loop Trail, Riparian Forest Overlook, Nisqually River Overlook, and the Estuary Boardwalk Trail.

Located in a sea of rushes next to the parking lot, the modern-looking visitor center is open Wednesday–Sunday, 9 a.m.–4 p.m., except holidays. Pay the day-use fee at a kiosk and

DISTANCE & CONFIGURATION:
4.7-mile balloon, including out-and-back on main boardwalk

DIFFICULTY: Easy–moderate

SCENERY: Wildlife, wetlands, tidelands, forest, old barns

EXPOSURE: Mostly exposed; a few shaded areas along the Nisqually River and near the visitor center

TRAFFIC: Busy on weekends and sunny days

TRAIL SURFACE: Mixture of gravel, dirt, and boardwalk

HIKING TIME: 2–3 hours, or longer with side trips

ACCESS: Hikable year-round, daily, sunrise–sunset (seasonal closures occur throughout the year); $3 daily fee per group (4 maximum)

WHEELCHAIR TRAVERSABLE: Yes, on the Twin Barns Loop Trail

FACILITIES: Toilets and water at the visitor center

DOGS: Not allowed

CONTACT: 360-753-9467; fws.gov/refuge /Billy_Frank_Jr_Nisqually

LOCATION: 100 Brown Farm Road NE, Olympia, WA 98516

pick up a park-information pamphlet with a map. Several display signs at an overlook outside the building describe some of the wildlife you may see on your trip, and volunteers are frequently available to answer questions. Free lectures from wildlife experts and naturalists are held in the auditorium on many evenings; check the schedule if you are interested.

The refuge is a patchwork of lands managed by the U.S. Department of Fish and Wildlife, the Washington Department of Fish and Wildlife, and the Nisqually Indian tribe, although you are unlikely to notice these divisions anywhere except on the map. What you will notice is the wide range of habitats throughout the area, including mudflats, shrubs, coniferous forests, freshwater marshes, saltwater marshes, open salt water, rivers and creeks, mixed grasslands, and riparian woodlands. This habitat diversity attracts a considerable assortment of birds, with waterfowl, songbirds, raptors, and waders all calling the refuge home.

The 1-mile Twin Barns Loop Trail is the central hub of this hike, with multiple side trails radiating outward. All the trails are worth exploring, but the main attraction at the refuge is the long Estuary Boardwalk Trail. Dedicated in February 2011, this boardwalk was the final stage of a giant restoration project undertaken over several years that included the dismantling of the Brown Farm Dike in 2009.

The dike had been disrupting the natural estuarine environment since it was built more than a century ago to develop this land into a working farm. Its removal returned 762 acres of tidal wetlands to their natural state and completely altered the refuge, to visitors' benefit.

Along with the physical changes brought by the removal of the dike, Nisqually also received a new name. To honor a local fisherman and tribal leader, the refuge officially became the Billy Frank Jr. Nisqually National Wildlife Refuge in December 2015. In conjunction, the Medicine Creek Treaty National Memorial was declared at the site of a historically significant stump along McAllister Creek.

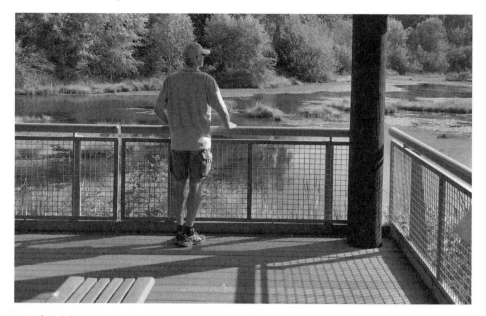

At the visitor center

That stump was the location for the signing of the Medicine Creek Treaty between the US government and various local American Indian tribes in 1854. The treaty consigned the tribes to reservations, but they were promised access to their traditional hunting and fishing grounds on the Nisqually River.

However, for more than 100 years, access to the grounds was prohibited, until tribal fisherman Billy Frank Jr. took up the cause. Frank brought the issue to public attention through a campaign of civil disobedience, and the case went before the US Supreme Court in 1974.

The court ruled in favor of the tribes, restoring their salmon fishing rights. Frank went on to be chairman of the Northwest Indian Fisheries Commission for more than three decades, helping comanage salmon fisheries with the State of Washington. After his death in 2014, Frank was awarded the Presidential Medal of Freedom, and now the refuge has been renamed in his honor as well.

Find the start of the Twin Barns Loop on the southeastern side of the visitor center and follow the boardwalk trail. Very soon a side branch heads to the Riparian Forest Overlook, where interpretive signs provide information on the flora and fauna to be seen, including otters, mink, and frogs. The deciduous woods here are thick and dark, with cottonwoods, big-leaf maples, and willows. Massive skunk cabbage with leaves several feet in length line the muddy creek. Several wooden benches grace the observation platform at the end of the short trail.

The boardwalk continues through the forest to where another spur leads north to the Nisqually River Overlook. Despite many side branches, which siphon off the flow, the broad, green river has a noticeable current and is the largest source of freshwater into the estuary.

Return from this dead end and follow the Nisqually Estuary Trail as it climbs onto a dirt levee and heads northwest, emerging from the trees. The gravel path is wide, flat, and straight, running through various bushes, reeds, and grasses. There is no shade, so in summer be prepared for the full force of the sun.

The Estuary Boardwalk Trail starts from the Estuary Trail about 0.5 mile farther along. What you will see from the boardwalk is in constant flux, varying by the season and even hourly during the day. At extreme low tide, the land below will be a vast mudflat; at high tide, you will be walking above several feet of water.

The boardwalk runs north along the eastern bank of McAllister Creek for almost exactly 1 mile. Several viewing platforms and blinds offer places to stop and study the surroundings along the way. The boardwalk ends at a covered viewing platform, styled like a gazebo and built on top of where the old Brown Farm Dike used to stand. The platform provides a commanding view over the heart of the refuge and the southern end of Puget Sound, known as Nisqually Reach. Photography from the platform tends to be best early or late in the day, when wildlife is typically more active and there is softer ambient light.

Return on the Estuary Trail to rejoin the Twin Barns Loop Trail, adjacent to its namesake barns. These two giant structures show the magnitude of the Brown Farm at its height; its facilities included a creamery, a meatpacking house, and an incubation and brooding house for chickens. The farm was huge for its day, and it seems more like a piece of modern, industrial agriculture than its historical roots would indicate.

The barns are now used only for storage, but countless swallows nest under the eaves, aided by mesh netting. The flocks whirling overhead are an impressive sight.

Complete the loop by following the Twin Barns Loop Trail on a boardwalk next to more wetlands. It's a pleasant 0.5-mile walk from the barns back to the parking lot.

Nearby Activities

The Luhr Beach boat ramp at Nisqually Reach Nature Center allows access to the northern end of the refuge and to Puget Sound. Canoeists, kayakers, and small boaters of all kinds can explore the bottom end of the wetlands from the surface of the water. The launch is located at the end of D'Milluhr Road NE, off 46th Avenue NE and Meridian Road NE.

GPS TRAILHEAD COORDINATES
N47° 4.377' W122° 42.815'

From I-5 south of Tacoma, take Exit 114 for Nisqually. Follow the exit ramp as it crosses over I-5 to an intersection with Nisqually Cut-Off Road. Turn right at the light onto Nisqually Cut-Off Road and cross under I-5. In 0.2 mile turn right again at a T-intersection onto Brown Farm Road. The road ends in 0.7 mile at the wildlife refuge visitor center, where there is ample parking.

54 Federation Forest State Park

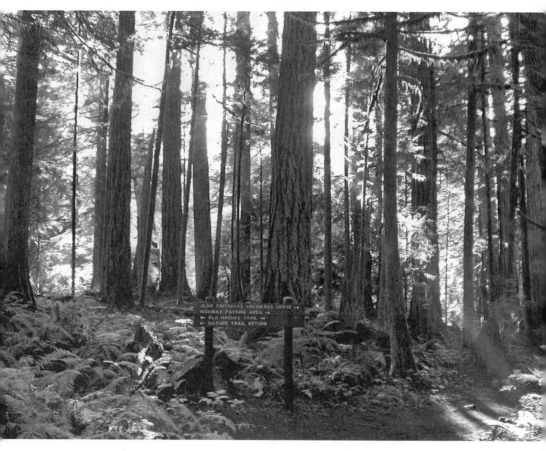

Trail junction in the forest

In Brief

A most unlikely oasis in a desert of clear-cuts, Federation State Forest is one of the last stands of significant old growth anywhere in the White River Valley. This thin stretch of protected land along WA 410 features a lush, lowland forest of Douglas fir, western hemlock, western red cedar, and the relatively uncommon Sitka spruce. Some of the largest trees reach from 5 to 7 feet in diameter and grow several hundred feet high.

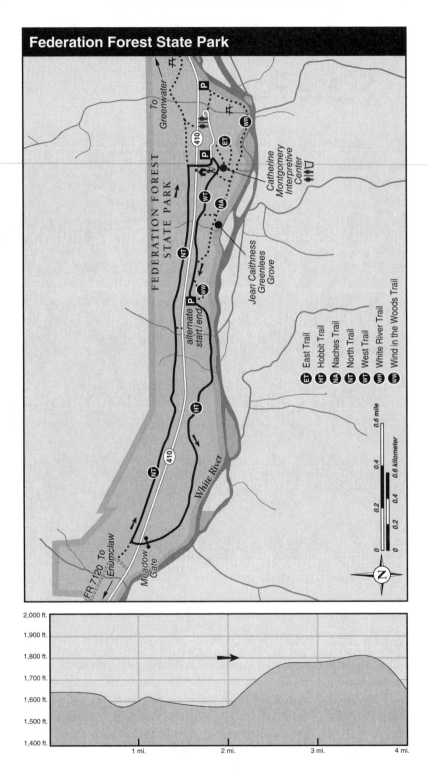

Federation Forest State Park

FEDERATION FOREST STATE PARK

To Greenwater

Catherine Montgomery Interpretive Center

Jean Caithness Greenlees Grove

alternate start/end

White River

Meadow Gate

FR 7120 To Enumclaw

ET East Trail
HT Hobbit Trail
NA Naches Trail
NT North Trail
WT West Trail
WR White River Trail
WW Wind in the Woods Trail

0.6 mile
0.6 kilometer

DISTANCE & CONFIGURATION: 4.0-mile loop	**ACCESS:** Hikable April 1–September 30, daily, 8 a.m.–sunset; Discover Pass required for parking
DIFFICULTY: Easy	
SCENERY: Plant life, old-growth forest, interpretive center and displays	**WHEELCHAIR TRAVERSABLE:** No
	MAP(S): USGS *Greenwater*
EXPOSURE: Shaded	**FACILITIES:** Toilet and water at interpretive center
TRAFFIC: Moderate in summer, low in off-season	**DOGS:** Allowed on-leash
	CONTACT: 360-663-2207; parks.state .wa.us/502/Federation-Forest
TRAIL SURFACE: Dirt	
HIKING TIME: 1–3 hours	**LOCATION:** Greenwater

Description

Federation Forest State Park was founded in 1949. But it was born centuries before, when many of its giant trees were only seedlings. Since then, the forest has miraculously survived storms, fire, and the chain saw to stand as an impressive reminder of what the entire region was like before modern civilization arrived.

Catherine Montgomery was a pioneer educator and is largely responsible for the preservation of this natural area, organizing and acquiring the park lands through her affiliation with the Washington State Federation of Women's Clubs and keeping the magnificent trees here from meeting the same fate as most of their brothers and sisters along the White River. The influence of women on the park can be easily seen in many of the features named in their honor, such as Ester Maltby Trail, Jean Caithness Greenlees Grove, and Ella Higginson Grove, a tribute to the one-time poet laureate of Washington State.

The park's interpretive center now bears Montgomery's name; the center has limited, seasonal hours. Inside, exhibits detail the various ecosystems visible across the state, from the coastal rain forest to the dry deserts of the east. In front of the building is a garden of plants from throughout the region with a helpful guide for any would-be naturalist.

The linear park consists of a number of easy trails, many short enough to be suitable for even the youngest children. Multiple hiking options are available, but the best extended hike is detailed here—a loop between the river and the southern side of WA 410 through some of the largest trees and then returning on the far side of the road.

The trailhead is located on the western side of the parking lot, where a wide gravel path leads into the dark woods. Stay to the right on West Trail and soon leave the gravel to enter an interpretive forest, where a wide array of plant species is identified. Orange honeysuckle, salal, and sword fern grow through the understory. Oregon grape, the Oregon state flower, also grows here; the plant bears blueberry-like fruit and has serrated leaves like holly. The traffic on WA 410 can generally be heard through the trees, but moss-laden vine maples and giant Douglas firs help create the illusion of deep wilderness.

Despite its status for many as the signature tree of the Pacific Northwest, the Douglas fir is not a true fir and can be identified because its cones hang down (true fir cones grow upward). Although that is difficult to gauge when looking at a tall tree with cones far above your head, this is the type of useful information the interpretive forest can provide.

Western hemlock (*Tsuga heterophylla*) is another false fir, with numerous small cones that hang from the end of its thin branches. It is also known as the Pacific hemlock, or West Coast hemlock, and is marked by a narrow, flexible crown with frequently droopy new growth. A shallow root system makes western hemlocks susceptible to blowdown in high winds, but the tree is also adaptable enough to grow directly on decaying wood.

The western hemlock narrowly beat out the western red cedar to be adopted as the state tree of Washington in 1947. The year before, the prominent Portland *Oregonian* newspaper had teased its neighbor to the north about not having a state tree and suggested the hemlock. Many proud Washingtonians did not want anyone from rival Oregon dictating their state tree and instead selected the red cedar. However, when the matter finally came to a vote in the legislature, the western hemlock won. Nonetheless, the red cedar holds a special place in the hearts of many Washingtonians, not least because it was used by George Pocock for some of his famed Seattle-built rowing shells, including the *Husky Clipper,* which a team of extraordinary University of Washington undergraduates rowed to the gold medal at the 1936 Berlin Olympic games and which now hangs in a place of honor at the university's Conibear Shellhouse.

Of particular interest are the large Sitka spruces, which you will pass as you continue west on the trail. This spruce is the tallest conifer in North America, often reaching 150–200 feet high, with an estimated life span of up to 800 years. Because of its high moisture requirements, it is typically confined to a narrow coastal fog belt. But it can also grow inland along low-elevation rivers and streams, like the ones here.

The fine grain, good strength-to-weight ratio, and long, straight trunk made the wood of the Sitka spruce particularly valuable in the manufacture of airplane wings in World War I, prior to the advent of aluminum, fiberglass, and other modern construction materials. Although the Seattle-based Boeing Corporation had pioneered the use of this local wood, it was rival Howard Hughes's famous *Spruce Goose* that probably did the most to advertise it as an aircraft construction material. However, Hughes's enormous floating plane was actually built primarily of laminated birch, not spruce, and was considered by many to be nothing more than a manifestation of Hughes's questionable sanity at the time.

At a major, signed junction, continue right, toward the Jean Caithness Greenlees Grove. Just past the sign is one of the finest collections of old-growth trees in the park. A huge fire swept through this area in 1846; this would have cleared out the understory and left only the biggest trees. Amazingly, some of the ancient trees here still show charred bark, scarred as the unlikely survivors of this epic event that took place more than 150 years ago.

The trail continues through Deadman Flat and eventually reaches the elevated bank of the White River. Below, the milky water reveals its glacial origins as it tumbles over a bed of smooth, white rocks. The path winds its way generally along the river, with a surprising series of short ups and downs. Expect some areas to be muddy and wet, although wooden boardwalks with attached metal laths help keep you above the worst of it.

The trail becomes carpeted with moss and then crosses an open area just before reaching the Meadow Gate to the right. Go through the gate and cross WA 410 to reenter the forest on the opposite side. Immediately turn right at a T-intersection to head back in the direction you came.

The trail on this side is elevated above the road and more exposed to its traffic and noise, although the forest here is still worth seeing. Fungi of all shapes, sizes, and colors line the route, a very different display than offered by the giant trees but impressive all the same.

After about 1.5 miles, turn right at a sign leading back to the interpretive center. Cross the road in front of the Federation Forest State Park sign and return to the parking lot and your vehicle.

Nearby Activities

The Muckleshoot tribe owns and operates the Muckleshoot Casino on their reservation in Auburn. The sprawling facility is located on WA 164, 2 miles south of the junction with WA 18. In addition to gaming, the casino offers a wide variety of amenities, food services, and lodging. For more information, call 800-804-4944 or visit muckleshootcasino.com.

GPS TRAILHEAD COORDINATES
N47° 9.124' W121° 41.299'

From I-5 between Seattle and Tacoma, take Exit 142A for WA 18 E. Travel 4.2 miles east on WA 18 into Auburn, then exit onto WA 164 E toward Enumclaw. Continue 14.7 miles on WA 164 through Enumclaw to a junction with WA 410/Roosevelt Avenue, and turn left (east). Stay on WA 410 E for 16.2 miles until just after milepost 4 and just before the town of Greenwater, then turn right into a well-signed parking area for the state park. If the parking area near the interpretive center is closed, drive back toward Enumclaw about 0.5 mile to a wide parking area pullout on the southern side of WA 410.

---

55 Flaming Geyser State Park

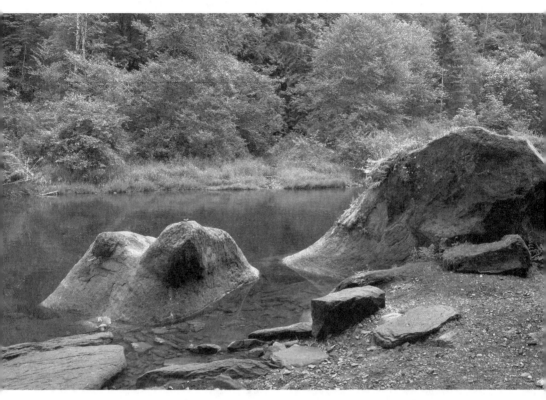

Boulders on the Green River

In Brief

A popular state park with a very impressive name, Flaming Geyser presents several basic hiking options on more than 4 miles of trails. Multiple short hikes explore a ridgeline in the forest, the edge of the Green River Gorge, and the unusual geological features advertised in the title.

Description

The words *Flaming Geyser* can't help but evoke images of the spectacular hydrothermal vents at Yellowstone National Park, or perhaps spurting columns of lava, a little more likely to be seen in the volcanically active Cascade Range. Unfortunately, the geysers here are small, misnamed methane seeps, and their glory is limited, to say the least. No

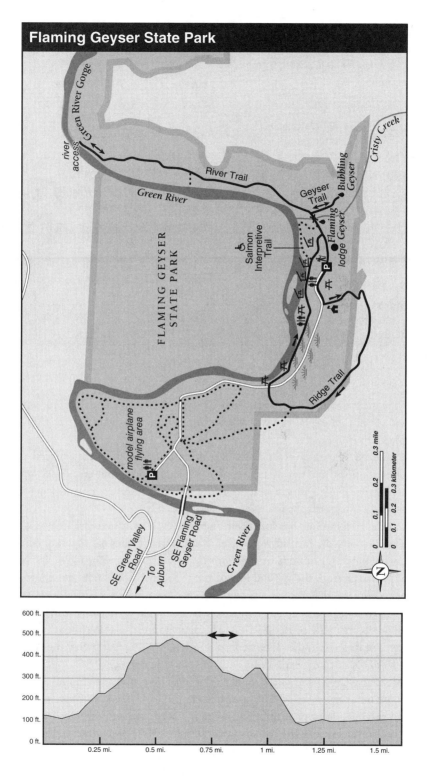

Flaming Geyser State Park

Green River Gorge

river access

River Trail

Green River

Cristy Creek

Geyser Trail

Bubbling Geyser

Flaming lodge Geyser

FLAMING GEYSER STATE PARK

Salmon Interpretive Trail

Ridge Trail

model airplane flying area

0.3 mile

0.3 kilometer

0.2

0.1

0.2

0.1

0

0

SE Green Valley Road

To Auburn

SE Flaming Geyser Road

Green River

N

600 ft.

500 ft.

400 ft.

300 ft.

200 ft.

100 ft.

0 ft.

0.25 mi.   0.5 mi.   0.75 mi.   1 mi.   1.25 mi.   1.5 mi.

DISTANCE & CONFIGURATION:
1.5-mile loop (Ridge Trail), 1.7-mile out-and-back (River Trail), 0.4-mile loop (Geyser Trail)

DIFFICULTY: Easy–moderate

SCENERY: Three hiking trails and an interpretive trail, Flaming and Bubbling Geysers, Green River Gorge

EXPOSURE: Mostly shaded

TRAFFIC: High visitation to park; only moderate traffic on trails (get an early start on sunny weekends or parking may fill up)

TRAIL SURFACE: Dirt

HIKING TIME: 1–2 hours

ACCESS: Hikable year-round, daily, 8 a.m.–sunset; Discover Pass required for parking

WHEELCHAIR TRAVERSABLE: Yes, on the Salmon Interpretive Trail and access to the Flaming Geyser site

MAP(S): USGS *Black Diamond*

FACILITIES: Toilet at trailhead in summer; no drinking water

DOGS: Allowed on-leash

CONTACT: 253-735-8839; parks.state.wa.us/504/Flaming-Geyser

LOCATION: 23700 SE Flaming Geyser Road, Auburn, WA 98092

COMMENTS: Flaming Geyser State Park gets very busy on summer weekends, and parking is sure to fill up unless you get there early! Make a point of arriving well before noon to avoid getting turned away at the entrance.

one but the most dedicated geologist is likely to be mesmerized by them for any length of time. At least that explains why visitors from around the world are not flocking to this modest destination.

Nonetheless, Flaming Geyser does hold some attractions for hikers who can explore a few different options, including a loop trail on the ridge and an out-and-back route along the Green River. The geysers, a unique natural phenomenon in the landscape, are also worth seeing, as long as expectations are set appropriately.

From the parking lot, head eastward next to the Environmental Learning Center Lodge (usually closed), just off to the right. The park's namesake Flaming Geyser lies behind two concrete fishponds used as imprinting tanks for steelhead smolts. Methane gas used to escape from the ground here through a concrete cylinder sunk into a stone basin. As recently as 2006, the gas was continuously consumed by a faint, flickering 6-inch flame, but now it has expired. Once, the flame stood much higher and probably deserved its name, but it largely faded in the 1960s. The most impressive thing about the seep now is the depth of its source; the gas rose from more than 1,400 feet below the surface, the by-product of coal-drilling explorations carried out here years ago.

Cross Cristy Creek and head uphill to the right on a stony singletrack. A quick 0.2 mile brings you up some stairs along a wooden fence. Cross back over the creek to reach a wooden viewing platform at Bubbling Geyser, where methane emerges from between some pebbles at the side of the stream, laying a milky-white precipitate in the creek bed. The gas can often be smelled in the air as well.

It used to be possible to complete a loop along the creek, but now it is necessary to go back the way you came. At the foot of the creek, you can head right, joining River Trail on a wide, muddy surface. A few spurs lead from the main trail down to the banks of the Green River, frequently used by fly-fishermen and others to reach the water's edge.

River Trail continues through a forest of alders, mossy maples, and some large yellow cedars as it climbs about 50 feet above the shoreline. The river itself becomes increasingly difficult to see down the slope to the left, and a high ridge climbs away to the right. Seams of sedimentary rock are exposed in a small cliff band on the right, with some obvious coal visible in the layered sandstone.

The trail eventually narrows to a muddy singletrack, running through some short climbs and drops, sometimes near the river's edge and sometimes farther above it. Eventually, emerge from the brush into some smooth rocks on the banks of the Green. This is the official end of the trail, although it is possible to boulder-hop farther upstream if the water level is low enough.

Across the water, steep rock walls rise 100 feet above the river, the western end of the steep and narrow Green River Gorge. The gorge is at its deepest and most impressive another few miles upstream near the Black Diamond Bridge, but the cliffs here give a small hint of what it's like. The setting on the bank makes a nice place to rest as the water flows by, surprisingly clear and clean. The return on River Trail is the same as the way you came, a total round-trip of approximately 0.9 mile.

Ridge Trail starts 0.25 mile away on the park road, at the entrance to the final parking lot. Look for the big bathroom building on the river side of the road and an AUTHO-RIZED VEHICLES ONLY sign on a white steel gate on the other side at small traffic turnout. The trail begins beyond the gate.

Cross the grass at the edge of the field, walk about 50 yards, and look for the TRAIL sign pointing to the left. Start to climb on a now-abandoned road that heads steeply uphill and begins to bear right. After ascending some 100 feet, the trail flattens out through some high brush, now heading west.

The road is slowly being reclaimed and turned into a trail, narrowing as it continues along the ridge. An easement allows passage here at the edge of some private property, so be sure to stay on the established track. Some very large maples populate the slope to the left, rising far above the trail, which never reaches the top of the ridge, despite its name. Some sandstone cliffs are visible up through the trees.

Although the park receives many visitors, who use the picnic facilities and playing fields below, up here on the ridge you are likely to have the trail all to yourself because very few people venture into the woods. You are also far enough above the crowds that the only sounds you typically hear are the singing of the birds in the trees and the gurgling of several small creeks that run down the slope.

Descend slightly to reach a junction, where a singletrack traverses left and a double-track continues down the hill. Follow the doubletrack past a small wetland area to reach a gravel pullout on the main park road. Cross the road and then pass through a picnic area to approach the river. A return trail runs along the bank to the right, skirting several more picnic areas and a playfield before returning to the parking lot, a total distance of about 1.5 miles around.

As a final option, a short, paved interpretive trail explaining local salmon habitat protection and restoration efforts runs for less than 0.25 mile on the northern side of the parking lot, near the riverbank.

Nearby Activities

If you should find yourself unable to get into Flaming Geyser because the park is full, there are some short trails you can explore at Kanaskat–Palmer State Park instead. To reach Kanaskat–Palmer, head east on SE Green Valley Road away from Flaming Geyser until you reach Enumclaw–Black Diamond Road SE (WA 169). Turn right on WA 169; after a few miles turn left onto SE 400th Street. This road bends left to become 272nd Avenue SE and then right to become SE 392nd Street before reaching SE Veazie–Cumberland Road. Turn left on Veazie-Cumberland and then follow this road about 7 miles to the park entrance, on the left. Check parks.state.wa.us/527/kanaskat-palmer for more information.

GPS TRAILHEAD COORDINATES
N47° 16.351' W122° 1.399'

From I-5 between Seattle and Tacoma, take Exit 142A for WA 18 E. Travel 6.1 miles east on WA 18 through Auburn, then exit onto Auburn–Black Diamond Road. Turn right, then immediately turn right again onto SE Green Valley Road. Continue 8.0 miles and pass 218th Avenue SE, then look for SE Flaming Geyser Road and the entrance to Flaming Geyser State Park on the right. Drive 1.3 miles to the parking lot at the end of the road.

56 Mount Rainier National Park:
MOWICH LAKE, EUNICE LAKE, AND TOLMIE PEAK LOOKOUT

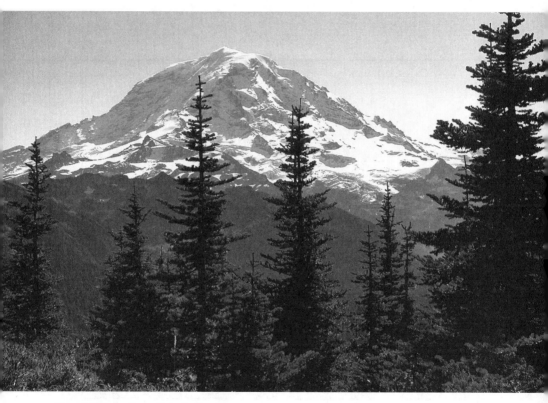

Mount Rainier from Tolmie Peak

In Brief

The panoramic view from Tolmie Peak is one of the finest in the entire northwest corner of Mount Rainier National Park. The summit lookout provides a great perspective for studying the giant volcano and its surroundings, while Eunice Lake shimmers in a steep alpine bowl directly below.

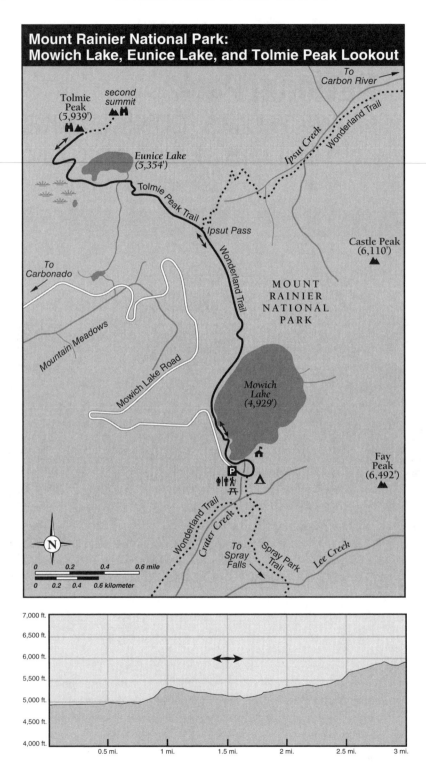

**Mount Rainier National Park:
Mowich Lake, Eunice Lake, and Tolmie Peak Lookout**

To
Carbon River

Tolmie
Peak
(5,939')

second
summit

Eunice Lake
(5,354')

Tolmie Peak Trail

Ipsut Creek

Wonderland Trail

Ipsut Pass

Castle Peak
(6,110')

To
Carbonado

Wonderland Trail

MOUNT
RAINIER
NATIONAL
PARK

Mountain Meadows

Mowich Lake Road

Mowich
Lake
(4,929')

Fay
Peak
(6,492')

P

Wonderland Trail

Crater Creek

To
Spray
Falls

Spray Park Trail

Lee Creek

N

0   0.2   0.4   0.6 mile

0   0.2   0.4   0.6 kilometer

7,000 ft.

6,500 ft.

6,000 ft.

5,500 ft.

5,000 ft.

4,500 ft.

4,000 ft.

0.5 mi.   1 mi.   1.5 mi.   2 mi.   2.5 mi.   3 mi.

DISTANCE & CONFIGURATION: 6.0-mile out-and-back	**ACCESS:** Hikable summer–fall (check road conditions and snowpack); $10 per person
DIFFICULTY: Moderate	
SCENERY: Plant life and wildflowers, scenic lakes, fire-lookout cabin; superb views of Mount Rainier	**WHEELCHAIR TRAVERSABLE:** No
	MAP(S): Green Trails *Mount Rainier West 269*; USGS *Mowich Lake* and *Golden Lakes*
EXPOSURE: Shaded on about half the route	**FACILITIES:** Toilet at trailhead; no drinking water
TRAFFIC: Heavy; get an early start to beat the crowds	**DOGS:** Not allowed
TRAIL SURFACE: Dirt	**CONTACT:** 360-569-2211; nps.gov/mora
HIKING TIME: 3–4 hours	**LOCATION:** Carbonado

Description

Most hikers leave Mowich Lake bound for Spray Park, lured up Rainier's northwest flank by the many attractions of the subalpine meadow. However, the best views of the mountain itself are found on some of the high ridges in the opposite direction, far enough away that the entire mountain can be taken in at once. Head up 5,900-foot Tolmie Peak to enjoy such a vista, and possibly escape some of the crowds as well.

Tolmie Peak is named for Dr. William Fraser Tolmie, who penetrated this area in 1833 in search of medicinal plants and herbs. Tolmie was likely the first non–American Indian man to explore this remote wilderness, less than 30 years after Lewis and Clark had reached the Pacific and long before the founding of either the State of Washington in 1889 or the national park 10 years later.

At the time of Tolmie's journey, the entire Pacific Northwest was part of the disputed Oregon Territory, claimed by both the United States and Britain. Legal ownership was not resolved until President James K. Polk signed the Treaty of Oregon in 1846, setting the boundary between the United States and Canada on the 49th parallel, where it remains today. The agreement with the British turned expansionist Polk into yet another politician unable to deliver on campaign promises; he had been elected in 1844 with the slogan "Fifty-four forty or fight!," pledging to annex the entire region between the California border and latitude 54°40', near the current Canadian city of Prince George. However, Polk was already facing war with Mexico, so he backed away from hostilities with Britain and agreed to divide the land.

Tolmie is believed to have reached a high point somewhere in the vicinity of Mowich Lake, but probably not on the peak that now bears his name. His botanical expedition would have to be considered a success, as he is credited with discovering Tolmie's saxifrage (*Saxifraga tolmiei*). Also known as alpine saxifrage, the hardy, flowering plant is typically found in high-elevation meadows or in loose rocks and scree throughout most of the mountainous West.

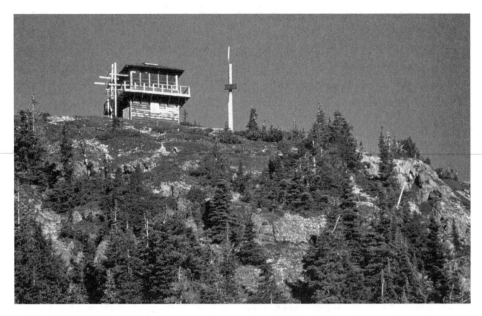

Tolmie Peak Lookout

There's a host of formal and informal trails that explore the southern end of Mowich Lake near the campground. Most of these eventually join Wonderland Trail, which runs along the western side of the lake and has a signed trailhead near the parking lot entrance. Head north along the shoreline, following signs to Ipsut Pass. Larger and larger sections of Mount Rainier become visible to the southeast as the mountain emerges from behind Fay Peak.

The trail climbs out of the lake bowl at the northern end and continues beneath a rocky ridge for another 0.5 mile. A view opens down a valley to the left, looking out over Mountain Meadows and Meadow Creek as the creek descends toward its confluence with the Mowich River.

Stay right at the next junction to explore a short detour to Ipsut Pass, well worth the negligible effort. The pass offers a great view down the steep Ipsut Creek Valley, bounded by the sharp spires of Castle Peak and Mother Mountain to the south. At one time legions of round-the-mountain hikers crossed through here on the Wonderland Trail, part of their long loop around Rainier. However, although this is still officially part of the route, most long-distance hikers choose to bypass this section by climbing up through Spray and Seattle Parks and then rejoining the Wonderland down along the Carbon River, to the east.

Return to the junction and go down the slope toward Tolmie Peak, heading northwest below some rocky cliffs. A 0.25-mile climb follows, leading uphill to Eunice Lake at an elevation of 5,354 feet. Be careful to stay on the trail as it passes through fragile subalpine meadows along the lake's southern shore. Camping used to be allowed here but has since been restricted due to excessive damage to plant growth. Expect a colorful display both in the spring from blooming wildflowers and in the autumn from fall colors among the stunted evergreens, mostly grand firs.

Tolmie Peak guards the northern side of Eunice Lake above steep cliffs of columnar basalt. The summit lookout can be seen perched on the western end of the high ridge, 600 feet above. Follow the path around to the western end of the lake to begin the hardest ascent of the entire route, unfortunately right at the end. Hikers accustomed to life at sea level are likely to feel the altitude, now more than 1 mile high.

The trail winds up several switchbacks to reach the summit ridge and the lookout about 0.5 mile beyond the lake. The grand view here stretches to all points of the compass and includes the Olympic Mountains, Glacier Peak, Mount Stuart, Mount Baker, and even an unusual glimpse right into the crater of Mount St. Helens to the south. Eunice Lake lies almost straight below and a corner of Mowich Lake, where you started, can be seen through the trees.

Nonetheless, it is Mount Rainier that dominates the skyline. There are few better places to study the mighty glaciers, cliffs, and ridges of the mountain's northwestern aspect than here, although the true summit, at Columbia Crest (14,410'), is hidden behind Liberty Cap (14,112') at the top of the Willis Wall. Arriving particularly early or late in the day will improve the view, as the lower-angle light from the sun will bring the crevasses and gullies into sharper relief.

For the adventurous, an easy scramble route continues eastward along the ridge to a second summit, slightly higher than the lookout. Otherwise, return the way you came.

GPS TRAILHEAD COORDINATES
N46° 55.970' W121° 51.839'

From I-5 between Seattle and Tacoma, take Exit 142A for WA 18 E. Travel 2.5 miles east on WA 18 toward Auburn, then take the W. Valley Highway exit toward WA 167 S and Puyallup. Turn right onto W. Valley Highway S, and go 0.5 mile. Turn left onto 15th Street and immediately turn right onto WA 167. In 6.8 miles, before reaching Puyallup, exit onto WA 410 toward Sumner and Mount Rainier National Park. Continue 11.8 miles on WA 410 to the town of Buckley. In Buckley, turn right (south) toward Wilkeson on WA 165 and immediately take another right to stay on WA 165. In 1.6 miles at a fork, bear left to stay on WA 165 and drive through the small towns of Wilkeson and Carbonado. In 8.7 miles at another fork, bear right to stay on WA 165, which is clearly signed for Mowich Lake (the road on the left is signed for Carbon River). Drive 10.9 miles to the national park boundary and fee station. After paying the required fees, drive 5.7 miles on this dirt road (now called Road 79 and Mowich Lake Road) to its end at the Mowich Lake Campground.

57 Mount Rainier National Park:
SPRAY FALLS AND SPRAY PARK

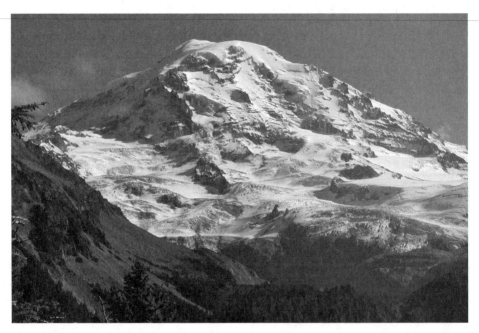

Mount Rainier from Eagle Cliffs viewpoint

In Brief

This deservedly popular hike consists of a moderate walk through the woods to one of the highest and most beautiful waterfalls in the state of Washington—or anywhere else, for that matter. Past the falls, a challenging 600-foot ascent in the next 0.5 mile leads to majestic Spray Park, a vast subalpine meadow on Mount Rainier's northwestern flank. In the spring, the meadow is a sea of wildflowers, complementing the wide views of the mountain and the surrounding landscape.

Description

Like most of nature's finest spectacles, words alone cannot adequately convey the power and beauty of the cascade at Spray Falls. There is simply no substitute for the direct

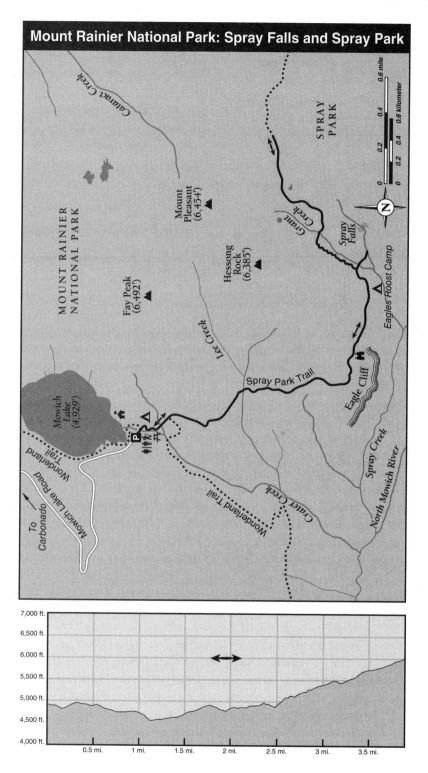

DISTANCE & CONFIGURATION:
4.5-mile out-and-back to Spray Falls; 7.0-mile out-and-back with optional hike up to Spray Park

DIFFICULTY: Moderate to Spray Falls, difficult to Spray Park

SCENERY: Stunning waterfall, meadows, and wildflowers (in Spray Park); views of Mount Rainier

EXPOSURE: Mostly shaded; exposed in Spray Park

TRAFFIC: Heavy; lower in off-season and beyond the falls

TRAIL SURFACE: Dirt

HIKING TIME: 3–8 hours

ACCESS: Hikable summer–fall (check road conditions and snowpack); $10 per person

WHEELCHAIR TRAVERSABLE: No

MAP(S): Green Trails *Mount Rainier West 269*; USGS *Mowich Lake*

FACILITIES: Toilet at trailhead; no drinking water

DOGS: Not allowed

CONTACT: 360-569-2211; nps.gov/mora

LOCATION: Carbonado

experience of standing below the torrent as it tumbles over the rocks, to hear its deafening roar, to feel the mist and wind, and to marvel at the ever-changing vista as the white water makes its way through countless alternate routes, like champagne spilling over a pyramid of glasses. A trip to the falls is an absolute must for anyone visiting this section of the national park, a truly outstanding natural feature even among the many for which the park is famous.

Spray Falls tends to attract a crowd; don't expect to have this place to yourself on a summer weekend. What is surprising is how many people ignore the falls altogether and pass right by on their way up to Spray Park, a testament to the true embarrassment of riches this trail has to offer. Nonetheless, the total foot traffic is still much less than it would be if the hike started from the popular and easily accessible visitor centers at Paradise or Sunrise on the southern and eastern sides of the mountain. Thanks to its lack of amenities and unpaved approach road, Mowich Lake sees far fewer park users than do the other major access points.

Start hiking at the trailhead on the southern side of the campground, behind some picnic tables. The trail unexpectedly starts downhill on some steps and reaches a junction in 0.4 mile, indicating that you have already been following a section of the Wonderland Trail. Although the Wonderland technically continues along Mowich Lake to descend toward the Carbon River through Ipsut Pass, the route up and over the Spray Park divide has become the de facto Wonderland for most round-the-mountain hikers, the same path you will be following. Stay left at the junction, signed for Eagles Roost and Spray Park.

The trail gradually descends to cross Lee Creek after another 0.5 mile, and then reaches its low point at just less than 4,600 feet, some 300 feet below the lake. Cross a boulder field and begin to gain back all of the elevation you have lost so far, as the trail heads uphill on a series of switchbacks, climbing through a mixed forest of young and old trees.

The trail skirts the top of Eagle Cliff, eventually reaching an excellent viewpoint on a marked spur to the right near the 1.5-mile mark. Be sure to make this short side trip for a

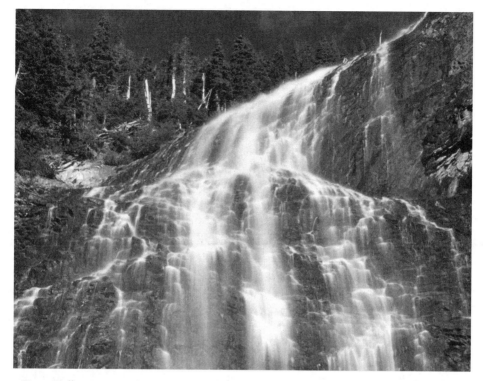

Spray Falls

commanding view. From the overlook, the mountain rises almost 10,000 feet in a horizontal distance of about 6 miles, and the steep walls of the Spray Creek Valley drop
another 1,500 feet straight down, for a total of about 11,500 feet of visible vertical relief.
Even with a good topographic map and a practiced eye, it can be a real challenge to posi-
tively identify every feature of the terrain in view, which includes seven major glaciers
and countless ridges and rocky points.

Another 0.5 mile yields first the Eagles Roost campsite (typically used by Wonderland thru-hikers) and then the Grant Creek crossing (a log footbridge over a pleasant
stream that flows down through a series of boulders in a small waterfall). This waterfall
is no match for what is to come, however, as the junction for Spray Falls lies just on the
other side of the creek.

Head right at the junction, cross another small bridge, and then traverse a talus field
of small white rocks to emerge, after 0.1 mile, below the mighty falls. It's easy to see where
the falls got its name, as curtains of spray and mist repeatedly sweep across everyone and
everything below. If the prevailing winds and volume of water are favorable, you may be
able to find a dry spot to relax and take a picture, but there is no guarantee. Scramble up
through the boulders to get a better sense of the true size of the 350-foot cascade, although
this is likely to expose you to an even greater wetness.

The stream sweeps around a broad curve, keeping the top essentially invisible from hikers at the base. However, the majesty of the falls lies in the 80-foot width across the fan and the white water contrasting against the reddish volcanic rock underneath.

For many hikers, the falls make a suitable day-hike destination, but additional rewards await anyone continuing uphill to Spray Park. To reach the subalpine meadow, return to the main trail and turn right to begin a tough uphill grind through a long chain of switchbacks. Your effort will be rewarded when you finally escape the trees near the 5,700-foot line.

Many hikers consider Spray Park the finest place to view wildflowers anywhere at Mount Rainier, as the fields are carpeted with white avalanche lilies through much of the late spring and summer. Less heralded but equally impressive is the view in autumn, when fiery reds, oranges, and yellows ignite the landscape and the biting insects have mostly disappeared.

The trail continues uphill for another mile to reach a saddle, at 6,400 feet, that separates Spray Park from Seattle Park. This high point is as far as most day hikers are likely to venture, about 4 miles total from the trailhead, but anyone with greater ambitions can continue eastward as far as they wish. More typically, hikers will be captivated by the many pleasures of Spray Park and seek to explore it on their own. Scramblers may pursue multiple peak-bagging opportunities to the northwest in the vicinity of Hessong Rock and Mount Pleasant, rock hounds might investigate the pumice and other volcanic rocks at the higher elevations, botanists and naturalists can enjoy the wildflower displays and other subalpine life, and many people may simply wish to relax and soak in the fantastic views of both Mount Rainier itself and the landscape stretching as far as the northern Cascades on a clear day.

GPS TRAILHEAD COORDINATES
N46° 55.97' W121° 51.839'

From I-5 between Seattle and Tacoma, take Exit 142A for WA 18 E. Travel 2.5 miles east on WA 18 toward Auburn, then take the W. Valley Highway exit toward WA 167 S and Puyallup. Turn right onto W. Valley Highway S, and go 0.5 mile. Turn left onto 15th Street and immediately turn right onto WA 167. In 6.8 miles, before reaching Puyallup, exit onto WA 410 toward Sumner and Mount Rainier National Park. Continue 11.8 miles on WA 410 to the town of Buckley. In Buckley, turn right (south) toward Wilkeson on WA 165 and immediately take another right to stay on WA 165. In 1.6 miles at a fork, bear left to stay on WA 165 and drive through the small towns of Wilkeson and Carbonado. In 8.7 miles at another fork, bear right to stay on WA 165, which is clearly signed for Mowich Lake (the road on the left is signed for Carbon River). Drive 10.9 miles to the national park boundary and fee station. After paying the required fees, drive 5.7 miles on this dirt road (now called Road 79 and Mowich Lake Road) to its end at the Mowich Lake Campground.

58 Mud Mountain Dam and White River Trail

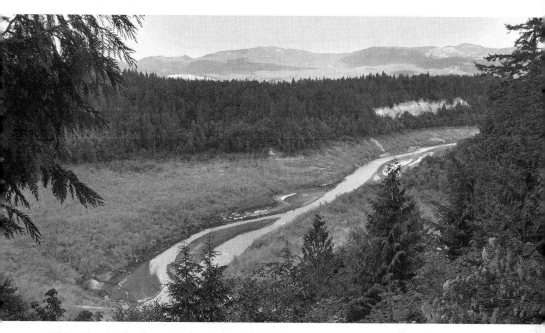

White River Valley from Mud Mountain Recreation Area

In Brief

This one-of-a-kind trail follows the White River above Mud Mountain Dam, first on a high bluff and then right along the water, providing the unique opportunity to walk on a part-time lake bed. This hike feels more like a riparian zone in eastern Washington than anything in the Cascades, making this trail, with year-round access and limited traffic, unlike any other in the region.

Description

Among such Pacific Northwest engineering marvels as the Grand Coulee and Bonneville Dams on the Columbia River, Mud Mountain Dam is something of an anomaly. Despite being the tallest dam in the world of its type when it was built in the 1940s, it was designed purely to prevent floods, generating no hydroelectric power and rarely even holding back any water. Instead, the dam acts like a regulator valve for the White River Valley, only

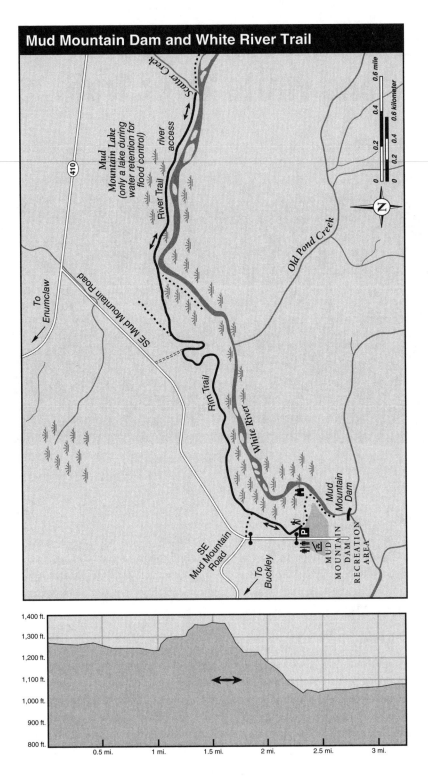

DISTANCE & CONFIGURATION:
6.5-mile out-and-back

DIFFICULTY: Moderate

SCENERY: Walking along the White River on a dry lake bed, viewpoints of valley from Rim Trail and Mud Mountain Dam when the park is open

EXPOSURE: Shaded on Rim Trail, exposed on River Trail

TRAFFIC: Low

TRAIL SURFACE: Dirt with some gravel

HIKING TIME: 3–4 hours

ACCESS: Hikable year-round (recreation area closed Saturday–Sunday, October 1– April 15; mid-September–mid-May, 9 a.m.–4 p.m.; mid-May–mid-September, 9 a.m.–8 p.m.); no fee for parking or trail access

WHEELCHAIR TRAVERSABLE: No, but the park has some accessible viewpoints

MAP(S): Green Trails *Enumclaw 237*; USGS *Enumclaw*

FACILITIES: None at trailhead; toilets and water in park when open

DOGS: Allowed off-leash

CONTACT: 206-316-3019; tinyurl.com /mudmountaindam

LOCATION: Enumclaw

allowing a certain volume to pass through and usually doing nothing to impede the river's standard flow. However, during occasional periods of flooding, the river gets backed up behind the dam to form a temporary reservoir, protecting development downstream.

This means that unless you happen to arrive during one of the infrequent periods of extreme high water, the Mud Mountain Dam will be essentially dormant, nothing more than a giant wall waiting to be put into service. Thankfully, it also means that the engaging lower section of the trail above the White River will be dry and accessible, rather than at the bottom of a temporary, man-made lake.

To begin the hike, head east from the parking lot on a gravel path next to the chain-link fence, just outside the park gate. Turn left at the edge of the gorge, several hundred feet above the White River, which is visible down the steep slope through the trees. Note that the dam itself is just downstream from this location, but it is not visible from here. Although one viewpoint farther along provides a glimpse of the dam, it is necessary to visit the interpretive site inside the adjacent park in order to get a good look at the impressive structure.

The trail quickly meets an unpaved road entering from the left, a secondary access for when the outer gates to the recreation area are closed. To find this alternate starting point, look for a bright-yellow metal gate marked MUD MOUNTAIN DAM TEST WELL on the left side of the main road, just before the big sign reading ENTERING MUD MOUNTAIN DAM AND RECREATION AREA.

Continue to follow the trail as it heads east along the top of the White River Valley rim. A few gaps in the trees provide views of the water churning far below, and Mount Rainier even makes a token appearance with the crest of Liberty Cap rising just above the ridgeline on the opposite side of the valley.

Turn right at a junction with a dirt road and follow the road until a left turn returns you to the singletrack at a sign marked with a hiking icon, two figures with walking sticks.

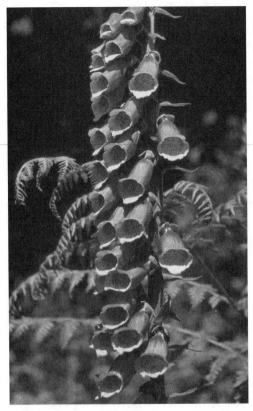

Foxglove

The trail descends about 40 feet into a forest of large Douglas firs and cedars. Amazingly, these massive and seemingly immovable trees are sometimes uprooted by high winds that howl through the valley during storms. Several sizable specimens lie on either side of the path as it heads through a flat swampy section, where thoughtfully laid wooden planks keep hikers mostly above the mud. Giant skunk cabbages are right at home here in the dampness and shade.

Meet a second dirt road at the end of the flats, and look for another sign with a hiking icon, just to the right. The trail runs next to the road for about 30 yards before bending back out along the valley rim. You are now much closer to the river than you were before, and the water, laden with the glacial silt that gives it a greenish color, can easily be heard flowing over the rocks. The silt has been carried from far up on Mount Rainier's northeastern flank, where five separate glaciers (including the giant Emmons and Winthrop Glaciers) drain into the White River watershed.

Split rail fencing helps to keep people back from the steep drop-off at a few places where the trail runs right out to the edge. One such point provides the only vantage on the entire trail of Mud Mountain Dam itself, with just a corner visible far downstream through the trees.

At the 2-mile mark, Rim Trail ends at a gravel road, used by equestrians for access. This is a good turnaround point for hikers seeking a shorter outing. However, the second part of the hike, on the banks of the river, is well worth the additional effort. To reach it, head downhill on the road to the right.

Follow the road as it loses elevation and bears left, dropping through a forest of bigleaf maples and then a mix of willows and alders before emerging into a broad clearing. This is, in fact, the footprint of Mud Mountain Lake, created when the water is sufficiently backed up by the dam, although the thick growth of grasses, bushes, and trees shows the relative rarity of such flooding events. A thick steel cable that spans the entire valley anchors a series of metal pontoons used to trap debris on the surface of the lake before it can reach the dam intake.

The road continues upstream just above the river where the limited shade keeps the footing from becoming too muddy and churned up, even in the winter. Owing to the open terrain, the hike seems more like something in the Yakima River Valley than on the western slope of the Cascades, right down to the abundant reeds and snake grass. The only thing missing is the fragrant sagebrush.

The trail narrows and eventually reaches a small sandy beach on the riverbank, where a creek flows in from the left. This spot provides easy access to the water and a few convenient boulders for sitting and relaxing. Although it is possible to continue exploring upstream, this is likely the best turnaround point for most hikers. From here, it is 3.25 miles back to the start for a 6.5-mile round-trip journey, including a 300-foot elevation gain back up to the rim.

Nearby Activities

The U.S. Army Corps of Engineers operates the Mud Mountain Recreation Area adjacent to the trailhead, offering a public park and playground facilities. An interpretive site at the eastern end of the park provides information about the design and construction of the dam, along with an excellent viewpoint of the rock-and-earth structure. A short walk into the canyon leads to a second vista with a much lower viewpoint, accenting the height of the dam. For more information, visit the Mud Mountain Dam website at tinyurl.com/mudmtndam.

GPS TRAILHEAD COORDINATES
N47° 8.705' W121° 56.035'

From I-5 between Seattle and Tacoma, take Exit 142A for WA 18 E. Travel 4.2 miles east on WA 18 into Auburn, then exit onto WA 164 E toward Enumclaw. Continue 14.7 miles on WA 164 through Enumclaw to a junction with WA 410/Roosevelt Avenue, and turn left (east). Stay on WA 410 E for 4.9 miles, and turn right onto SE Mud Mountain Road. Follow this road 2.1 miles to Mud Mountain Recreation Area and park in the lot outside the park gate.

59 Pinnacle Peak County Park: CAL MAGNUSSON TRAIL

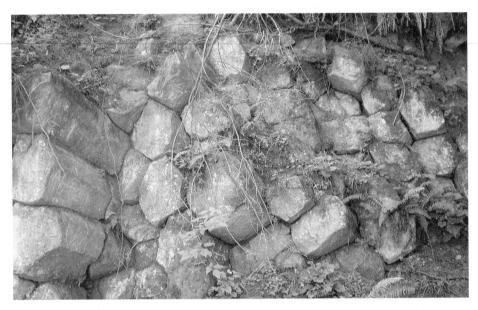

Columns of extruded volcanic rock

In Brief

Pinnacle Peak is an old favorite of southeast King County hikers that deserves wider attention. The geologically unusual mountain rises straight up from the surrounding farmland, thrust upward like a monument to the powerful volcanic forces that shape the Washington landscape. Although views are limited, the quick climb to the top still makes a worthy outing.

Description

Despite having several alternate names, or perhaps because of it, Pinnacle Peak remains mostly obscure to many Puget Sound hikers. Yet whether it is called Mount Pete, Mount Peak, or Pinnacle Peak (as shown on the USGS topographic map), this singular mountain is worth knowing about.

Pinnacle Peak is just as striking and abrupt in the landscape as some of the cinder cones outside of Bend in central Oregon, although its volcanic origins are not as obvious. Where well-known landmarks like Black Butte and Lava Butte leave no doubt about their

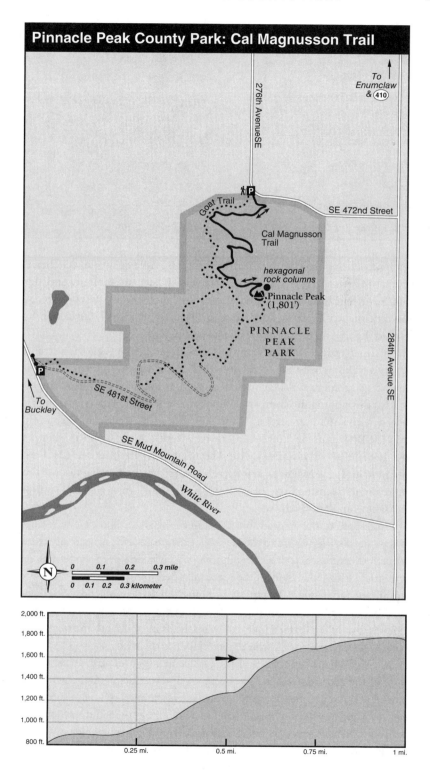

Pinnacle Peak County Park: Cal Magnusson Trail

276th AvenueSE

To Enumclaw & (410)

Goat Trail

SE 472nd Street

Cal Magnusson Trail

hexagonal rock columns

Pinnacle Peak (1,801')

PINNACLE PEAK PARK

284th Avenue SE

P

To Buckley

SE 481st Street

SE Mud Mountain Road

White River

N

0   0.1   0.2   0.3 mile
0   0.1   0.2   0.3 kilometer

2,000 ft.
1,800 ft.
1,600 ft.
1,400 ft.
1,200 ft.
1,000 ft.
800 ft.

0.25 mi.   0.5 mi.   0.75 mi.   1 mi.

DISTANCE & CONFIGURATION: 2.0-mile out-and-back, with a loop option	**ACCESS:** Hikable year-round; no fee for parking or trail access
DIFFICULTY: Moderate	**WHEELCHAIR TRAVERSABLE:** No
SCENERY: Steep hike through dense forest on a stand-alone mountain, unique rock formations, modest views of country-side along the trail	**MAP(S):** Green Trails *Enumclaw 237*; USGS *Enumclaw*
	FACILITIES: None at trailhead
EXPOSURE: Shaded	**DOGS:** Allowed on-leash
TRAFFIC: Medium–high	**CONTACT:** 206-477-4527; tinyurl.com /pinnaclepeak
TRAIL SURFACE: Dirt	
HIKING TIME: 1–2 hours	**LOCATION:** Enumclaw

fiery beginnings from beneath the Earth's crust, the evidence at Pinnacle Peak is more subtle, found in interesting columns of extruded rock near the summit. And although at only 1,800 feet it hardly qualifies as a significant climb, its visibility and prominence in the Enumclaw region give Pinnacle Peak a certain "because it's there" satisfaction to all who have reached the top, no matter how easy the trip might be.

Two distinct trails originate from the parking area, the wide main trail heading uphill to the left, known as Cal Magnusson Trail, and a narrower one to the right. Long-time Enumclaw resident Cal Magnusson worked as an engineer for Boeing and then later for REI, developing the company's first quality-control program through a friend-ship he had with mountaineer Jim Whittaker, the first American to summit Mount Everest in 1963. Magnusson later helped revive interest in backcountry-ski touring and climbing through his involvement with The Mountaineers in the 1960s. Despite the similarity in names, Cal Magnusson is no relation to Warren G. Magnuson, who served as a congressman from the State of Washington for more than 40 years and for whom Seattle's Magnuson Park is named.

Both trails lead to the summit, but the trail to the right follows a more rugged and circuitous path, looping around to the far side of the peak before eventually reaching the top. The main Magnusson trail zigzags up the northern side of the mountain and is far more commonly traveled, making it the recommended route.

Start hiking up the steep hill, rapidly climbing above the trailhead at 760 feet. Several long switchbacks cut back and forth across the slope, with an extended traverse leading to a major left turn in the first 0.5 mile. A few use trails head off into the trees to the right, connecting to the alternate trail, which runs farther to the west.

Pinnacle Peak has been logged in the past, and a web of abandoned roads covers most parts of the mountain, especially on the southern side. Nonetheless, a few larger trees remain, including some substantial Douglas firs standing right along the trail.

Reach a major intersection near 1,550 feet with an old road and stay left. Unmarked social trails abound in this section, but it is always easy to figure out which way to go. Just as in proverbial Rome, virtually every path here heading uphill eventually leads to the top.

Most potential viewpoints are obscured by the trees, which are surprisingly thick. Occasional glimpses of the farmland to the north do appear, however, including King County Fairgrounds just over a mile away on the opposite side of 284th Avenue SE.

Watch for some distinctive hexagonal rock columns protruding from the short, steep rise on the right. The viscous stone is molded by great heat and pressure below the surface of the Earth, then it crystallizes and solidifies into these remarkable patterns. Formations like this are generally referred to as columnar basalt, but there are actually four different types of volcanic rock that can be extruded in this way: basalt, andesite, dacite, and rhyolite. Basalt is the most common in the Pacific Northwest and is marked by its dark gray color. The columns at Pinnacle Peak are much lighter, resembling sandstone, and are likely composed of one of the other kinds of rock, which contain more silica.

The volcanic rocks are about 0.75 mile from the trailhead and only 0.25 mile short of the top. Make a quick orbit around to the other side of the peak and emerge at the summit, where some more volcanic columns stand below, with their geometric ends poking straight up out of the dirt.

A fire lookout once stood here, but all that remain are the four concrete blocks that anchored the foundation. The structure was removed in the 1960s, likely because increasing development in the White River Valley made the area much less remote, and wildfires would generally be spotted by other means. Unfortunately, there is now almost no view from the top to speak of, as the trees have all grown up around the clearing. It is worth exploring the side trails on the southern and eastern sides of the summit, where better viewpoints can be found looking out toward Mount Rainier and some of the nearby managed forests. These side trails connect to the top of the alternate trail, which provides a good optional descent route and allows for completion of a loop.

Thankfully, although some of the land on Pinnacle Peak was once threatened by real estate developers, King County Parks purchased several parcels on the mountain's southwest flank in late 2007, securing the area for public use for the foreseeable future. An alternate trail starting from the intersection of SE 481st Street and SE Mud Mountain Road follows an old gated road to provide access from that side.

GPS TRAILHEAD COORDINATES
N47° 10.719' W121° 58.425'

From I-5 between Seattle and Tacoma, take Exit 142A for WA 18 E. Travel 4.2 miles east on WA 18 into Auburn, then exit onto WA 164 E toward Enumclaw. Continue 14.7 miles on WA 164 through Enumclaw to a junction with WA 410/Roosevelt Avenue, and turn left (east). In 0.8 mile, turn right onto 284th Avenue SE and proceed 1.5 miles past King County Fairgrounds to SE 472nd Street on the right. Stay on SE 472nd Street 0.5 mile to reach the parking area and trailhead, where the road turns north and becomes 276th Avenue SE. Park in the designated head-in spots or along the road out of traffic flow.

60 Point Defiance Park

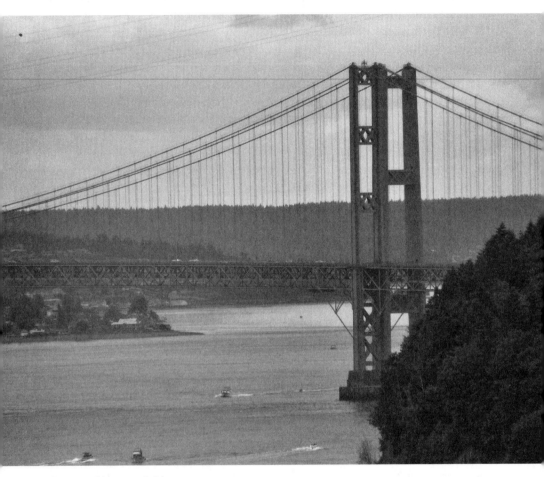

Tacoma Narrows Bridge

In Brief

Considered Tacoma's backyard playground by many local residents, Point Defiance offers just about everything any hiker could want: historical sites, great views, deep forest, and sandy beaches, all accessible via an extensive network of trails. A loop around Outside Perimeter Trail will confirm the park as one of the finest urban green spaces anywhere, a natural treasure not far from Tacoma's downtown core.

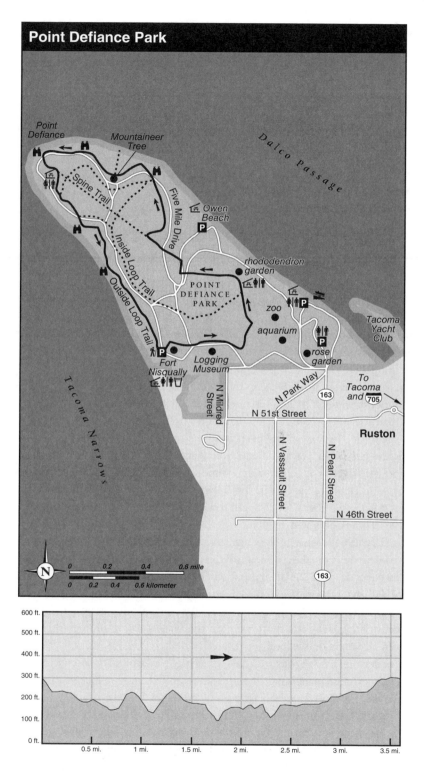

DISTANCE & CONFIGURATION: 4.3-mile loop	**ACCESS:** Hikable year-round, daily, 30 minutes before sunrise–30 minutes after sunset; no fee for parking or trail access
DIFFICULTY: Easy	
SCENERY: Urban trail through old-growth forest, historical Fort Nisqually, rhododendron garden, sandy beaches; views across Puget Sound	**WHEELCHAIR TRAVERSABLE:** No, but Owen Beach Promenade is accessible
	MAP(S): USGS *Gig Harbor*
	FACILITIES: Toilets and water throughout the park
EXPOSURE: Mostly shaded	
TRAFFIC: Medium on trails, high at beaches and viewpoints	**DOGS:** Allowed on-leash
	CONTACT: 253-305-1088; metroparks tacoma.org/point-defiance-park
TRAIL SURFACE: Dirt	
	LOCATION: 5400 N. Pearl St., Tacoma, WA 98407
HIKING TIME: 2–3 hours	

Description

Point Defiance got its name when an early explorer noted that the prominent peninsula held such an advantageous position that a fort on the site could stand against any conceivable invading force. The federal government agreed with that assessment, and in 1866 the land was appropriated for defense of the young Washington Territory, which had been carved out of the larger Oregon Territory in 1853. The land remained a military installation for many decades as the city of Tacoma grew to the south.

By the time Washington had been admitted to the Union as the 42nd state in 1889, however, the possibility of war in Puget Sound against the British or any other significant foreign power was growing increasingly remote, and the need for the continuing fortification of Point Defiance became far less apparent. In a victory for local citizens, the land was turned over to the city in 1905 and reborn as a public park, whose first century of existence Tacoma celebrated in 2005.

Ironically, Point Defiance now attracts rather than repels invaders, the multitudes who come every day to take advantage of the park's 700 acres of attractions. On a typical summer weekend, Point Defiance is particularly popular, which can make parking difficult, especially near the main entrance. However, there is usually ample space available in the interior along Five Mile Drive. The lot at Fort Nisqually is a good starting point for a hike because it typically has room even on the busiest days, although it is possible to begin from anywhere on the loop.

Outer Perimeter Trail runs atop the bluff all the way around the peninsula and can be hiked in either direction, although it is typically traveled counterclockwise, mirroring the general flow of traffic on Five Mile Drive, which follows a similar route.

Look for the start of the trail on the eastern side of the parking lot, away from the water, in the trees beyond the bathrooms and picnic area. The trail is generally well marked with short wooden posts, particularly useful at many points where the hike

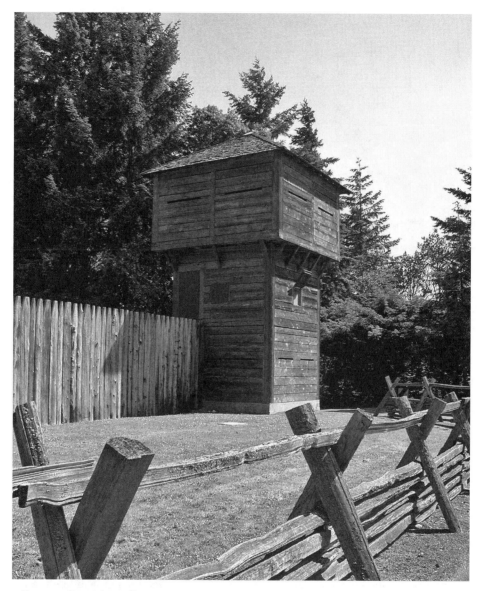

Tower at Fort Nisqually

crosses the road, although some of the posts are concealed by underbrush. Watch for posts with blue squares and arrows to show the way. Alternate symbols will also appear, a circle for Spine Trail and a triangle for Inside Perimeter Trail, both of which intersect Outer Perimeter Trail and frequently share sections of the route.

After leaving Fort Nisqually, the trail runs gradually downhill through a shady forest of big trees, majestic examples of many signature species of the Pacific Northwest,

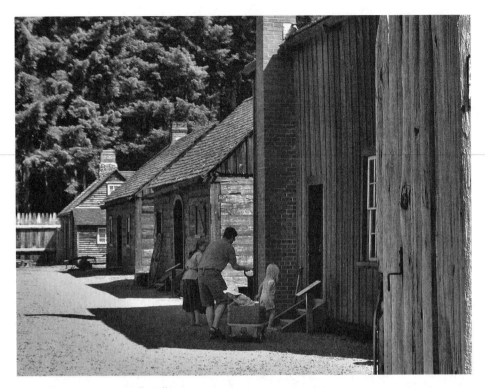

Visitors at Fort Nisqually Village

including hemlocks, cedars, and firs, with a carpet of ferns underneath. After 0.5 mile, pass through the rhododendron garden, where a multitude of azaleas and rhododendrons generously donated by private citizens is on display. The garden is particularly stunning in spring when the plants are in bloom.

A quarter mile past the rhododendrons, cross the Owen Beach access road, which heads down the hill to the right. The beach is a long stretch of sand and driftwood with a waterfront promenade and a grassy picnic area, invariably busy on sunny days.

Continue along the eastern side of the peninsula to a view of Vashon Island, just across the stretch of water known as Dalco Passage. Some of the finest old-growth forest in the park stands along this section of the trail, culminating in the impossible-to-miss Mountaineer Tree, a massive, 400-year-old Douglas fir rising more than 200 feet into the sky. Just before the giant tree, watch for a side trail, marked with a green square, heading down the bluff. It leads to a secluded beach below that is great for exploring when the tide is out.

Pass several more viewpoints around the northern tip of the peninsula and then cross the road to head inland toward the south. Amazingly, although Point Defiance is less than a mile across for most of its length, there is a noticeable difference between the environments on either side. The eastern bluff (which actually faces northeast) is wetter than the western bluff, which has considerable southern exposure. The trail surface underfoot reflects the difference, changing from frequently muddy to more sandy and dry as the trail heads around the point. The plant growth changes as well, with the western side featuring thinner forest and a higher density of the distinctive red-barked madrones.

Outer Perimeter Trail crosses the road again to the outside and then follows the edge of the bluff on the western side more closely than it does on the eastern, providing many views over Puget Sound and the Narrows. The Tacoma Narrows Bridge is visible to the south, gracefully spanning the waters between Tacoma and Gig Harbor. A second bridge parallel to the first was completed in the summer of 2007. It is a safe bet that neither the new concrete structure nor the older steel one will suffer the fate of the infamous original Tacoma Narrows Bridge, affectionately known as Galloping Gertie, which collapsed from a spectacular torsional failure brought on by high winds in November 1940. Engineering students around the world now study the structure as a lesson in how not to design a suspension bridge.

Finish the loop by hiking along the bluff and reach Fort Nisqually, where you began.

Nearby Activities

Point Defiance Park has a host of additional popular attractions, including the Tacoma Zoo and Aquarium, the reconstructed Fort Nisqually site, the Camp Six Logging Museum, an award-winning rose garden, and a boathouse and marina on Commencement Bay. For more information, visit the Point Defiance Park website at metroparks tacoma.org/point-defiance-park.

GPS TRAILHEAD COORDINATES
N47° 18.200' W122° 31.981'

From Tacoma, take I-5 to Exit 132B. Travel 3.0 miles on WA 16 W, and before the Tacoma Narrows bridge, take Exit 3 for Sixth Avenue. At the bottom of the ramp, continue straight onto Bantz Boulevard, and in 0.2 mile turn right onto Pearl Street/WA 163. Continue on Pearl Street 3.0 miles, all the way to the main entrance of Point Defiance Park. Drive straight into the park and follow the counterclockwise loop roads 1.5 miles to Fort Nisqually. Park in the large lot there.

Appendix A:
HIKING STORES

Feathered Friends
119 Yale Ave. N
Seattle, WA 98109
206-292-2210
featheredfriends.com

Outdoor Emporium
1701 Fourth Ave. S
Seattle, WA 98134
206-624-6550
sportco.com

REI
rei.com

Seattle
222 Yale Ave. N
Seattle, WA 98109
206-223-1944

Alderwood
3000 184th St. SW, Ste. 952
Lynnwood, WA 98037
425-640-6200

Issaquah
735 NW Gilman Blvd.
Issaquah, WA 98027
425-313-1660

Redmond
7500 166th Ave. NE
(Redmond Town Center)
Redmond, WA 98052
425-882-1158

Silverdale/Bremerton
10903 Myhre Place NW
Silverdale, WA 98383
360-337-1938

Southcenter/Tukwila
240 Andover Park W
Tukwila, WA 98188
206-248-1938

Tacoma
3825 S. Steele St.
Tacoma, WA 98409
253-671-1938

Second Ascent
5209 Ballard Ave. NW
Seattle, WA 98107
206-545-8810
secondascent.com

Sportco Warehouse Sporting Goods
4602 20th St. E
Fife, WA 98424
253-922-2222
sportco.com

Appendix B:
PLACES TO BUY MAPS

Metsker Maps of Seattle
1511 First Ave.
(Pike Place Market)
Seattle, WA 98101
206-623-8747
800-727-4430
metskers.com

University Bookstore
4326 University Way NE
Seattle, WA 98105
206-634-3400
www.bookstore.washington.edu

World Wide Books and Maps
4411 Wallingford Ave. N
Seattle, WA 98103
206-634-3453
888-534-3453
wideworldtravelstore.com

Green Trails Maps
greentrailsmaps.com

National Forest Map Store
nationalforestmapstore.com

USGS Map Store
store.usgs.gov

REI (see Appendix A)

Appendix C:
HIKING CLUBS

The Mountaineers–Seattle Branch
7700 Sand Point Way NE
Seattle, WA 98115
206-521-6000
mountaineers.org

The Mountaineers–Everett Branch
everettmountaineers.org

The Mountaineers–Foothills Branch (Eastside and I-90)
mountaineers.org/about/branches-committees/foothills-branch

The Mountaineers–Kitsap Branch
mountaineers.org/about/branches-committees/kitsap-branch

The Mountaineers–Olympia Branch
olympiamountaineers.org

The Mountaineers–Tacoma Branch
mountaineers.org/about/branches-committees/tacoma-branch

Issaquah Alps Trail Club
PO Box 351
Issaquah, WA 98027
issaquahalps.org

Washington Trails Association
705 Second Ave., Ste. 300
Seattle, WA 98104
206-625-1367
wta.org

Index

About the Authors

ANDREW WEBER

Thanks to a family scattered around the globe, Andrew Weber grew up a world traveler for life, counting the Canadian Rockies, the beaches of New Zealand, and the deserts of southern Africa among his favorite places. He has been exploring the great outdoors of the Pacific Northwest for more than 20 years, including a successful climb of Mount Rainier in 2005 and a solo circumnavigation of the Wonderland Trail around the mountain in 2002. Working as a freelance journalist and photographer, Andrew has written about a wide range of topics, including cultural events, the arts, and professional sports. He currently resides with his wife, Heather, and two sons, Bennett and Russell, who come along on his adventures whenever they can.

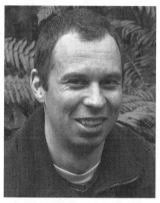

photographed by Heather Kovich

BRYCE STEVENS

A lifelong Washingtonian, Bryce Stevens grew up in the Yakima area, graduated from the University of Washington, and has lived in Seattle for about three decades. He has thoroughly explored the Cascade Range, the Olympic Mountains, and the lowlands of Puget Sound, all while hiking, backpacking, climbing, mountain biking, backcountry snowboarding, and sea kayaking. He discovered his love of outdoor photography while canyoneering in southeastern Utah in 2001 and has returned to the spectacular region many times since. In 1999 he cofounded Trails.com, a leading trail information resource and mapping service. He continues to own and operate many outdoor and travel-related websites. Bryce lives in the Maple Leaf neighborhood of Seattle with his wife, Julie, and their two sons, Kyle and Andrew.

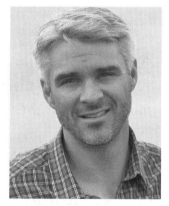

DEAR CUSTOMERS AND FRIENDS,

SUPPORTING YOUR INTEREST IN OUTDOOR ADVENTURE, travel, and an active lifestyle is central to our operations, from the authors we choose to the locations we detail to the way we design our books. Menasha Ridge Press was incorporated in 1982 by a group of veteran outdoorsmen and professional outfitters. For many years now, we've specialized in creating books that benefit the outdoors enthusiast.

Almost immediately, Menasha Ridge Press earned a reputation for revolutionizing outdoors- and travel-guidebook publishing. For such activities as canoeing, kayaking, hiking, backpacking, and mountain biking, we established new standards of quality that transformed the whole genre, resulting in outdoor-recreation guides of great sophistication and solid content. Menasha Ridge Press continues to be outdoor publishing's greatest innovator.

The folks at Menasha Ridge Press are as at home on a whitewater river or mountain trail as they are editing a manuscript. The books we build for you are the best they can be, because we're responding to your needs. Plus, we use and depend on them ourselves.

We look forward to seeing you on the river or the trail. If you'd like to contact us directly, visit us at menasharidge.com. We thank you for your interest in our books and the natural world around us all.

SAFE TRAVELS,

Bob Sehlinger

BOB SEHLINGER
PUBLISHER